Pocketbook of Drug Eruptions and Interactions

Pocketbook of Drug Eruptions and Interactions

Jerome Z. Litt, MD
Assistant Clinical Professor of Dermatology
Case Western Reserve University School of Medicine
Cleveland, Ohio

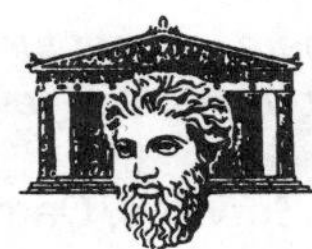

The Parthenon Publishing Group
International Publishers in Medicine, Science & Technology

NEW YORK LONDON

Published in the USA by
The Parthenon Publishing Group Inc.
One Blue Hill Plaza
PO Box 1564, Pearl River
New York 10965, USA

Published in the UK and Europe by
The Parthenon Publishing Group Limited
Casterton Hall, Carnforth
Lancs. LA6 2LA, UK

ISBN 1-85070-077-X

Typeset by Martin Lister Publishing Services, Carnforth, UK

Printed and bound by J.W. Arrowsmith Ltd., Bristol, UK

Contents

DEDICATIONS

To Vel:
Everything!

To Walter Pawlak:
for his untiring help when help was needed
and for his continuing friendship and loyalty

Introduction

More and more people – primarily the older population – are taking more and more prescription and over-the-counter medications. New drugs are appearing in the medical marketplace on an almost daily basis. More and more drug reactions – in the form of cutaneous eruptions – are developing from all drugs.

Dermatologists and primary care physicians are often perplexed by the nature of some of these problems. The few sources that are available to identify the causes of many of these side effects cannot be accessed by proprietary (trade) names.

This Pocketbook is a drug eruption reference guide that describes and catalogues the adverse cutaneous side effects of more than 600 commonly prescribed and over-the-counter American generic drugs. The drugs have been listed and indexed by both their generic and trade (brand) names for easy accessibility. More than 1,100 trade name drugs have been catalogued.

The first part of the Pocketbook lists in alphabetical order all the generic drugs that have been accessed. Then in alphabetical order, and in columns, follows the listing of all the 1,100-plus trade name drugs and their generic counterparts. Following this is a section devoted to the various classes of drugs.

The major portion of the Pocketbook – the body of the work – lists the more than 600 generic drugs and the adverse reactions that can arise from their use. For each drug, I have listed all the known adverse side effects – in the form of drug reactions – that can develop from the use of that drug. These side effects include those that primarily involve the skin, the hair, the nails and the mucous membranes.

The last sections of the Pocketbook include a description of the 29 most common reaction patterns and a listing of those medications that have been reported to occasion 80 common reaction patterns, including **acne, acute generalized exanthematous pustulosis, alopecia, aphthous stomatitis, bullous eruptions, bullous pemphigoid, erythema multiforme, erythema nodosum, exanthems, exfoliative dermatitis, fixed eruptions, lichenoid eruptions, lupus erythematosus, onycholysis, pemphigus, photosensitivity, pityriasis rosea, pruritus, psoriasis, purpura, Stevens- Johnson syndrome, taste disturbances, toxic epidermal necrolysis, urticaria, vasculitis,** and others.

USAGE, STYLE & CONVENTIONS EMPLOYED IN THIS MANUAL

The **generic** drug name is at the top of each page.

The most common American **trade name(s),** along with the names of the pharmaceutical companies that manufacture them are then listed alphabetically. Following this is a one-line listing of other common **trade-name** drugs – American and foreign. Then follows the **type** or **class** or **group** in which the drug belongs. This is followed by a list of clinically important, potentially serious drug **interactions**. On occasion, an important or pertinent **note** will follow.

Reactions: these are the **adverse reaction patterns** to the particular **generic drug**. They are classified in four **categories: skin, hair, nails,** and **other**. (**Other** refers to **mucous membranes, teeth, muscle** and various other forms of **reactions**.) The **reactions** are listed alphabetically in each **category**.

There are occasions when there are very few adverse reactions to a specific drug. These drugs are still included in the Pocketbook since there is often a **positive significance in negative findings.**

Notes

(sic) means **just so.** This is how the authors designated the **reaction.** For example, **rash** (sic); **dermatitis** (sic); **skin rash** (sic). [The term **skin rash** is a deplorable and reprehensible idiotism adored by non-dermatologists and the writers of the PDR (read package inserts). Can you have a **rash** on any other organ?]

I have simplified the references to the many **reaction patterns** by eliminating, for the most part, tags such as "-like" as in psoriasis-like, "-reactivation," "-syndrome," "-dissemination," "-iform," etc.

I have taken the liberty to lump **anaphylaxis, anaphylactic reactions** and **anaphylactoid reactions** under the general rubric of **anaphylactoid reaction**.

I have also incorporated **hypersensitivity reaction, hypersensitivity reactions** and **hypersensitivity** under the general heading of **hypersensitivity**.

Enjoy!

Jerome Z. Litt, M.D.

ALPHABETICAL LIST OF GENERIC NAMES

Abciximab
Acebutolol
Acetaminophen
Acetazolamide
Acetohexamide
Acitretin
Acyclovir
Albendazole
Albuterol
Aldesleukin
Alendronate
Allopurinol
Alprazolam
Alprostadil
Alteplase
Altretamine
Amantadine
Amikacin
Amiloride
Aminocaproic acid
Aminoglutethimide
Aminophylline
Aminosalicylate sodium
Amiodarone
Amitriptyline
Amlodipine
Amobarbital
Amoxapine
Amoxicillin
Amphotericin B
Ampicillin
Apraclonidine
Aprobarbital
Ascorbic acid
Asparaginase
Aspartame
Aspirin
Astemizole
Atenolol
Atorvastatin
Atovaquone
Atropine sulfate
Auranofin
Aurothioglucose
Azatadine
Azathioprine
Azelastine
Azithromycin
Aztreonam
Benactyzine
Benazepril
Bendroflumethiazide
Benzthiazide
Benztropine
Bepridil
Beta-carotene
Betaxolol
Bethanechol
Bicalutamide
Biperiden
Bisacodyl
Bisoprolol
Bleomycin
Bromfenac
Bromocriptine
Brompheniramine
Buclizine
Bumetanide
Bupropion
Buspirone
Busulfan
Butabarbital
Butalbital
Butorphanol
Cabergoline
Calcitonin
Captopril
Carbamazepine
Carbenicillin
Carbidopa
Carboplatin
Carisoprodol
Carmustine
Carteolol
Carvedilol
Cefaclor
Cefadroxil
Cefamandole
Cefazolin
Cefdinir
Cefepime
Cefixime
Cefotaxime
Cefoxitin
Cefpodoxime
Ceftazidime
Ceftibuten
Ceftriaxone
Cefuroxime
Cephalexin
Cephalothin
Cephradine
Cerivastatin
Cetirizine
Chloral hydrate
Chlorambucil
Chloramphenicol
Chlordiazepoxide
Chlormezanone
Chloroquine
Chlorothiazide
Chlorotrianisene
Chlorpromazine
Chlorpropamide
Chlorthalidone
Chlorzoxazone
Cholestyramine
Cimetidine
Ciprofloxacin
Cisapride
Cisplatin
Cladribine
Clarithromycin
Clemastine
Clidinium
Clindamycin
Clofazimine
Clofibrate
Clomiphene
Clomipramine
Clonazepam
Clonidine
Clopidogrel
Clorazepate
Cloxacillin
Clozapine
Cocaine
Codeine
Colchicine
Colestipol
Corticosteroids
Cortisone
Cotrimoxazole
Cromolyn
Cyanocobalamin
Cyclamate
Cyclobenzaprine
Cyclophosphamide
Cycloserine
Cyclosporine
Cyclothiazide
Cyproheptadine
Cytarabine

Dacarbazine
Dactinomycin
Dalteparin
Danazol
Dantrolene
Dapsone
Daunorubicin
Deferoxamine
Delavirdine
Demeclocycline
Desipramine
Desmopressin
Dexfenfluramine
Dextroamphetamine
Dextromethorphan
Diazepam
Diazoxide
Diclofenac
Dicloxacillin
Dicumarol
Dicyclomine
Didanosine
Dideoxycytidine
Diethylpropion
Diethylstilbestrol
Diflunisal
Digoxin
Dihydrotachysterol
Diltiazem
Dimenhydrinate
Diphenhydramine
Diphenoxylate
Dipyridamole
Dirithromycin
Disopyramide
Disulfiram
Divalproex
Docetaxel
Docusate
Dolasetron
Donepezil
Dopamine
Doxapram
Doxazosin
Doxepin
Doxorubicin
Doxycycline
Dronabinol
Edrophonium
Enalapril
Enoxacin
Enoxaparin
Ephedrine
Epinephrine
Epoetin alfa
Ergocalciferol
Erythromycin
Esmolol
Estazolam
Estramustine
Ethacrynic acid
Ethambutol
Ethanolamine
Ethchlorvynol
Ethionamide
Ethosuximide
Ethotoin
Etidronate
Etodolac
Etoposide
Famciclovir
Famotidine
Felbamate
Felodipine
Fenfluramine
Fenofibrate
Fenoprofen
Fentanyl
Fexofenadine
Finasteride
Flavoxate
Flecainide
Fluconazole
Flucytosine
Flumazenil
Fluorouracil
Fluoxetine
Fluoxymesterone
Fluphenazine
Flurazepam
Flurbiprofen
Flutamide
Fluvastatin
Fluvoxamine
Folic acid
Foscarnet
Fosfomycin
Fosinopril
Furazolidone
Furosemide
Gabapentin
Ganciclovir
Gemcitabine
Gemfibrozil
Gentamicin
Glimepiride
Glipizide
Glucagon
Glyburide
Gold
Granisetron
GCSF
Grepafloxacin
Griseofulvin
Guanabenz
Guanadrel
Guanethidine
Guanfacine
Haloperidol
Halothane
Heparin
Heroin
Hydralazine
Hydrochlorothiazide
Hydroflumethiazide
Hydromorphone
Hydroxychloroquine
Hydroxyurea
Hydroxyzine
Ibuprofen
Idarubicin
Ifosfamide
Imipenem/cilastatin
Imipramine
Indapamide
Indinavir
Indomethacin
Insulin
Interferons, alfa
Interleukin-2
Ipodate
Ipratropium
Irbesartan
Isocarboxazid
Isoniazid (INH)
Isoproterenol
Isosorbide
Isotretinoin
Isradipine
Itraconazole
Ivermectin
Kanamycin
Ketamine
Ketoconazole
Ketoprofen
Ketorolac
Labetalol
Lamivudine
Lamotrigine
Lansoprazole
Latanoprost
Letrozole
Leuprolide
Levamisole
Levobunolol
Levodopa
Levofloxacin
Levothyroxine
Lidocaine
Lincomycin
Liothyronine
Lisinopril
Lithium
Lomefloxacin

Lomustine
Loperamide
Loracarbef
Loratadine
Lorazepam
Losartan
Lovastatin
Loxapine
Maprotiline
Marihuana
Mazindol
Mebendazole
Mechlorethamine
Meclizine
Meclofenamate
Medroxyprogesterone
Mefenamic acid
Mefloquine
Melphalan
Meperidine
Mephenytoin
Mephobarbital
Meprobamate
Mercaptopurine
Mesalamine
Mesna
Mesoridazine
Metaxalone
Metformin
Methadone
Methamphetamine
Methantheline
Methazolamide
Methenamine
Methicillin
Methimazole
Methocarbamol
Methohexital
Methotrexate
Methoxsalen
Methsuximide
Methyclothiazide
Methyldopa
Methylphenidate
Methyltestosterone
Methysergide
Metoclopramide
Metolazone
Metoprolol
Metronidazole
Mexiletine
Mezlocillin
Mibefradil
Miconazole
Midazolam
Minocycline
Minoxidil
Misoprostol
Mitomycin
Mitotane
Moexipril
Molindone
Montelukast
Moricizine
Nabumetone
Nadolol
Nafarelin
Nafcillin
Nalidixic acid
Naloxone
Naproxen
Naratriptan
Nefazodone
Nelfinavir
Neomycin
Nevirapine
Niacin; niacinamide
Nicardipine
Nifedipine
Nimodipine
Nisoldipine
Nitrofurantoin
Nitroglycerin
Nizatidine
Norfloxacin
Nortriptyline
Nystatin
Octreotide
Ofloxacin
Olanzapine
Olsalazine
Omeprazole
Ondansetron
Oral contraceptives
Orphenadrine
Oxacillin
Oxaprozin
Oxazepam
Oxytetracycline
Paclitaxel
Pamidronate
Papaverine
Para-aminosalicylic acid
Paramethadione
Paroxetine
Pemoline
Penbutolol
Penicillamine
Penicillins
Pentagastrin
Pentamidine
Pentazocine
Pentobarbital
Pentostatin
Pentoxifylline
Pergolide
Perphenazine
Phenazopyridine
Phendimetrazine
Phenelzine
Phenindamine
Phenobarbital
Phenolphthalein
Phensuximide
Phentermine
Phentolamine
Phenytoin
Phytonadione
Pimozide
Pindolol
Piperacillin
Piroxicam
Plicamycin
Polythiazide
Potassium iodide
Pramipexole
Pravastatin
Prazepam
Praziquantel
Prazosin
Primaquine
Primidone
Probenecid
Procainamide
Procarbazine
Prochlorperazine
Procyclidine
Progestins
Promazine
Promethazine
Propafenone
Propantheline
Propofol
Propoxyphene
Propranolol
Propylthiouracil
Protamine
Protriptyline
Pseudoephedrine
Psoralens
Pyrazinamide
Pyridoxine
Pyrilamine
Pyrimethamine
Quazepam
Quetiapine
Quinacrine
Quinapril
Quinestrol
Quinethazone
Quinidine
Quinine
Raloxifene
Ramipril

Ranitidine
Repaglinide
Reserpine
Ribavirin
Riboflavin
Rifabutin
Rifampin
Rimantadine
Risperidone
Ritonavir
Ritordine
Ropinirole
Saccharin
Salmeterol
Salsalate
Saquinavir
Scopolamine
Secobarbital
Secretin
Selegiline
Sertraline
Sibutramine
Sildenafil
Simvastatin
Sotalol
Sparfloxacin
Spectinomycin
Spironolactone
Stanozolol
Streptokinase
Streptomycin
Streptozocin
Succinylcholine
Sucralfate
Sulfadoxine
Sulfamethoxazole
Sulfasalazine
Sulfinpyrazone
Sulfisoxazole
Sulindac
Sumatriptan
Tacrine
Tacrolimus
Tamoxifen
Temazepam
Terazosin
Terbinafine
Terbutaline
Terfenadine
Testosterone
Tetracycline
Thalidomide
Thiabendazole
Thiamine
Thioguanine
Thiopental
Thioridazine
Thiotepa
Thiothixene
Tiagabine
Ticarcillin
Ticlopidine
Timolol
Tiopronin
Tizanidine
Tobramycin
Tolazamide
Tolazoline
Tolbutamide
Tolcapone
Tolmetin
Tolterodine
Topiramate
Topotecan
Toremifene
Torsemide
Tramadol
Trandolapril
Tranylcypromine
Trazodone
Triamterene
Triazolam
Trichlormethiazide
Trientine
Trifluoperazine
Trihexyphenidyl
Trimeprazine
Trimethadione
Trimethoprim
Trimetrexate
Trimipramine
Trioxsalen
Tripelennamine
Triprolidine
Troglitazone
Troleandomycin
Trovafloxacin
Urokinase
Ursodiol
Valproic acid
Valsartan
Vancomycin
Vasopressin
Venlafaxine
Verapamil
Vinblastine
Vincristine
Vinorelbine
Vitamin A
Vitamin B_1
Vitamin B_2
Vitamin B_3
Vitamin B_6
Vitamin B_{12}
Vitamin C
Vitamin D
Vitamin E
Vitamin K
Warfarin
Yohimbine
Zafirlukast
Zalcitabine
Zidovudine
Zileuton
Zolmitriptan
Zolpidem

ALPHABETICAL LIST OF TRADE/GENERIC NAMES

Trade name	Generic name
8-MOP	methoxsalen
8-MOP	psoralens
Abbokinase	urokinase
Accolate	zafirlukast
Accupril	quinapril
Accutane	isotretinoin
Achromycin V	tetracycline
Actagen	triprolidine
Actibine	yohimbine
Actidil	triprolidine
Actifed	pseudoephedrine
Actifed	triprolidine
Actigall	ursodiol
Activase	alteplase
Acular	ketorolac
Adalat	nifedipine
Adipex-P	phentermine
Adrenalin	epinephrine
Adriamycin	doxorubicin
Adrucil	fluorouracil
Advil	ibuprofen
Aerolate	aminophylline
Afrinol	pseudoephedrine
Ak-Chlor	chloramphenicol
Akineton	biperiden
Ala-Tet	tetracycline
Albenza	albendazole
Aldactazide	hydrochlorothiazide
Aldactone	spironolactone
Aldomet	methyldopa
Aldoril	hydrochlorothiazide
Aldoril	methyldopa
Aleve	naproxen
Alferon N	interferons, alfa
Alka-Seltzer	aspirin
Alkeran	melphalan
Allegra	fexofenadine
Allerid	pseudoephedrine
Allermax	diphenhydramine
Allerphed	triprolidine
Alophen	phenolphthalein
Altace	ramipril
Alurate	aprobarbital
Amaryl	glimepiride
Ambien	zolpidem
Ambisome	amphotericin B
Amen	medroxyprogesterone
Amen	progestins
Amerge	naratriptan
Amicar	aminocaproic acid
Amikin	amikacin
Aminophyllin	aminophylline
Amoxil	amoxicillin
Amoxil	penicillins
Amphocin	amphotericin B
Amytal	amobarbital
Anacin	aspirin
Anacin-3	acetaminophen
Anafranil	clomipramine
Ancef	cefazolin
Ancobon	flucytosine
Androderm	testosterone
Android	methyltestosterone
Android-F	fluoxymesterone
Anectine	succinylcholine
Anergan	promethazine
Anestacon	lidocaine
Anhydron	cyclothiazide
Ansaid	flurbiprofen
Antabuse	disulfiram
Antivert	meclizine
Antiviral	lamivudine
Anturane	sulfinpyrazone
Anzemet	dolasetron
Aphrodyne	yohimbine
Apresazide	hydralazine
Apresazide	hydrochlorothiazide
Apresoline	hydralazine
Aquachloral	chloral hydrate
Aquamephyton	phytonadione
Aquasol A	vitamin A
Aquasol E	vitamin E
Aralen	chloroquine
Aredia	pamidronate
Aricept	donepezil
Aristocort	corticosteroids
Aristospan	corticosteroids
Artane	trihexyphenidyl
Arthrotec	diclofenac
Arthrotec	misoprostol
Asacol	mesalamine
Ascorbicap	ascorbic acid
Ascriptin	aspirin
Asendin	amoxapine
Aspergum	aspirin
Astelin	azelastine
Atabrine	quinacrine
Atarax	hydroxyzine
Ativan	lorazepam
Atromid-S	clofibrate
Atrovent	ipratropium
Augmentin	amoxicillin
Augmentin	penicillins
Avapro	irbesartan

Aventyl	nortriptyline	**Capozide**	hydrochlorothiazide
Axid	nizatidine	**Carafate**	sucralfate
Aygestin	progestins	**Carbatrol**	carbamazepine
Azactam	aztreonam	**Cardene**	nicardipine
Azlin	penicillins	**Cardioquin**	quinidine
Azo-Gantrisin	sulfisoxazole	**Cardizem**	diltiazem
AZT, Retrovir	zidovudine	**Cardura**	doxazosin
Azulfidine	sulfasalazine	**Cartrol**	carteolol
Bactocill	oxacillin	**Casodex**	bicalutamide
Bactocill	penicillins	**Cataflam**	diclofenac
Bactrim	cotrimoxazole	**Catapres**	clonidine
Banflex	orphenadrine	**Caverject**	alprostadil
Banthine	methantheline	**Cebid**	ascorbic acid
Baycol	cerivastatin	**Ceclor**	cefaclor
Beepen	penicillins	**Cecon**	ascorbic acid
Belladenal	atropine sulfate	**Cedax**	ceftibuten
Bellergal-S	atropine sulfate	**CeeNU**	lomustine
Benadryl	diphenhydramine	**Cefanex**	cephalexin
Benemid	probenecid	**Ceftin**	cefuroxime
Bentyl	dicyclomine	**Celestone**	corticosteroids
Benylin	dextromethorphan	**Celontin**	methsuximide
Benylin	diphenhydramine	**Cemill**	ascorbic acid
Betagan	levobunolol	**Cenafed**	pseudoephedrine
Betalin S	thiamine	**Cenafed**	triprolidine
Betapace	sotalol	**Centrax**	prazepam
Betapen	penicillins	**Ceptaz**	ceftazidime
Betimol	timolol	**Cerubidine**	daunorubicin
Betoptic	betaxolol	**Cetane**	ascorbic acid
Biaxin	clarithromycin	**Cevalin**	ascorbic acid
Bicillin	penicillins	**Cheracol**	codeine
Bicnu	carmustine	**Cheracol-D**	dextromethorphan
Bilivist	ipodate	**Chibroxin**	norfloxacin
Biltricide	praziquantel	**Chloromycetin**	chloramphenicol
Blenoxane	bleomycin	**Chloroptic**	chloramphenicol
Blocadren	timolol	**Choledyl**	aminophylline
Bontril	phendimetrazine	**Cibacalcin**	calcitonin
Brethaire	terbutaline	**Ciloxan**	ciprofloxacin
Brethine	terbutaline	**Cipro**	ciprofloxacin
Brevibloc	esmolol	**Claforan**	cefotaxime
Brevicon	oral contraceptives	**Claritin**	loratadine
Brevital	methohexital	**Cleocin**	clindamycin
Bricanyl	terbutaline	**Cleocin-T**	clindamycin
Bromo-Seltzer	acetaminophen	**Clinoril**	sulindac
Bronkodyl	aminophylline	**Clomid**	clomiphene
Bucladin-S	buclizine	**Cloxapen**	cloxacillin
Bufferin	aspirin	**Cloxapen**	penicillins
Bumex	bumetanide	**Clozaril**	clozapine
Buspar	buspirone	**Cocaine**	cocaine
Butibel	atropine sulfate	**Cogentin**	benztropine
Butisol	butabarbital	**Cognex**	tacrine
Calan	verapamil	**Colbemid**	colchicine
Calcidrine	codeine	**Colemid**	probenecid
Calciferol	ergocalciferol	**Colase**	docusate
Calcimar	calcitonin	**Colestid**	colestipol
Calciparine	heparin	**Combipres**	chlorthalidone
Calm-X	dimenhydrinate	**Combipres**	clonidine
Capoten	captopril	**Combivent**	albuterol
Capozide	captopril	**Combivent**	ipratropium

Combivir	lamivudine	**Depakote**	divalproex
Compazine	prochlorperazine	**Depen**	penicillamine
Compoz	diphenhydramine	**Depo-Medrol**	corticosteroids
Cordarone	amiodarone	**Depo-Provera**	medroxyprogesterone
Coreg	carvedilol	**Deprol**	benactyzine
Corgard	nadolol	**Desferal**	deferoxamine
Coricidin D	aspirin	**Desogen**	oral contraceptives
Cortef	corticosteroids	**Desoxyn**	methamphetamine
Cortone	corticosteroids	**Desyrel**	trazodone
Cortone	cortisone	**Detrol**	tolterodine
Corzide	bendroflumethiazide	**Dexameth**	corticosteroids
Corzide	nadolol	**Dexedrine**	dextroamphetamine
Cosmegen	dactinomycin	**DHT**	dihydrotachysterol
Cotrim	cotrimoxazole	**Diabeta**	glyburide
Coumadin	warfarin	**Diabinese**	chlorpropamide
Cozaar	losartan	**Dialose**	docusate
Crixivan	indinavir	**Diamox**	acetazolamide
Crysticillin	penicillins	**Diastat**	diazepam
Cuprimine	penicillamine	**Dicumarol**	dicumarol
Curretab	medroxyprogesterone	**Didronel**	etidronate
Curretab	progestins	**Diethylstilbestrol**	diethylstilbestrol
Cyanoject	cyanocobalamin	**Diflucan**	fluconazole
Cycrin	medroxyprogesterone	**Dilacor XR**	diltiazem
Cycrin	progestins	**Dilantin**	phenytoin
Cylert	pemoline	**Dilatrate-SR**	isosorbide
Cyomin	cyanocobalamin	**Dilaudid**	hydromorphone
Cytadren	aminoglutethimide	**Dimetabs**	dimenhydrinate
Cytomel	liothyronine	**Dimetane**	brompheniramine
Cytosar-U	cytarabine	**Diovan**	valsartan
Cytotec	misoprostol	**Dipentum**	olsalazine
Cytovene	ganciclovir	**Diprivan**	propofol
Cytoxan	cyclophosphamide	**Disalcid**	salsalate
Dalmane	flurazepam	**Diucardin**	hydroflumethiazide
Danocrine	danazol	**Diuril**	chlorothiazide
Dantrium	dantrolene	**Dolobid**	diflunisal
Dapsone	dapsone	**Dolophine**	methadone
Daraprim	pyrimethamine	**Donnagel**	atropine sulfate
Darvocet-N	acetaminophen	**Donnatal**	atropine sulfate
Darvocet-N	propoxyphene	**Donnazyme**	atropine sulfate
Darvon	propoxyphene	**Dopar**	levodopa
Darvon Compound	aspirin	**Dopram**	doxapram
Darvon Compound	propoxyphene	**Doral**	quazepam
Datril	acetaminophen	**Dostinex**	cabergoline
Daunoxome	daunorubicin	**Doxinate**	docusate
Daypro	oxaprozin	**Dramamine**	dimenhydrinate
DDAVP	desmopressin	**Drisdol**	ergocalciferol
Decadron	corticosteroids	**Dristan**	acetaminophen
Declomycin	demeclocycline	**Drixoral**	dextromethorphan
Decofed	pseudoephedrine	**Drixoral**	pseudoephedrine
Del-Vi-A	vitamin A	**DTIC**	dacarbazine
Delta-Cortef	corticosteroids	**Dulcolax**	bisacodyl
Delta-Lutin	progestins	**Duract**	bromfenac
Deltalin	ergocalciferol	**Duragesic**	fentanyl
Deltasone	corticosteroids	**Duralutin**	progestins
Demadex	torsemide	**Duricef**	cefadroxil
Demerol	meperidine	**Dyazide**	hydrochlorothiazide
Demulen	oral contraceptives	**Dyazide**	triamterene
Depakene	valproic acid	**Dycil**	penicillins

Dycill dicloxacillin
Dymelor acetohexamide
Dynabac dirithromycin
Dynacin minocycline
Dynacirc isradipine
Dynapen dicloxacillin
Dynapen penicillins
Dyrenium triamterene
E-Mycin erythromycin
E-Vitamin Succinate vitamin E
E-Zide hydrochlorothiazide
E.E.S. erythromycin
Ecotrin aspirin
Ectasule ephedrine
Edecrin ethacrynic acid
Edex alprostadil
Efedron ephedrine
Effexor venlafaxine
Efudex fluorouracil
Elavil amitriptyline
Eldepryl selegiline
Elixophyllin aminophylline
Elspar asparaginase
Emcyt estramustine
Empirin aspirin
Endep amitriptyline
Enduron methyclothiazide
Enlon edrophonium
Enovid oral contraceptives
Entex pseudoephedrine
Ephedsol ephedrine
Epifrin epinephrine
Epipen epinephrine
Epitol carbamazepine
Epivir lamivudine
Epogen epoetin alfa
Eprolin vitamin E
Equagesic aspirin
Equal aspartame
Equanil meprobamate
Ergamisol levamisole
Ery-Ped erythromycin
Ery-Tab erythromycin
Eryc erythromycin
Erypar erythromycin
Erythrocin erythromycin
Erythropoietin epoetin alfa
Eryzole erythromycin
Esidrix hydrochlorothiazide
Eskalith lithium
Espotabs phenolphthalein
Estrostep oral contraceptives
Estrovis quinestrol
Ethamolin ethanolamine
Ethmozine moricizine
Eulexin flutamide
Evista raloxifene
Ex-Lax phenolphthalein
Excedrin acetaminophen
Excedrin aspirin
Exna benzthiazide
Famvir famciclovir
Fansidar pyrimethamine
Fansidar sulfadoxine
Fareston toremifene
Fastin phentermine
Feen-A-Mint phenolphthalein
Felbatol felbamate
Feldene piroxicam
Femara letrozole
Fiorinal aspirin
Fiorinal butalbital
Flagyl metronidazole
Fleet Laxative bisacodyl
Flexeril cyclobenzaprine
Floxin ofloxacin
Flumadine rimantadine
Fluoroplex fluorouracil
Fluothane halothane
Folex methotrexate
Folvite folic acid
Fortaz ceftazidime
Fortovase saquinavir
Fosamax alendronate
Foscavir foscarnet
Fragmin dalteparin
Fulvicin griseofulvin
Fungizone amphotericin B
Furadantin nitrofurantoin
Furoxone furazolidone
Gabitril tiagabine
Gantanol sulfamethoxazole
Gantrisin sulfisoxazole
Garamycin gentamicin
Gastrocrom cromolyn
Gelprin aspirin
Gemzar gemcitabine
Genac triprolidine
Geocillin carbenicillin
Geopen penicillins
Gesterol 50 progestins
Glucagon Emergency Kit glucagon
Glucophage metformin
Glucotrol glipizide
Glynase glyburide
Grifulvin griseofulvin
Gris-Peg griseofulvin
Grisactin griseofulvin
Guaituss AC codeine
Halcion triazolam
Haldol haloperidol
Halotensin fluoxymesterone
Halotussin codeine
Hep-Flush heparin
Hep-Lock heparin
Heroin heroin

Hexabetalin	pyridoxine
Hexadrol	corticosteroids
Hexalen	altretamine
Hiprex	methenamine
Hismanal	astemizole
Hivid	zalcitabine
Humulin	insulin
Hycamtin	topotecan
Hycodan	atropine sulfate
Hydeltrasol	corticosteroids
Hydrea	hydroxyurea
Hydro-Chlor	hydrochlorothiazide
Hydro-D	hydrochlorothiazide
Hydro-Par	hydrochlorothiazide
Hydrodiuril	hydrochlorothiazide
Hydromox	quinethazone
Hygroton	chlorthalidone
Hylorel	guanadrel
Hylutin	progestins
Hyperstat	diazoxide
Hytakerol	dihydrotachysterol
Hytrin	terazosin
Hyzaar	losartan
Idamycin	idarubicin
Ifex	ifosfamide
Iletin Lente	insulin
Ilosone	erythromycin
Ilotycin	erythromycin
Imdur	isosorbide
Imitrex	sumatriptan
Imodium	loperamide
Imuran	azathioprine
Inderal	propranolol
Indocin	indomethacin
Infergen	interferons, alfa
Intal	cromolyn
Interleukin-2	aldesleukin
Intron A	interferons, alfa
Intropin	dopamine
Invirase	saquinavir
Ionamin	phentermine
Iopidine	apraclonidine
Ismelin	guanethidine
Ismo	isosorbide
Isoptin	verapamil
Isopto Atropine	atropine sulfate
Isordil	isosorbide
Isuprel	isoproterenol
Janimine	imipramine
Jenest	oral contraceptives
Kabikinase	streptokinase
Kantrex	kanamycin
Keflet	cephalexin
Keflex	cephalexin
Keflin	cephalothin
Kefzol	cefazolin
Kefzol	cephalothin
Kemadrin	procyclidine
Kenalog	corticosteroids
Kerlone	betaxolol
Ketalar	ketamine
Klonopin	clonazepam
Kytril	granisetron
Lamictal	lamotrigine
Lamisil	terbinafine
Lamprene	clofazimine
Laniazid	isoniazid
Lanoxicaps	digoxin
Lanoxin	digoxin
Lariam	mefloquine
Larodopa	levodopa
Larotid	penicillins
Lasix	furosemide
Ledercillin	penicillins
Legatrin	quinine
Lescol	fluvastatin
Leukeran	chlorambucil
Leustatin	cladribine
Levaquin	levofloxacin
Levatol	penbutolol
Levlen	oral contraceptives
Levothyroid	levothyroxine
Levoxyl	levothyroxine
Lexxel	enalapril
Lexxel	felodipine
Librax	clidinium
Libritabs	chlordiazepoxide
Librium	chlordiazepoxide
Limbitrol	amitriptyline
Limbitrol	chlordiazepoxide
Lincocin	lincomycin
Lipitor	atorvastatin
Lipoxide	chlordiazepoxide
Liquaemin	heparin
Liquiprin	acetaminophen
Lithobid	lithium
Lithonate	lithium
Lithotabs	lithium
Lo/Ovral	oral contraceptives
Lodine	etodolac
Loestrin	oral contraceptives
Lofene	atropine sulfate
Logen	atropine sulfate
Lomanate	atropine sulfate
Lomotil	atropine sulfate
Lomotil	diphenoxylate
Loniten	minoxidil
Lopid	gemfibrozil
Lopressor	metoprolol
Lopurin	allopurinol
Lorabid	loracarbef
Lorcet	acetaminophen
Lotensin	benazepril
Lotrel	amlodipine
Lotrel	benazepril
Lovenox	enoxaparin

Loxitane	loxapine	**Minocin**	minocycline
Lozol	indapamide	**Mintezol**	thiabendazole
Ludiomil	maprotiline	**Mirapex**	pramipexole
Luminal	phenobarbital	**Mithracin**	plicamycin
Lupron	leuprolide	**Moban**	molindone
Luvox	fluvoxamine	**Modane**	docusate
Lymphocin	vancomycin	**Modane**	phenolphthalein
Lysodren	mitotane	**Modicon**	oral contraceptives
Macrobid	nitrofurantoin	**Moduretic**	amiloride
Macrodantin	nitrofurantoin	**Monistat**	miconazole
Mandelamine	methenamine	**Mono-Gesic**	salsalate
Mandol	cefamandole	**Monodox**	doxycycline
Marihuana	marihuana	**Monoket**	isosorbide
Marinol	dronabinol	**Monopril**	fosinopril
Marmine	dimenhydrinate	**Monurol**	fosfomycin
Marplan	isocarboxazid	**Motrin**	ibuprofen
Matulane	procarbazine	**Mustargen**	mechlorethamine
Mavik	trandolapril	**Mutamycin**	mitomycin
Maxaquin	lomefloxacin	**Myambutol**	ethambutol
Maxipime	cefepime	**Mycifradin**	neomycin
Maxzide	hydrochlorothiazide	**Mycobutin**	rifabutin
Maxzide	triamterene	**Mycostatin**	nystatin
Mazanor	mazindol	**Myidil**	triprolidine
Measurin	aspirin	**Mykrox**	metolazone
Mebaral	mephobarbital	**Myleran**	busulfan
Meclomen	meclofenamate	**Myochrysine**	gold
Medihaler-ISO	isoproterenol	**Mysoline**	primidone
Medipren	ibuprofen	**Nafcil**	nafcillin
Medrol	corticosteroids	**Nalfon**	fenoprofen
Mefoxin	cefoxitin	**Nallpen**	nafcillin
Megace	progestins	**Naprosyn**	naproxen
Mellaril	thioridazine	**Naqua**	trichlormethiazide
Mephyton	phytonadione	**Narcan**	naloxone
Mepron	atovaquone	**Nardil**	phenelzine
Meridia	sibutramine	**Nasalcrom**	cromolyn
Mesantoin	mephenytoin	**Nascobal**	cyanocobalamin
Mesnex	mesna	**Naturetin**	bendroflumethiazide
Metahydrin	trichlormethiazide	**Navane**	thiothixene
Meticorten	corticosteroids	**Navelbine**	vinorelbine
Metrocream	metronidazole	**Nebcin**	tobramycin
Metrogel	metronidazole	**Nebupent**	pentamidine
Mevacor	lovastatin	**Neggram**	nalidixic acid
Mexate	methotrexate	**Nembutal**	pentobarbital
Mexitil	mexiletine	**Neoral**	cyclosporine
Mezlin	mezlocillin	**Neosar**	cyclophosphamide
Mezlin	penicillins	**Neptazane**	methazolamide
Miacalcin	calcitonin	**Neurontin**	gabapentin
Micronase	glyburide	**Neutrexin**	trimetrexate
Micronor	progestins	**Niaspan**	niacin; niacinamide
Microzide	hydrochlorothiazide	**Nico-Vert**	dimenhydrinate
Midamor	amiloride	**Nicolar**	niacin; niacinamide
Midol	ibuprofen	**Nicotinamide**	niacin; niacinamide
Milontin	phensuximide	**Nilstat**	nystatin
Miltown	meprobamate	**Nimotop**	nimodipine
Minipress	prazosin	**Niong**	nitroglycerin
Minitran	nitroglycerin	**Nipent**	pentostatin
Minizide	polythiazide	**Nitrocap**	nitroglycerin
Minizide	prazosin	**Nitrocine**	nitroglycerin

Nitrodisc	nitroglycerin
Nitrodur	nitroglycerin
Nitroglyn	nitroglycerin
Nitroject	nitroglycerin
Nitrol	nitroglycerin
Nitronet	nitroglycerin
Nitrong	nitroglycerin
Nitrospan	nitroglycerin
Nitrostat	nitroglycerin
Nizoral	ketoconazole
Noctec	chloral hydrate
Nolahist	phenindamine
Nolvadex	tamoxifen
Nor-QD	progestins
Nordette	oral contraceptives
Norflex	orphenadrine
Norgesic	aspirin
Norinyl	oral contraceptives
Norisodrine	isoproterenol
Noritate	metronidazole
Norlestrin	oral contraceptives
Norlutate	progestins
Norlutin	progestins
Normodyne	labetalol
Noroxin	norfloxacin
Norpace	disopyramide
Norphyl	aminophylline
Norpramin	desipramine
Norvasc	amlodipine
Norvir	ritonavir
Novafed	pseudoephedrine
Novahistine DH	codeine
Novolin R	insulin
NPH	insulin
Nucofed	codeine
Nuprin	ibuprofen
Nutrasweet	aspartame
Nydrazid	isoniazid
Nystex	nystatin
Octamide	metoclopramide
Ocuflox	ofloxacin
Ocupress	carteolol
Olycillin	penicillins
Omnicef	cefdinir
Omnipen	ampicillin
Omnipen	penicillins
Oncovin	vincristine
Ophthochlor	chloramphenicol
Optimine	azatadine
Oragrafin	ipodate
Orap	pimozide
Orasone	corticosteroids
Oretic	hydrochlorothiazide
Oreton	methyltestosterone
Orinase	tolbutamide
Ortho Tri-Cyclen	oral contraceptives
Ortho-Cept	oral contraceptives
Ortho-Cyclen	oral contraceptives
Ortho-Novum	oral contraceptives
Orudis	ketoprofen
Oruvail	ketoprofen
Osteocalcin	calcitonin
Ovcon	oral contraceptives
Ovral	oral contraceptives
Ovrette	progestins
Oxsoralen	methoxsalen
Oxsoralen	psoralens
Palmitate A	vitamin A
Pamelor	nortriptyline
Pamprin	ibuprofen
Panadol	acetaminophen
Panmycin	tetracycline
Paradione	paramethadione
Paraflex	chlorzoxazone
Parafon Forte DSC	chlorzoxazone
Paraplatin	carboplatin
Parlodel	bromocriptine
Parnate	tranylcypromine
Pathocil	penicillins
Pavabid	papaverine
Paxil	paroxetine
PBZ	tripelennamine
PCE	erythromycin
Pediazole	erythromycin
Peganone	ethotoin
Pen Vee K	penicillins
Penetrex	enoxacin
Pentam 300	pentamidine
Pentasa	mesalamine
Pentothal Sodium	thiopental
Pepcid	famotidine
Peptavlon	pentagastrin
Percodan	aspirin
Percogesic	acetaminophen
Percoset	acetaminophen
Periactin	cyproheptadine
Permax	pergolide
Permitil	fluphenazine
Persantine	dipyridamole
Pertussin	dextromethorphan
Phenaphen	acetaminophen
Phenolax	phenolphthalein
Pheryl-E	vitamin E
Phyllocontin	aminophylline
Phytomenadione	phytonadione
Pima	potassium iodide
Pipracil	penicillins
Pipracil	piperacillin
Pitressin	vasopressin
Placidyl	ethchlorvynol
Plaquenil	hydroxychloroquine
Platinol	cisplatin
Plavix	clopidogrel
Plegine	phendimetrazine
Plendil	felodipine
Polycillin	ampicillin

Polymox	amoxicillin	**Rebetron**	ribavirin
Polymox	penicillins	**Redux**	dexfenfluramine
Pondimin	fenfluramine	**Regitine**	phentolamine
Ponstel	mefenamic acid	**Reglan**	metoclopramide
Posicor	mibefradil	**Regutol**	docusate
Prandin	repaglinide	**Rela**	carisoprodol
Pravachol	pravastatin	**Relafen**	nabumetone
Prevacid	lansoprazole	**Renese**	polythiazide
Prilosec	omeprazole	**Reopro**	abciximab
Primaquine	primaquine	**Requip**	ropinirole
Primaxin	imipenem/cilastatin	**Rescriptor**	delavirdine
Principen	ampicillin	**Restoril**	temazepam
Principen	penicillins	**Reversol**	edrophonium
Prinivil	lisinopril	**Rezulin**	troglitazone
Prinizide	hydrochlorothiazide	**Rheumatrex**	methotrexate
Prinizide	lisinopril	**Riboflavin**	riboflavin
Priscoline	tolazoline	**Ridaura**	gold
Pro-Banthine	propantheline	**Rifadin**	rifampin
Pro-Depo	progestins	**Rifampicin**	rifampin
Procan	procainamide	**Rimactane**	rifampin
Procardia	nifedipine	**Riobin**	riboflavin
Procrit	epoetin alfa	**Risperdal**	risperidone
Prodrox	progestins	**Ritalin**	methylphenidate
Profen	ibuprofen	**Robaxin**	methocarbamol
Progestaject	progestins	**Robaxisal**	aspirin
Prograf	tacrolimus	**Robimycin**	erythromycin
Proleukin	aldesleukin	**Robitet**	tetracycline
Prolixin	fluphenazine	**Robitussin**	dextromethorphan
Proloprim	trimethoprim	**Robitussin AC**	codeine
Pronestyl	procainamide	**Rocephin**	ceftriaxone
Propecia	finasteride	**Roferon-A**	interferons, alfa
Propulsid	cisapride	**Rogaine**	minoxidil
Propylthiouracil	propylthiouracil	**Romazicon**	flumazenil
Proscar	finasteride	**Rowasa**	mesalamine
Prosom	estazolam	**Rubex**	doxorubicin
Prostaphlin	oxacillin	**Rubramin**	cyanocobalamin
Prostaphlin	penicillins	**Rufen**	ibuprofen
Prostin VR	alprostadil	**Rythmol**	propafenone
Protamine	insulin	**Saccharin**	saccharin
Protamine Sulfate	protamine	**Salflex**	salsalate
Proventil	albuterol	**Salsitab**	salsalate
Provera	medroxyprogesterone	**Saluron**	hydroflumethiazide
Provera	progestins	**Sandimmune**	cyclosporine
Prozac	fluoxetine	**Sandostatin**	octreotide
Purinethol	mercaptopurine	**Sanorex**	mazindol
Pyrazinamide	pyrazinamide	**Sansert**	methysergide
Pyridium	phenazopyridine	**Seconal**	secobarbital
Quarzan	clidinium	**Secretin-Ferring**	secretin
Quelicin	succinylcholine	**Sectral**	acebutolol
Questran	cholestyramine	**Seldane**	terfenadine
Quibron	aminophylline	**Seldane-D, Sudafed**	pseudoephedrine
Quinaglute	quinidine	**Septra**	cotrimoxazole
Quinidex	quinidine	**Ser-Ap-Es**	hydralazine
Quiphile	quinine	**Ser-Ap-Es**	reserpine
Rauzide	bendroflumethiazide	**Ser-Ap-Es**	hydrochlorothiazide
Raxar	grepafloxacin	**Serax**	oxazepam
Razepam	temazepam	**Serentil**	mesoridazine
Rebetron	interferons, alfa	**Serevent**	salmeterol

Seromycin	cycloserine
Serophene	clomiphene
Seroquel	quetiapine
Serpasil	reserpine
Serzone	nefazodone
Sinemet	carbidopa
Sinemet	levodopa
Sinequan	doxepin
Singulair	montelukast
Sinutab	acetaminophen
Skelaxin	metaxalone
Slo-Bid	aminophylline
Sodium P.A.S.	aminosalicylate sodium
Solatene	beta-carotene
Solfoton	phenobarbital
Solganal	gold
Solu-Cortef	corticosteroids
Solu-Medrol	corticosteroids
Soma	carisoprodol
Soma Compound	aspirin
Sominex 2	diphenhydramine
Somophyllin	aminophylline
Sorbitrate	isosorbide
Soriatane	acitretin
Sparine	promazine
Spectrobid	penicillins
Sporanox	itraconazole
SSKI	potassium iodide
Stadol	butorphanol
Staphcillin	methicillin
Staphcillin	penicillins
Stelazine	trifluoperazine
Streptase	streptokinase
Streptomycin	streptomycin
Stromectol	ivermectin
Sucaryl	cyclamate
Sucrets	dextromethorphan
Sular	nisoldipine
Sulfalax	docusate
Sumycin	tetracycline
Sunkist	ascorbic acid
Suppress	dextromethorphan
Suprax	cefixime
Surfak, etc.	docusate
Surmontil	trimipramine
Sus-Phrine	epinephrine
Sweet 'n Low	saccharin
Symmetrel	amantadine
Synarel	nafarelin
Synthroid	levothyroxine
Syprine	trientine
Tace	chlorotrianisene
Tagamet	cimetidine
Talwin	pentazocine
Talwin Compound	aspirin
Tambocor	flecainide
TAO	troleandomycin
Tapazole	methimazole
Tarabine	cytarabine
Tarka	trandolapril
Tarka	verapamil
Tasmar	tolcapone
Tavist	clemastine
Taxol	paclitaxel
Taxotere	docetaxel
Tazicef	ceftazidime
Tazidime	ceftazidime
Teczem	diltiazem
Teczem	enalapril
Tega-Cert	dimenhydrinate
Tega-Vert	dimenhydrinate
Tegopen	cloxacillin
Tegopen	penicillins
Tegretol	carbamazepine
Temaril	trimeprazine
Tenex	guanfacine
Tenoretic	atenolol
Tenormin	atenolol
Tensilon	edrophonium
Tenuate	diethylpropion
Terramycin	oxytetracycline
Testoderm	testosterone
Testred	methyltestosterone
Thalidomide	thalidomide
Thalitone	chlorthalidone
Theo-Dur	aminophylline
Thioguanine	thioguanine
Thiola	tiopronin
Thioplex	thiotepa
Thorazine	chlorpromazine
Tiazac	diltiazem
Ticar	penicillins
Ticar	ticarcillin
Ticlid	ticlopidine
Timoptic	timolol
Tobrex	tobramycin
Tofranil	imipramine
Tolectin	tolmetin
Tolinase	tolazamide
Topamax	topiramate
Toposar	etoposide
Toprol	metoprolol
Toradol	ketorolac
Totacillin	ampicillin
Trancopal	chlormezanone
Trandate	labetalol
Transderm-Nitro	nitroglycerin
Transderm-Scop	scopolamine
Tranxene	clorazepate
Trecator-SC	ethionamide
Trental	pentoxifylline
Tri-Levlen	oral contraceptives
Tri-Norinyl	oral contraceptives
Triaminic	pyrilamine
Tricor	fenofibrate
Tridil	nitroglycerin

Tridione	trimethadione
Trifed	triprolidine
Trilafon	perphenazine
Trimox	amoxicillin
Trimox	penicillins
Trimpex	trimethoprim
Trinalin	pseudoephedrine
Triofed	triprolidine
Triphasil	oral contraceptives
Triposed	triprolidine
Triptone	dimenhydrinate
Trisoralen	psoralens
Trisoralen	trioxsalen
Trobicin	spectinomycin
Trovan	trovafloxacin
Truphylline	aminophylline
Tussar-2	codeine
Tussi-Organidin	codeine
Tylenol	acetaminophen
Ultracef	cefadroxil
Ultram	tramadol
Unasyn	penicillins
Unipen	nafcillin
Unipen	penicillins
Uniretic	moexipril
Univasc	moexipril
Urecholine	bethanechol
Urex	methenamine
Urised	atropine sulfate
Urised	methenamine
Urispas	flavoxate
Uroqid	methenamine
V-Cillin	penicillins
Valadol	acetaminophen
Valdrene	diphenhydramine
Valium	diazepam
Vancocin	vancomycin
Vancoled	vancomycin
Vanquish	aspirin
Vantin	cefpodoxime
Vascor	bepridil
Vasotec	enalapril
Vazepam	diazepam
Vectrin	minocycline
Velban	vinblastine
Velosef	cephradine
Velosulin	insulin
Ventolin	albuterol
VePesid	etoposide
Verelan	verapamil
Vermox	mebendazole
Versed	midazolam
Vertab	dimenhydrinate
Viagra	sildenafil
Vibra-Tabs	doxycycline
Vibramycin	doxycycline
Vicks Formula 44	dextromethorphan
Vicks Vatronol	ephedrine
Vicodin	acetaminophen
Videx	didanosine
Vincasar	vincristine
Viracept	nelfinavir
Viramune	nevirapine
Virazole	ribavirin
Virilon	methyltestosterone
Visken	pindolol
Vistaril	hydroxyzine
Vita Plus E	vitamin E
Vitamin B_1	thiamine
Vitamin B_2	riboflavin
Vitamin B_6	pyridoxine
Vitamin B_{12}	cyanocobalamin
Vitamin D	ergocalciferol
Vitamin K_1	phytonadione
Vitec	vitamin E
Vivactil	protriptyline
Volmax	albuterol
Voltaren	diclofenac
Wehamine	dimenhydrinate
Wellbutrin	bupropion
Winstrol	stanozolol
Wintrocin	erythromycin
Wycillin	penicillins
Wymox	amoxicillin
Wymox	penicillins
Wytensin	guanabenz
Xalatan	latanoprost
Xanax	alprazolam
Xylocaine	lidocaine
Yocon	yohimbine
Yohimex	yohimbine
Yutopar	ritordine
Zagam	sparfloxacin
Zanaflex	tizanidine
Zanosar	streptozocin
Zantac	ranitidine
Zarontin	ethosuximide
Zaroxolyn	metolazone
Zebeta	bisoprolol
Zestril	lisinopril
Ziac	bisoprolol
Zithromax	azithromycin
Zocor	simvastatin
Zofran	ondansetron
Zolicef	cefazolin
Zoloft	sertraline
Zomig	zolmitriptan
Zonalon	doxepin
Zosyn	piperacillin
Zovirax	acyclovir
Zyban	bupropion
Zyflo	zileuton
Zyloprim	allopurinol
Zyprexa	olanzapine
Zyrtec	cetirizine

Classes of drugs

ACE-inhibitors
- benazepril
- captopril
- cilazapril
- enalapril
- fosinopril
- lisinopril
- moexipril
- perindopril
- quinapril
- ramipril
- spirapril
- trandolapril

Alpha adrenergic receptor inhibitors
- doxazosin
- phentolamine
- prazosin
- tamsulosin
- terazosin

Alpha adrenoreceptor agonists
- clonidine
- guanabenz
- guanfacine
- tizanidine

Aminoglycosides
- amikacin
- ceftazidime
- gentamicin
- kanamycin
- neomycin
- netilmicin
- streptomycin
- tobramycin

Amphetamines
- amphetamine sulfate
- dexfenfluramine
- dextroamphetamine
- diethylpropion
- fenfluramine
- mazindol
- methamphetamine
- methylphenidate
- phendimetrazine
- phentermine

Antiarrhythmic agents
- adenosine
- amiodarone
- atropine
- belladonna
- bretylium
- chlorothiazide
- disopyramide
- edrophonium
- esmolol
- flecainide
- isoproterenol
- lidocaine
- magnesium sulfate
- metoprolol
- mexiletine
- minoxidil
- moricizine
- procainamide
- propafenone
- propranolol
- quinidine
- sotalol
- tocainide
- verapamil

Anticholinergic agents
- albuterol
- amantadine
- atropine
- belladonna
- benztropine
- biperiden
- bromocriptine
- carbidopa
- clidinium
- dicyclomine
- diphenhydramine
- glycopyrrolate
- homatropine
- ipratropium
- levodopa
- methantheline
- orphenadrine
- pergolide
- physostigmine
- procyclidine
- propantheline
- scopolamine
- selegiline
- tacrine
- trihexiphenidyl

Anticonvulsants
- acetazolamide
- carbamazepine
- chlorpromazine
- clonazepam
- diazepam
- divalproex
- ethosuximide
- ethotoin
- felbamate
- gabapentin
- hydroxyzine
- lamotrigine
- mephenytoin
- mephobarbital
- methsuximide
- paraldehyde
- paramethadione
- pentobarbital
- phenobarbital
- phensuximide
- phenytoin
- primidone
- topiramate
- trimethadione
- valproic acid

Antidepressants

[T]=tricyclic
[H]=heterocyclic
[TE]=tetracyclic

- amitriptyline [T]
- amoxapine [T]
- benactyzine
- bupropion [H]
- clomipramine [T]
- desipramine [T]
- divalproex
- doxepin [T]
- fluoxetine
- fluvoxamine
- imipramine [T]
- isocarboxazid
- lithium
- loxapine [T]
- maprotiline [TE]
- methylphenidate
- nefazodone
- nortriptyline [T]
- paroxetine
- perphenazine
- phenelzine
- protriptyline [T]
- sertraline
- thioridazine
- tranylcypromine
- trazodone [H]
- trimipramine [T]

venlafaxine [H]

Antidiabetic agents

acarbose
acetohexamide
chlorpropamide
glimepiride
glipizide
glucagon
glyburide
insulin
metformin
tolazamide
tolbutamide
troglitazone

Antifungals

amphotericin B
clotrimazole
fluconazole
flucytosine
griseofulvin
itraconazole
ketoconazole
metronidazole
miconazole
nystatin
terbinafine

Antihypertensives

acebutolol
amiloride
amlodipine
atenolol
benazepril
bendroflumethiazide
benzthiazide
betaxolol
bisoprolol
captopril
carteolol
chlorothiazide
chlorthalidone
clonidine
cyclothiazide
diazoxide
diltiazem
doxazosin
enalapril
ethacrynic acid
felodipine
fosinopril
guanabenz
guanethidine
guanfacine
hydralazine
hydrochlorothiazide
hydroflumethiazide
indapamide
isradipine
labetalol
lisinopril
losartan
meclofenamate
methyclothiazide
methyldopa
methylphenidate
metolazone
metoprolol
minoxidil
moexipril
nadolol
nicardipine
nifedipine
nimodipine
nisoldipine
nitroglycerin
penbutolol
phentolamine
pindolol
polythiazide
prazosin
propantheline
propranolol
quinapril
ramipril
reserpine
spironolactone
terazosin
timolol
torsemide
triamterene
trichlormethiazide
verapamil
yohimbine

Antimalarial agents

chloroquine
hydroxychloroquine
mefloquine
primaquine
pyrimethamine
quinacrine
quinine

Antimycobacterial agents

aminosalicylic acid
capreomycin
clofazimine
cycloserine
dapsone
ethambutol
ethionamide
isoniazid
kanamycin
pyrazinamide
rifampin
streptomycin

Antineoplastics

azathioprine
aldesleukin
asparaginase
bleomycin
busulfan
carboplatin
carmustine
chlorambucil
chlorotrianisene
cisplatin
cyclophosphamide
cytarabine
dacarbazine
dactinomycin
daunorubicin
diethylstilbestrol
docetaxel
doxorubicin
estradiol
estramustine
etoposide
fluorouracil
fluoxymesterone
flutamide
hydroxyprogesterone
hydroxyurea
idarubicin
interferon
leucovorin
leuprolide
levamisole
lomustine
masoprocol
mechlorethamine
medroxyprogesterone
megestrol
melphalan
mercaptopurine
mesna
methotrexate
methyltestosterone
mitomycin
mitotane
paclitaxel
plicamycin
procarbazine
progesterone
streptozocin
tamoxifen
testosterone
thioguanine
thiotepa
topotecan
trimetrexate
vinblastine
vincristine
vinorelbine

Anxiolytics, sedatives, & hypnotics

alprazolam

amobarbital
aprobarbital
buspirone
butabarbital
chloral hydrate
chlordiazepoxide
chlormezanone
chlorzoxazone
clonazepam
clorazepate
diazepam
droperidol
estazolam
ethchlorvynol
fentanyl
flurazepam
glutethimide
hydroxzine
ketamine
lorazepam
mephobarbital
meprobamate
methohexital
midazolam
opium alkaloids
oxazepam
paraldehyde
paroxetine
pentobarbital
phenobarbital
prazepam
prochlorperazine
promethazine
propofol
quazepam
secobarbital
sertraline
temazepam
thiopental
triazolam
trifluoperazine
zolpidem

Benzodiazepines

alprazolam
amitriptyline
chlordiazepoxide
clorazepate
diazepam
estazolam
flurazepam
lorazepam
midazolam
olanzapine
oxazepam
prazepam
quazepam
temazepam
triazolam

Beta-blockers

acebutolol
atenolol
betaxolol
bisoprolol
carteolol
carvedilol
esmolol
labetalol
levobunolol
metipranolol
metoprolol
nadolol
penbutolol
pindolol
propranolol
sotalol
timolol

Beta-lactam antibiotics

aztreonam
cefixime
cefoxitin
imipenen/cilastin
loracarbef
meropenem
moxalactam
tazobactam

Calcium channel blockers

amlodipine
bepridil
diltiazem
felodipine
isradipine
nicardipine
nifedipine
nimodipine
nisoldipine
verapamil

Cephalosporins

cefaclor
cefadroxil
cefamandole
cefazolin
cefdinir
cefepime
cefixime
cefmetazole
cefonicid
cefoperazone
ceforanide
cefotaxime
cefotetan
cefoxitin
cefpodoxime
cefprozil
ceftazidime
ceftibuten
ceftizoxime
ceftriaxone
cefuroxime
cephalexin
cephalothin
cephapirin
cephradine

Diuretics

acetazolamide
amiloride
bendroflumethiazide
benzthiazide
bumetanide
chlorthalidone
chorothiazide
cyclothiazide
ethacrynic acid
furosemide
hydrochlorothiazide
hydroflumethiazide
indapamide
isosorbide
mannitol
methyclothiazide
metolazone
polythiazide
potassium chloride
quinethazone
spironolactone
torsemide
triamterene
trichlormethiazide
urea

Diuretics, loop

bumetanide
ethacrynic acid
furosemide
torsemide

HMG-CoA reductase inhibitors

atorvastatin
fluvastatin
lovastatin
pravastatin
simvastatin

Hypnotics

aprobarbital
ethchlorvynol
flurazepam
glutethimide
l-tryptophan
methohexital
opium alkaloids
pentobarbital
phenobarbital
propofol
quazepam
secobarbital
temazepam
thiopental

triazolam
zolpidem

Hypolipidemic agents

atorvastatin
cerivastatin
cholestyramine
clofibrate
colestipol
dextrothyroxine
fenofibrate
fluvastatin
gemfibrozil
lovastatin
niacin
pravastatin
probucol
simvastatin

Macrolides

azithromycin
clarithromycin
dirithromycin
erythromycin
rifabutin

Monamine oxidase inhibitors

isocarboxazid
pargyline
phenelzine
tranylcypromine

Neuroleptics

amitriptyline
chlorpromazine
fluphenazine
haloperidol
lithium
loxapine
molindone
prochlorperazine
thioridazine
thiothixene
tranylcypromine
trifluoperazine

NSAIDs

aspirin
diclofenac
diflunisal
etodolac
fenoprofen
flurbiprofen
ibuprofen
indomethacin
ketoprofen
ketorolac
meclofenamate
mefenamic acid
mesalamine
methotrexate
nabumetone
naproxen
olsalazine
oxaprozin
oxyphenbutazone
phenylbutazone
piroxicam
salsalate
sulindac
tolmetin

Selective serotonin reuptake inhibitors (SSRIs)

fluoxetine
fluvoxamine
nefazodone
paroxetine
sertraline
trazodone
venlafaxine

Tranquilizers

amitriptyline
buspirone
chlordiazepoxide
chlormezanone
chlorpromazine
clorazepate
diazepam
doxepin
droperidol
fluphenazine
haloperidol
hydroxyzine
lorazepam
loxapine
meprobamate
mesoridazine
molindone
oxazepam
perphenazine
pimozide
prochlorperazine
promazine
promethazine
reserpine
risperidone
thioridazine
thiothixene
trifluoperazine

ABCIXIMAB

Trade name: Reopro (Lilly)
Category: Platelet aggregation inhibitor
Half-life: 10–30 minutes
Clinically important, potentially serious interactions with: no data

REACTIONS

SKIN
- Cellulitis (0.3%)
- Peripheral edema (1.6%)
- Petechiae (0.3%)
- Pruritus (0.3%)

OTHER
- Hypesthesia (1%)
- Myalgia (0.3%)
- Myopathy (0.3%)

ACEBUTOLOL

Trade name: Sectral (Wyeth)
Other common trade names: Acecor; Acetanol; Alol; Monitan; Neptal; Prent; Rhodiasectral
Category: Beta-adrenergic blocking agent; antiarrhythmic; antihypertensive
Clinically important, potentially serious interactions with: calcium channel blockers, clonidine, reserpine

REACTIONS

SKIN
- Dermatitis (sic)
- Edema (1–10%)
- Erythema multiforme (<1%)
- Exanthems (4%)
- Facial edema (<1%)
- Hyperhidrosis
- Hyperkeratosis (palms & soles)
- Lichenoid eruption
- Lupus erythematosus (<1%)
- Pityriasis rubra pilaris
- Pruritus (<2%)
- Psoriasis
- Rash (sic) (2%)
- Raynaud's phenomenon
- Toxic epidermal necrolysis
- Urticaria
- Vasculitis
- Xerosis

HAIR
- Hair – alopecia

NAILS
- Nails – bluish
- Nails – dystrophy
- Nails – onycholysis

OTHER
- Hyperesthesia (<2%)
- Hypesthesia (<2%)
- Myalgia (2%)
- Oculo-mucocutaneous syndrome
- Oral lichenoid eruption
- Peyronie's disease
- Xerostomia (<1%)

ACETAMINOPHEN

Trade names: Anacin-3; Bromo-Seltzer; Darvocet-N; Datril; Dristan; Excedrin; Liquiprin; Lorcet; Panadol; Percogesic; Percoset; Phenaphen; Sinutab; Tylenol; Valadol; Vicodin; etc. (Various pharmaceutical companies.)
Other common trade names: Abenol; Anaflon; Ben-U-Ron; Doliprane; Geluprane; Panadol
Category: Antipyretic analgesic
Clinically important, potentially serious interactions with: alcohol

REACTIONS

SKIN
- Acute generalized exanthematous pustulosis (AGEP)
- Angioedema (<1%)
- Contact dermatitis
- Dermatitis (sic)
- Erythema (sic)
- Erythema multiforme
- Erythema nodosum (<1%)
- Exanthems (rare)
- Exfoliative dermatitis
- Fixed eruption (<1%)
- Flushing
- Hyperhidrosis
- Neutrophilic eccrine hidradenitis
- Pemphigus
- Penile edema
- Pityriasis rosea
- Progressive pigmentary purpura (Schamberg's disease)
- Pruritus
- Purpura
- Purpura fulminans
- Rash (sic) (<1%)
- Sensitivity (sic)
- Stevens-Johnson syndrome
- Toxic epidermal necrolysis
- Urticaria
- Vasculitis

HAIR
- Hair – alopecia

NAILS
- Nails – disorder (sic)

OTHER
- Anaphylactoid reaction
- Dysgeusia
- Hypersensitivity (<1%)

ACETAZOLAMIDE

Trade name: Diamox (Storz)
Other common trade names: Acetazolam; Defiltran; Diuramid
Category: Anticonvulsant; carbonic anhydrase inhibitor; diuretic
Clinically important, potentially serious interactions with: cyclosporine

REACTIONS

SKIN
- Acute generalized exanthematous pustulosis (AGEP)
- Bullous eruption (<1%)
- Erythema multiforme
- Exanthems
- Lupus erythematosus
- Photosensitivity
- Pruritus
- Purpura
- Pustular eruption
- Pustular psoriasis
- Rash (sic) (<1%)
- Rosacea
- Stevens-Johnson syndrome
- Toxic epidermal necrolysis (<1%)
- Urticaria

HAIR
- Hair – hirsutism

OTHER
- Ageusia
- Anosmia
- Dysgeusia (>10%) (metallic taste)
- Extravasation
- Paresthesias (<1%)
- Xerostomia (<1%)

ACETOHEXAMIDE

Trade name: Dymelor (Lilly)
Other common trade names: Dimelin; Dimelor
Category: Sulfonylurea antidiabetic
Clinically important, potentially serious interactions with: beta-blockers, hydantoin, NSAIDs, phenylbutazones, thiazides

REACTIONS

SKIN
- Eczema
- Erythema (<1%)
- Exanthems (<1%)
- Lichenoid eruption
- Photosensitivity (1–10%)
- Pruritus (<1%)
- Rash (sic) (1–10%)
- Urticaria (1–10%)

HAIR
- Hair – alopecia

OTHER
- Porphyria cutanea tarda

ACITRETIN

Trade name: Soriatane (Roche)
Other common trade name: Neotigason
Category: Retinoid for psoriasis
Clinically important, potentially serious interactions with: antidiabetics, estrogens, methotrexate, vitamin A

REACTIONS

SKIN
- Bullous eruption (1–10%)
- Cheilitis (>75%)
- Cold/clammy skin (1–10%)
- Dermatitis (sic) (1–10%)
- Erythema (sic)
- Exanthems (10–25%)
- Fissures (1–10%)
- Hyperhidrosis (1–10%)
- Milia
- Palmoplantar desquamation
- Peeling
- Pruritus (25–50%)
- Psoriasis (1–10%)
- Purpura (1–10%)
- Pyogenic granuloma (1–10%)
- Rash (sic) (>10%)
- Seborrhea (1–10%)
- Skin atrophy (sic) (10–25%)
- Stickiness (10–25%)
- Sunburn (1–10%)
- Ulceration (1–10%)
- Urticaria
- Xerosis (25–50%)

HAIR
- Hair – alopecia (50–75%)

NAILS
- Nails – disorder (sic) (25–50%)
- Nails – fragility (sic)
- Nails – paronychia (10–25%)
- Nails – periungual granuloma

OTHER
- Bromhidrosis (1–10%)
- Gingival bleeding (1–10%)
- Gingivitis (1–10%)
- Hyperesthesia (10–25%)
- Myopathy
- Oral mucosal lesions
- Paresthesias (10–25%)
- Sialorrhea (1–10%)
- Stomatitis (1–10%)
- Ulcerative stomatitis (1–10%)
- Vulvovaginal candidiasis
- Xerostomia (10–25%)

ACYCLOVIR

Trade name: Zovirax (Glaxo Wellcome)
Other common trade names: Acyclo-V; Acyvir; Herpefug; Zyclir
Category: Antiviral, antiherpes drug
Clinically important, potentially serious interactions with: meperidine, phenytoin, probenecid, valproic acid

REACTIONS

SKIN
- Acne (<3%)
- Contact dermatitis
- Dermatitis (sic)
- Edema
- Erythema nodosum
- Exanthems (1–5%)
- Fixed eruption
- Herpes zoster (recurrent)
- Hyperhidrosis
- Lichenoid eruption
- Peripheral edema
- Pruritus (1–10%)
- Rash (sic) (<3%)
- Stevens-Johnson syndrome
- Urticaria (1–5%)
- Vasculitis
- Vesicular eruption

HAIR
- Hair – alopecia (<3%)

OTHER
- Anaphylactoid reaction (<1%)
- Dysgeusia (0.3%)
- Injection-site inflammation (>10%)
- Injection-site necrosis
- Injection-site thrombophlebitis (9%)
- Injection-site vesicular eruption
- Paresthesias (<1%)
- Vaginitis (candidal)

ALBENDAZOLE

Trade name: Albenza (SmithKline Beecham)
Other common trade names: ABZ; Albezole; Alzol; Bendex; Eskazole; Vermin; Zentel
Category: Anthelmintic
Clinically important, potentially serious interactions with: carbamazepine, praziquantel

REACTIONS

SKIN
- Allergic reactions (sic) (<1%)
- Contact dermatitis
- Pruritus (<1%)
- Rash (sic) (<1%)
- Stevens-Johnson syndrome
- Urticaria

HAIR
- Hair – alopecia (<1%)

OTHER
- Xerostomia (<1%)

ALBUTEROL

Trade names: Combivent (Boehringer Ingelheim); Proventil (Schering); Ventolin (Glaxo Wellcome); Volmax (Muro)
Other common trade names: Asmaven; Broncho-Spray; Cobutolin; Salbulin; Ventoline
Category: $Beta_2$ adrenergic agonist; bronchodilator (sympathomimetic)
Clinically important, potentially serious interactions with: MAO inhibitors, sympathomimetic agents, tricyclic antidepressants

Combivent is albuterol & ipratropium

REACTIONS

SKIN
- Contact dermatitis
- Erythema (palmar) (with infusion)
- Flushing (1–10%)
- Hyperhidrosis (1–10%)
- Lupus erythematosus (pseudo-lupus)
- Pruritus
- Urticaria

OTHER
- Dysgeusia (1–10%)
- Xerostomia (1–10%)

ALDESLEUKIN

Trade names: Interleukin-2; Proleukin (Chiron Thera)
Other common trade names: Aerovent; Atem; Atronase; Narilet
Category: Antineoplastic; biological response modulator
Clinically important, potentially serious interactions with: beta-blockers, psychotropics

REACTIONS

SKIN
- Allergic granulomatous angiitis (Churg-Strauss syndrome)
- Allergic reactions (sic) (<1%)
- Angioedema
- Bullous eruption
- Bullous pemphigoid
- Dermatitis (sic)
- Eczema reactivation
- Edema (47%)
- Erythema (sic) (41%)
- Erythema nodosum
- Erythroderma
- Exanthems
- Exfoliative dermatitis (14%)
- Graft-versus-host reaction
- Intertriginous cutaneous eruption
- Kaposi's sarcoma
- Linear IgA bullous dermatosis
- Pemphigus
- Peripheral edema (1–10%)
- Photosensitivity
- Pruritus (48%)
- Psoriasis
- Purpura (4%)
- Rash (sic) (26%)
- Scleroderma
- Toxic epidermal necrolysis
- Urticaria
- Vitiligo
- Xerosis (15%)

HAIR
- Hair – alopecia (<1%)

OTHER
- Aphthous stomatitis
- Dysgeusia (7%)
- Glossitis
- Injection-site nodules
- Injection-site panniculitis
- Injection-site reactions (sic) (3%)
- Myalgia (6%)
- Necrosis
- Oral mucosal eruption
- Oral ulceration
- Stomatitis (32%)

ALENDRONATE

Trade name: Fosamax (Merck)
Other common trade name: Fosalan
Category: Inhibitor of bone resorption; biphosphonate
Clinically important, potentially serious interactions with: none

REACTIONS

SKIN
- Erythema (<1%)
- Fixed eruption
- Petechiae
- Pruritus (0.6%)
- Rash (sic) (<1%)

OTHER
- Dysgeusia (0.6%)
- Hypersensitivity

ALLOPURINOL

Trade names: Lopurin (Knoll); Zyloprim (Glaxo Wellcome)
Other common trade names: Allo 300; Allo-Puren; Bleminol; Caplenal; Hamarin; Zyloric
Category: Antihyperuricemic, anti-gout
Clinically important, potentially serious interactions with: amoxicillin, azathioprine, dicumarol, mercaptopurine, theophylline

REACTIONS

SKIN
- Acute generalized exanthematous pustulosis (AGEP)
- Angiitis (<1%)
- Angioedema
- Ecchymoses (<1%)
- Edema (periorbital)
- Erythema multiforme (<1%)
- Exanthems (1–5%)
- Exfoliative dermatitis (>10%)
- Fixed eruption (<1%)
- Graft-versus-host reaction
- Granuloma annulare (disseminated)
- Hyperhidrosis (<1%)
- Ichthyosis
- Lichen planus (<1%)
- Lupus erythematosus
- Lymphocytoma cutis
- Perforating foot ulceration
- Petechiae
- Photosensitivity
- Pruritus (<1%)
- Purpura (>10%)
- Pustuloderma
- Rash (sic) (>10%)
- Stevens-Johnson syndrome (>10%)
- Toxic epidermal necrolysis
- Toxic erythema
- Toxic pustuloderma
- Urticaria (>10%)
- Vasculitis (<1%)

HAIR
- Hair – alopecia (1–10%)

NAILS
- Nails – onycholysis (<1%)

OTHER
- Hypersensitivity
- Mucocutaneous eruption
- Myalgia
- Myopathy (<1%)
- Oral ulceration
- Paresthesias (<1%)
- Polyarteritis nodosa
- Stomatitis
- Thrombophlebitis (<1%)
- Tongue edema (<1%)

ALPRAZOLAM

Trade name: Xanax (Pharmacia & Upjohn)
Other common trade names: Alprox; Cassadan; Kalma; Ralozam; Tafil
Category: Benzodiazepine anxiolytic tranquilizer
Clinically important, potentially serious interactions with: alcohol, cimetidine, clarithromycin, CNS depressants, dextropropoxyphene, digoxin, fluconazole, fluoxetine, itraconazole, ketoconazole, lithium, oral contraceptives, propoxyphene, ritonavir. Also grapefruit

REACTIONS

SKIN
- Acne
- Allergic reactions (sic)
- Dermatitis (sic) (3.8%)
- Edema (4.9%)
- Exanthems
- Hyperhidrosis (15.8%)
- Photosensitivity
- Phototoxic reaction
- Pruritus
- Purpura
- Rash (sic) (10.8%)
- Urticaria
- Xerosis

OTHER
- Dysgeusia
- Galactorrhea
- Gynecomastia
- Oral ulceration
- Paresthesias (2.4%)
- Pseudolymphoma
- Sialopenia (32.8%)
- Sialorrhea (4.2%)
- Xerostomia (14.7%)

ALPROSTADIL

Trade names: Caverject (Pharmacia & Upjohn); Edex (Schwarz); Prostin VR (Pharmacia & Upjohn)
Other common trade names: Lyple; Minprog; Palux; Prostine VR; Prostivas
Category: Prostaglandin; erectile dysfunction agent
Clinically important, potentially serious interactions with: none

REACTIONS

SKIN
- Balanitis (<1%)
- Diaphoresis (<1%)
- Ecchymoses
- Edema (1%)
- Flushing (10%)
- Penile edema (1%)
- Penile pain
- Penile rash (1–10%)
- Rash (sic) (<1%)
- Toxic epidermal necrolysis

OTHER
- Hypesthesia (<1%)
- Injection-site ecchymoses (1–10%)
- Injection-site hematoma (3%)
- Injection-site inflammation (<1%)
- Injection-site pain (2%)
- Injection-site pruritus (<1%)
- Priapism (4%)
- Xerostomia (<1%)

ALTEPLASE

Trade name: Activase (Genentech)
Other common trade names: Actilyse; Activacin
Category: Thrombolytic (tissue plasminogen activator)
Clinically important, potentially serious interactions with: nitroglycerin

REACTIONS

SKIN
- Angioedema
- Ecchymoses (1–10%)
- Rash (sic) (<0.02%)
- Purpura (<1%)
- Urticaria (<1%)

OTHER
- Anaphylactoid reaction (<0.02%)
- Gingival bleeding (<1%)

ALTRETAMINE

Trade name: Hexalen (US Bioscience)
Other common trade names: Hexamethylmelamin; Hexastat; Hexinawas
Category: Antineoplastic
Clinically important, potentially serious interactions with: antidepressants, cimetidine, MAO inhibitors, pyridoxine

REACTIONS

SKIN
- Dermatitis (sic)
- Exanthems
- Pruritus (<1%)
- Rash (sic) (<1%)

HAIR
- Hair – alopecia (<1%)

OTHER
- Mucocutaneous side effects

AMANTADINE

Trade name: Symmetrel (Dupont Pharma)
Other common trade names: Amixx; Grippin-Merz; Mantadix; PK-Merz; Protexin; Tregor
Category: Antiviral, antidyskinetic & antifatigue
Clinically important, potentially serious interactions with: amiloride, hydrochlorothiazide, trimethoprim

REACTIONS

SKIN
- Ankle edema
- Contact dermatitis
- Dermatitis (sic) (0.1%)
- Discoloration (sic)
- Eczematous eruption (sic)
- Edema
- Exanthems
- Livedo reticularis (50–90%)
- Peripheral edema (1–10%)
- Photosensitivity
- Pruritus (<1%)
- Rash (sic) (<1%)
- Urticaria

HAIR
- Hair – alopecia
- Hair – hypertrichosis

NAILS
- Nails – increased growth

OTHER
- Xerostomia (1–10%)

AMIKACIN

Trade name: Amikin (Mead Johnson)
Other common trade names: Amicacina; Amicasil; Amikan; Biklin; Kanbine; Lukadin; Miacin
Category: Aminoglycoside antibiotic
Clinically important, potentially serious interactions with: aminoglycosides, amphotericin, bumetanide, ethacrynic acid, furosemide, indomethacin, loop diuretics, succinylcholine, torsemide, vancomycin

REACTIONS

SKIN
- Dermatitis (sic)
- Exanthems
- Rash (sic) (<1%)
- Pruritus
- Urticaria

OTHER
- Injection-site necrosis
- Paresthesias (<1%)

AMILORIDE

Trade names: Midamor (Merck); Moduretic (Merck)
Other common trade names: Amikal; Kaluril; Medamor; Midoride; Modamide; Nirulid; Ride
Category: Potassium-sparing antihypertensive diuretic
Clinically important, potentially serious interactions with: ACE-inhibitors, amantadine, indomethacin, lithium, potassium salts, spironolactone

Moduretic is amiloride & hydrochlorothiazide

REACTIONS

SKIN
- Exanthems
- Flushing (>1%)
- Hyperhidrosis
- Photosensitivity
- Pruritus (<1%)
- Purpura
- Rash (sic) (<1%)
- Urticaria
- Vasculitis

HAIR
- Hair – alopecia (<1%)

OTHER
- Anaphylactoid reaction
- Dysgeusia (<1%)
- Gynecomastia (1–10%)
- Paresthesias (<1%)
- Xerostomia (<1%)

AMINOCAPROIC ACID

Trade name: Amicar (Lederle; Immunex)
Other common trade names: Capramol; Caproamin; Caprolisin; Ipron; Ipsilon; Resplamin
Category: Antifibrinolytic; antihemorrhagic
Clinically important, potentially serious interactions with: estrogens, oral contraceptives

REACTIONS

SKIN
- Bullous eruption
- Contact dermatitis
- Eczematous eruption
- Exanthems
- Kaposi's sarcoma
- Pruritus
- Purpura
- Rash (sic) (1–10%)
- Urticaria

OTHER
- Injection-site erythema
- Injection-site phlebitis
- Muscle necrosis
- Myopathy

AMINOGLUTETHIMIDE

Trade name: Cytadren (Novartis)
Other common trade names: Orimeten; Orimetene; Rodazol
Category: Antiadrenal & antineoplastic
Clinically important, potentially serious interactions with: propranolol

REACTIONS

SKIN
- Angioedema
- Erythema
- Exanthems
- Exfoliative dermatitis
- Lupus erythematosus (>10%)
- Pruritus (5%)
- Purpura
- Pustular psoriasis
- Rash (>10%)
- Urticaria

HAIR
- Hair – hirsutism (1–10%)

OTHER
- Anaphylactoid reaction
- Myalgia (3%)
- Oral mucosal eruption
- Oral ulceration

AMINOPHYLLINE

Trade names: Aerolate; Aminophyllin; Bronkodyl; Choledyl; Elixophyllin; Norphyl; Phyllocontin; Quibron; Slo-Bid; Somophyllin; Theo-Dur; Truphylline (Various pharmaceutical companies.)
Other common trade names: Corophyllin; Euphyllin; Palaron; Phyllotemp; Planphylline;
Category: Xanthine bronchodilator
Clinically important, potentially serious interactions with: allopurinol, cimetidine, ciprofloxacin, erythromycin, halothane, lithium, oral contraceptives, phenytoin, propranolol, rifampin

REACTIONS

SKIN
- Allergic reactions (sic) (<1%)
- Contact dermatitis
- Cutaneous side effects (sic)
- Dermatitis (sic)
- Exanthems
- Exfoliative dermatitis
- Flushing
- Hyperhidrosis
- Pruritus
- Rash (sic) (<1%)
- Stevens-Johnson syndrome
- Urticaria

HAIR
- Hair – alopecia

OTHER
- Hypersensitivity

AMINOSALICYLATE SODIUM (PAS)

Trade name: Sodium P.A.S. (Lannett; Palisades)
Other common trade names: Aminox; Eupasal; Nemasol
Category: Antimycobacterial; anti-inflammatory
Clinically important, potentially serious interactions with: digoxin, rifampin

REACTIONS

SKIN
- Allergic reactions (sic)
- Angioedema
- Bullous eruption
- Eczematous eruption (<1%)
- Erythema multiforme
- Exanthems
- Exfoliative dermatitis

Fixed eruption
Lichenoid eruption
Lupus erythematosus
Lymphoma (benign)
Photosensitivity
Pruritus
Purpura
Toxic epidermal necrolysis
Urticaria
Vasculitis (<1%)

HAIR
Hair – alopecia

OTHER
Oral lichenoid eruption
Oral mucosal eruption

AMIODARONE

Trade name: Cordarone (Wyeth)
Other common trade names: Aratac; Corbionax; Cordarex; Cordarone X; Tachydaron
Category: Class III antiarrhythmic
Clinically important, potentially serious interactions with: anticoagulants, astemizole, digoxin, diltiazem, fentanyl, methotrexate, quinidine, ritonavir, verapamil

REACTIONS

SKIN
Allergic reactions (sic)
Basal cell carcinoma
Ecchymoses (<1%)
Edema (1–10%)
Erythema nodosum (<1%)
Exanthems
Exfoliative dermatitis
Facial erythema (3.1%)
Flushing (1–10%)
Hyperhidrosis
Iododerma
Linear IgA bullous dermatosis
Lupus erythematosus
Photosensitivity (10–30%)
Pigmentation
Pruritus (1–5%)
Psoriasis
Purpura (2%)
Pustular psoriasis
Rash (sic) (<1%)
Rosacea
Stevens-Johnson syndrome (<1%)
Toxic epidermal necrolysis
Urticaria
Vasculitis (<1%)

HAIR
Hair – alopecia (<1%)
Hair – hypertrichosis

OTHER
Dysgeusia (1–10%)
Paresthesias (4–9%)
Parosmia (1–10%)
Pseudoporphyria
Pseudotumor cerebri (<1%)
Sialorrhea (1–3%)

AMITRIPTYLINE

Trade names: Elavil (Stuart); Endep (Roche); Limbitrol (Roche)
Other common trade names: Amineurin; Domical; Laroxyl; Lentizol; Levate; Saroten; Tryptizol
Category: Tricyclic antidepressant
Clinically important, potentially serious interactions with: clonidine, epinephrine, guanethidine, MAO inhibitors

Limbitrol is amitriptyline & chlordiazepoxide

REACTIONS

SKIN
Acne
Allergic reactions (sic) (<1%)
Angioedema

Bullous eruption (<1%)
Dermatitis (sic)
Dermatitis herpetiformis
Exanthems
Exfoliative dermatitis
Facial edema
Fixed eruption
Flushing
Hyperhidrosis (1–10%)
Lupus erythematosus
Petechiae
Photosensitivity (<1%)
Pigmentation
Pruritus
Purpura
Rash (sic)
Urticaria
Vasculitis

HAIR
Hair – alopecia (<1%)

OTHER
Ageusia
Anaphylactoid reaction
Black tongue
Bromhidrosis
Dysgeusia (>10%)
Galactorrhea (<1%)
Glossitis
Gynecomastia (<1%)
Lymphoid hyperplasia
Oral mucosal eruption
Paresthesias
Pseudolymphoma
Sialorrhea
Stomatitis
Stomatopyrosis
Tongue edema
Vaginitis
Xerostomia (>10%)

AMLODIPINE

Trade names: Lotrel (Novartis); Norvasc (Pfizer)
Other common trade names: Amdepin; Amlodin, Amlogard; Amlopin; Amlor; Istin; Norvas
Category: Calcium channel blocker; antianginal, antihypertensive
Clinically important, potentially serious interactions with: ACE-inhibitors, delavirdine, ibuprofen

Lotrel is amlodipine & benazepril

REACTIONS

SKIN
Dermatitis (sic) (1–10%)
Discoloration (sic) (<1%)
Edema (5–14%)
Erythema multiforme
Exanthems (2–4%)
Flushing (1–10%)
Hyperhidrosis (<1%)
Peripheral edema (>10%)
Petechiae (<1%)
Pruritus (2–4%)
Purpura (<1%)
Rash (sic) (1–10%)
Telangiectases (facial)
Urticaria (<1%)
Vasculitis
Xerosis (<0.1%)

HAIR
Hair – alopecia (<1%)

OTHER
Acute intermittent porphyria
Dysgeusia (<1%)
Gingival hyperplasia (<1%)
Gynecomastia
Hypesthesia (<1%)
Paresthesias (<1%)
Parosmia (<0.1%)
Xerostomia (<1%)

AMOBARBITAL

Trade name: Amytal (Lilly)
Other common trade names: Amytal Sodium; Isoamitil Sedante; Neur-Amyl; Sodium Amytal
Category: Intermediate-acting barbiturate; anticonvulsant; hypnotic; sedative
Clinically important, potentially serious interactions with: acetaminophen, anticoagulants, bepridil, diltiazem, felbamate, felodipine, isradipine, MAO inhibitors, verapamil

REACTIONS

SKIN
- Angioedema
- Erythema
- Exanthems
- Exfoliative dermatitis (<1%)
- Purpura
- Rash (sic) (<1%)
- Stevens-Johnson syndrome (<1%)
- Toxic epidermal necrolysis
- Urticaria (<1%)

OTHER
- Injection-site pain (>10%)
- Serum sickness
- Thrombophlebitis (<1%)

AMOXAPINE

Trade name: Asendin (Lederle)
Other common trade names: Amoxan; Asendis; Defanyl; Demolox
Category: Heterocyclic antidepressant
Clinically important, potentially serious interactions with: epinephrine, guanethidine, MAO inhibitors, tricyclic antidepressants

REACTIONS

SKIN
- Acne
- Acute generalized exanthematous pustulosis (AGEP)
- Allergic reactions (sic) (<1%)
- Cutaneous side effects (sic) (5.1%)
- Dermatitis (sic)
- Edema (>1%)
- Erythema multiforme (observation)
- Exanthems
- Flushing
- Hyperhidrosis (1–10%)
- Petechiae (rare)
- Photosensitivity (<1%)
- Pruritus (<1%)
- Purpura (rare)
- Rash (sic) (>1%)
- Toxic epidermal necrolysis
- Urticaria (<1%)
- Vasculitis (<1%)
- Xerosis

HAIR
- Hair – alopecia (<1%)

OTHER
- Black tongue
- Bromhidrosis
- Dysgeusia (>10%)
- Galactorrhea (<1%)
- Glossitis
- Gynecomastia (<1%)
- Paresthesias (<1%)
- Sialorrhea
- Stomatitis
- Vaginitis
- Xerostomia (14%)

AMOXICILLIN

Trade names: Amoxil (SmithKline Beecham); Augmentin (SmithKline Beecham); Polymox (Mead Johnson); Trimox (Bristol-Myers Squibb); Wymox (Wyeth)
Other common trade names: A-Gram; Almodan; Amodex; Clamoxyl; Eupen; Fisamox
Category: Aminopenicillin antibiotic
Clinically important, potentially serious interactions with: allopurinol, anticoagulants, cyclosporine, methotrexate

Augmentin is amoxicillin & clavulanate

REACTIONS

SKIN
- Acute generalized exanthematous pustulosis (AGEP)
- Angioedema
- Baboon syndrome
- Bullous pemphigoid
- Contact dermatitis
- Cutaneous side effects (sic)
- Diaper rash
- Ecchymoses
- Edema
- Erythema multiforme
- Exanthems (>5%)
- Exfoliative dermatitis
- Fixed eruption
- Hematomas
- Intertrigo
- Jarisch-Herxheimer reaction
- Keratosis pilaris
- Pemphigus
- Perleche
- Petechiae (Rumpel-Leede sign)
- Pruritus
- Psoriasis
- Pustular eruption
- Pustular psoriasis
- Rash (sic) (1–10%)
- Stevens-Johnson syndrome
- Toxic epidermal necrolysis
- Toxic pustuloderma
- Urticaria (1–5%)

OTHER
- Anaphylactoid reaction
- Black hairy tongue
- Dysgeusia
- Glossitis
- Glossodynia
- Hypersensitivity
- Injection-site pain
- Oral candidiasis
- Serum sickness
- Stomatitis
- Stomatodynia
- Vaginitis (1%)
- Xerostomia

AMPHOTERICIN B

Trade names: Ambisome (Fujisawa); Amphocin (Pharmacia & Upjohn); Fungizone (Bristol-Myers Squibb)
Other common trade names: Ampho-Moronal; Fungilin; Fungizone
Category: Antifungal; antiprotozoal
Clinically important, potentially serious interactions with: aminoglycosides, corticosteroids, cyclosporine, digoxin

REACTIONS

SKIN
- Exanthems (<1%)
- Exfoliative dermatitis
- Fixed eruption
- Flushing (1–10%)
- Pruritus
- Purpura
- Rash (sic)
- Raynaud's phenomenon (cyanotic)
- Red man syndrome
- Urticaria

OTHER
- Anaphylactoid reaction
- Infusion-site pain
- Infusion-site thrombophlebitis
- Paresthesias (1–10%)
- Thrombophlebitis (1–10%)

AMPICILLIN

Trade names: Omnipen (Wyeth); Polycillin (Mead Johnson); Principen (Bristol-Myers Squibb); Totacillin (SmithKline Beecham)
Other common trade names: Amfipen; Binotal; Penbritin; Penstabil; Totapen; Vidopen
Category: Aminopenicillin antibiotic
Clinically important, potentially serious interactions with: allopurinol, anticoagulants, atenolol, cyclosporine

REACTIONS

SKIN
- Acute generalized exanthematous pustulosis (AGEP)
- Allergic reactions (sic)
- Angioedema (<1%)
- Baboon syndrome
- Bullous eruption (<1%)
- Bullous pemphigoid
- Candidiasis
- Contact dermatitis
- Diaper rash
- Erythema annulare centrifugum
- Erythema multiforme (<1%)
- Exanthems (>10%)
- Exfoliative dermatitis
- Fixed eruption
- Linear IgA bullous dermatosis
- Pemphigus
- Pityriasis rosea
- Pruritus (1–5%)
- Psoriasis
- Purpura
- Pustular eruption
- Pustular psoriasis
- Rash (sic)
- Stevens-Johnson syndrome
- Toxic epidermal necrolysis (<1%)
- Urticaria
- Vasculitis

OTHER
- Anaphylactoid reaction
- Black hairy tongue
- Glossitis
- Hypersensitivity
- Oral candidiasis
- Oral mucosal eruption
- Serum sickness
- Stomatitis

APRACLONIDINE

Trade name: Iopidine (Alcon)
Category: $Alpha_2$-adrenergic agonist; sympathomimetic ophthalmic solution; vasoconstrictor
Clinically important, potentially serious interactions with: topical beta-blockers; MAO inhibitors

REACTIONS

SKIN
- Allergic reactions (<1%)
- Burning
- Contact dermatitis (<1%)
- Dermatitis (sic) (<1%)
- Edema (eyelids) (<3%)
- Facial edema (<1%)
- Pruritus (10%)

OTHER
- Dysgeusia (3%)
- Myalgia (0.2%)
- Paresthesias (<1%)
- Parosmia (0.2%)
- Xerostomia (1–10%)

APROBARBITAL

Trade name: Alurate (Roche)
Category: Intermediate-acting barbiturate
Clinically important, potentially serious interactions with: no data

REACTIONS

SKIN
- Angioedema
- Exanthems
- Exfoliative dermatitis
- Purpura
- Rash (sic)
- Stevens-Johnson syndrome
- Urticaria

OTHER
- Serum sickness

ASCORBIC ACID

Trade names: Ascorbicap; Cebid; Cetane; Cecon; Cevalin (Lilly); Cemill; Sunkist
Other common trade names: Cebion; Cetebe; Laroscorbine; Potent C; Pro-C; Redoxon
Category: Water-soluble nutritional supplement
Clinically important, potentially serious interactions with: iron, oral contraceptives, propranolol

REACTIONS

SKIN
- Angioedema
- Cutaneous side effects (sic)
- Eczema (sic)
- Erythema
- Flushing (<1%)

ASPARAGINASE

Trade name: Elspar (Merck)
Other common trade names: Crasnitin; Erwinase; Kidrolase; Laspar; Leunase
Category: Antineoplastic; protein synthesis inhibitor
Clinically important, potentially serious interactions with: methotrexate, prednisone, vincristine

REACTIONS

SKIN
- Angioedema
- Aphthous stomatitis (1–10%)
- Edema
- Exanthems
- Flushing
- Pruritus (<1%)
- Rash (sic) (<1%)
- Toxic epidermal necrolysis
- Urticaria (<1%)

HAIR
- Hair – alopecia

OTHER
- Anaphylactoid reaction (10–40%)
- Hypersensitivity (10–40%)
- Injection-site erythema
- Oral mucosal lesions (26%)
- Serum sickness

ASPARTAME

Trade names: Equal; Nutrasweet
Category: Low-calorie artificial sweetener
Clinically important, potentially serious interactions with: no data

REACTIONS

SKIN
- Allergic reactions (sic)
- Angioedema
- Dermatitis (sic)
- Exanthems
- Pruritus
- Pruritus ani
- Purpura
- Rash (sic)
- Urticaria

OTHER
- Anaphylactoid reaction
- Panniculitis

ASPIRIN

Trade names: Alka-Seltzer; Anacin; Ascriptin; Aspergum; Bufferin; Coricidin D; Darvon Compound; Ecotrin; Empirin; Equagesic; Excedrin; Fiorinal; Gelprin; Measurin; Norgesic; Percodan; Robaxisal; Soma Compound; Talwin Compound; Vanquish; etc. (Various Pharmaceutical Companies.)
Other common trade names: ASS; Aspro; Bex; Caprin; Claragine; Disprin; Ecotrin; Rhonal
Category: Nonsteroidal anti-inflammatory (NSAID)
Clinically important, potentially serious interactions with: anticoagulants, heparin, hypoglycemics, methotrexate, NSAIDs, valproic acid, warfarin

REACTIONS

SKIN
- Acute generalized exanthematous pustulosis (AGEP)
- Angioedema (1–5%)
- Aphthous stomatitis
- Bullous eruption (<1%)
- Dermatitis herpetiformis
- Dermatomyositis
- Erythema multiforme (<1%)
- Erythema nodosum (<1%)
- Erythroderma
- Exanthems
- Exfoliative dermatitis
- Fixed eruption (<1%)
- Flushing
- Herpes progenitalis
- Hyperhidrosis
- Lichenoid eruption
- Parapsoriasis
- Pemphigus (rare)
- Periorbital edema
- Petechiae
- Pityriasis rosea
- Pruritus
- Psoriasis
- Purpura
- Pustular psoriasis
- Rash (sic) (1–10%)
- Stevens-Johnson syndrome
- Toxic epidermal necrolysis (<1%)
- Urticaria (1–10%)
- Vasculitis

HAIR
- Hair – alopecia

OTHER
- Anaphylactoid reaction (1–10%)
- Dysgeusia
- Oral lichen planus
- Oral mucosal eruption
- Oral ulceration

ASTEMIZOLE

Trade name: Hismanal (Janssen)
Other common trade names: Alestol; Astimal; Astizol; Histamen; Pollon-Eze; Simprox; Stemiz
Category: Histamine H_1-receptor antagonist
Clinically important, potentially serious interactions with: amiodarone, azithromycin, bepridil, bretylium, clarithromycin, disopyramide, diuretics, erythromycin, fluconazole, fluoxetine, fluvoxamine, indinavir, itraconazole, ketoconazole, metronidazole, miconazole, nefazodone, probucol, procainamide, quinidine, quinine, ritonavir, saquinavir, sotalol, terfenadine, troleandomycin

REACTIONS

SKIN
- Angioedema (<1%)
- Dermatitis (sic)
- Eczema (sic)
- Edema (<1%)
- Exanthems (1.2%)
- Photosensitivity (<1%)
- Pityriasis lichenoides et varioliformis acuta (PLEVA)
- Pruritus
- Rash (sic) (<1%)
- Stevens-Johnson syndrome
- Urticaria

HAIR
- Hair – alopecia
- Hair – color change (sic)

OTHER
- Dysgeusia
- Myalgia (<1%)
- Oral mucosal eruption (5–15%)
- Paresthesias (<1%)
- Sore nipples (sic)
- Xerostomia (5.2%)

ATENOLOL

Trade names: Tenormin (Zeneca); Tenoretic (Zeneca)
Other common trade names: Antipressan; AteHexal; Atendol; Evitocor; Noten; Tenormine
Category: Beta-adrenergic blocking agent; antianginal; antihypertensive
Clinically important, potentially serious interactions with: calcium channel blockers, clonidine, flecainide, nifedipine, oral contraceptives, reserpine

Tenoretic is atenolol & chlorthalidone

REACTIONS

SKIN
- Dermatitis (sic)
- Erythema multiforme
- Exanthems
- Grinspan's syndrome*
- Hyperhidrosis
- Hyperkeratosis (palms & soles)
- Lichenoid eruption
- Lupus erythematosus
- Necrosis
- Papular & nodular eruption
- Photosensitivity
- Pityriasis rubra pilaris
- Pruritus (1–5%)
- Psoriasis
- Purpura
- Pustular psoriasis
- Rash (sic) (rare)
- Raynaud's phenomenon
- Toxic epidermal necrolysis
- Urticaria
- Vasculitis
- Vitiligo
- Xerosis

HAIR
- Hair – alopecia

NAILS
- Nails – bluish
- Nails – dystrophy
- Nails – onycholysis

Nails – splinter hemorrhages

OTHER

Acrocyanosis
Anaphylactoid reaction
Oculo-mucocutaneous syndrome
Oral lichenoid eruption
Peyronie's disease
Pseudolymphoma

*Grinspan's syndrome: the triad of oral lichen planus, diabetes mellitus, and hypertension.

ATORVASTATIN

Trade name: Lipitor (Parke-Davis)
Category: A statin; HMG-CoA reductase inhibitor; lipid lowering agent
Clinically important, potentially serious interactions with: digoxin, erythromycin

Reactions

SKIN

Acne (<2%)
Allergic reactions (<2%)
Cheilitis (<2%)
Contact dermatitis (<2%)
Ecchymoses (<2%)
Eczema (sic) (<2%)
Edema (<2%)
Exanthems
Facial edema (<2%)
Hyperhidrosis (<2%)
Petechiae (<2%)
Photosensitivity (<2%)
Pruritus (<2%)
Rash (sic) (>3%)
Seborrhea (<2%)
Toxic epidermal necrolysis
Ulceration (<2%)
Urticaria (<2%)
Xerosis (<2%)

HAIR

Hair – alopecia (<2%)

OTHER

Ageusia (<2%)
Dysgeusia (<2%)
Glossitis (<2%)
Gynecomastia (<2%)
Myalgia (>3%)
Oral ulceration (<2%)
Paresthesias (<2%)
Parosmia (<2%)
Stomatitis (<2%)

ATOVAQUONE

Trade name: Mepron (Glaxo Wellcome)
Other common trade name: Wellvone
Category: Antiprotozoal
Clinically important, potentially serious interactions with: rifampin, zidovudine

Reactions

SKIN

Exanthems
Hyperhidrosis (10%)
Pruritus (11%)
Rash (sic) (23%)

OTHER

Dysgeusia (3%)
Oral candidiasis (1–10%)

ATROPINE SULFATE

Trade names: Belladenal; Bellergal-S; Butibel; Donnagel; Donnatal; Donnazyme; Hycodan; Isopto Atropine; Lofene; Logen; Lomanate; Lomotil; Urised; etc. (Various Pharmaceutical Companies.)
Other common trade names: Atropine Martinet; Atropt; Chibro-Atropine; Isopto; Vitatropine
Category: Anticholinergic & antispasmodic
Clinically important, potentially serious interactions with: amantadine, anticholinergics, atenolol, digoxin

REACTIONS

SKIN
- Allergy (sic)
- Bullous eruption
- Contact dermatitis
- Eccrine hidrocystomas
- Erythema multiforme (<1%)
- Exanthems
- Exfoliative dermatitis
- Fixed eruption
- Flushing
- Hypohidrosis (>10%)
- Pruritus
- Rash (sic) (<1%)
- Sheet-like erythema
- Stevens-Johnson syndrome
- Urticaria

OTHER
- Dry mucous membranes (sic)
- Xerostomia (>10%)

AURANOFIN (See GOLD)

AUROTHIOGLUCOSE (See GOLD)

AZATADINE

Trade name: Optimine (Schering)
Other common trade names: Idulamine; Idulian; Lergocil; Nalomet; Verben; Zadine
Category: H_1-receptor antihistamine
Clinically important, potentially serious interactions with: alcohol, MAO inhibitors, procarbazine, tricyclic antidepressants

REACTIONS

SKIN
- Angioedema (<1%)
- Exanthems
- Flushing
- Hyperhidrosis
- Photosensitivity (<1%)
- Purpura
- Rash (sic) (<1%)
- Urticaria

OTHER
- Myalgia (<1%)
- Paresthesias (<1%)
- Xerostomia (1–10%)

AZATHIOPRINE

Trade name: Imuran (Glaxo Wellcome)
Other common trade names: Azamedac; Azamune; Imuprin, Imurek; Imurel; Thioprine
Category: Immunosuppressant & cytostatic
Clinically important, potentially serious interactions with: ACE-inhibitors, allopurinol, chlorambucil, cotrimoxazole, cyclophosphamide, methotrexate

REACTIONS

SKIN
- Acanthosis nigricans
- Acne
- Allergic reactions (sic)

Angioedema
Aphthous stomatitis (<1%)
Cancer (sic)
Contact dermatitis
Cutaneous infections (sic)
Erythema multiforme
Erythema nodosum
Exanthems (<1%)
Fixed eruption
Fungal infection
Herpes simplex
Herpes zoster
Kaposi's sarcoma
Keratoacanthoma
Lichenoid eruption
Pellagra
Photosensitivity
Pigmentation (sun-exposed skin)
Porokeratosis
Purpura
Pyoderma gangrenosum
Rash (sic) (1–10%)
Raynaud's phenomenon
Sarcoma
Scabies
Scleroderma
Skin peeling syndrome (sic)
Squamous cell carcinoma
Tinea corporis
Tinea versicolor
Toxic epidermal necrolysis
Tumors (sic)
Urticaria
Vasculitis
Viral infections
Warts

HAIR
Hair – alopecia (<1%)
Hair – curly

NAILS
Nails – discoloration (red lunulae)
Nails – onychomycosis

OTHER
Anaphylactoid reaction
Formication
Hypersensitivity (<1%)
Lymphoproliferative disease
Oral ulceration
Rheumatoid nodules
Stomatitis
Xerostomia

AZELASTINE

Trade name: Astelin (Wallace)
Other common trade names: Allergodil; Azeptin
Category: Antihistamine
Clinically important, potentially serious interactions with: alcohol, cimetidine, CNS depressants

REACTIONS

SKIN
Allergic reactions (sic) (<2%)
Aphthous stomatitis (<2%)
Contact dermatitis (<2%)
Eczema (sic) (<2%)
Exanthems
Flushing (<2%)
Folliculitis (<2%)
Furunculosis (<2%)
Herpes simplex (<2%)

OTHER
Ageusia (<2%)
Dysgeusia (bitter taste)
Glossitis (<2%)
Hypesthesia (<2%)
Mastodynia (<2%)
Myalgia (1.5%)
Oral dryness
Oral mucosal eruption
Stomatitis (ulcerative) (<2%)
Xerostomia (2.8%)

AZITHROMYCIN

Trade name: Zithromax (Pfizer)
Other common trade names: Azenil; Azitrocin; Azitromax; Zeto; Zitromax
Category: Macrolide antibiotic
Clinically important, potentially serious interactions with: astemizole, bromocriptine, carbamazepine, cyclosporine, digoxin, disopyramide, loratadine, pimozide, terfenadine, triazolam

REACTIONS

SKIN
- Allergic granulomatous angiitis (Churg-Strauss syndrome)
- Allergic reactions (sic) (<1%)
- Angioedema (<1%)
- Cutaneous side effects
- Diaper rash
- Edema
- Erythema
- Exanthems
- Facial edema
- Photosensitivity (1%)
- Pustular eruption
- Rash (sic) (<1%)
- Toxic pustuloderma
- Urticaria

OTHER
- Anaphylactoid reaction
- Infusion-site erythema
- Infusion-site tenderness
- Vaginitis (2%)

AZTREONAM

Trade name: Azactam (Bristol-Myers Squibb)
Other common trade names: Primbactam; Urobactam
Category: Synthetic narrow spectrum antibacterial (monobactam)
Clinically important, potentially serious interactions with: furosemide, probenecid

REACTIONS

SKIN
- Angioedema
- Erythema multiforme
- Exanthems
- Exfoliative dermatitis
- Hyperhidrosis
- Petechiae
- Pruritus
- Purpura
- Rash (sic) (1–10%)
- Toxic epidermal necrolysis
- Urticaria

OTHER
- Anaphylactoid reaction (<1%)
- Dysgeusia (<1%)
- Foetor ex ore (halitosis) (<1%)
- Injection-site phlebitis (1–10%)
- Mastodynia (<1%)
- Oral ulceration
- Paresthesias
- Tongue numb (sic) (<1%)
- Vaginal candidiasis
- Vaginitis (<1%)

BENACTYZINE

Trade name: Deprol (Wallace)
Category: Antidepressant
Clinically important, potentially serious interactions with: no data

Deprol is benactyzine & meprobamate

REACTIONS

SKIN
- Angioedema
- Bullous eruption
- Ecchymoses
- Edema
- Erythema multiforme
- Exanthems
- Exfoliative dermatitis
- Fixed eruption
- Petechiae
- Pruritus
- Urticaria

OTHER
- Anaphylactoid reaction
- Paresthesias
- Stomatitis
- Xerostomia

BENAZEPRIL

Trade names: Lotensin (Novartis); Lotrel (Novartis)
Other common trade names: Cibace; Cibacen; Cibacene
Category: Angiotensin-converting enzyme (ACE) inhibitor; antihypertensive & vasodilator
Clinically important, potentially serious interactions with: thiazide diuretics

Lotrel is benazepril & amlodipine

REACTIONS

SKIN
- Angioedema (<1%)
- Ankle edema
- Dermatitis (sic)
- Exanthems
- Flushing
- Hyperhidrosis (<1%)
- Peripheral edema
- Photosensitivity (<1%)
- Pruritus
- Rash (sic) (<1%)
- Urticaria

OTHER
- Dysgeusia
- Myalgia
- Paresthesias (<1%)

BENDROFLUMETHIAZIDE

Trade names: Corzide (Bristol-Myers Squibb); Naturetin (Bristol-Myers Squibb); Rauzide (Bristol-Myers Squibb)
Other common trade names: Aprinox; Berkozide; Centyl; Naturine; Neo-Naclex; Pluryle
Category: Thiazide diuretic; antihypertensive
Clinically important, potentially serious interactions with: digoxin, lithium, MAO inhibitors

Corzide is bendroflumethiazide & nadolol

REACTIONS

SKIN
- Allergic reactions (sic)
- Contact dermatitis
- Exanthems
- Exfoliative dermatitis
- Facial edema
- Grinspan's syndrome*
- Hyperhidrosis
- Pemphigoid (sic)
- Photosensitivity

Phototoxic reaction
Pruritus
Purpura
Rash (sic)
Urticaria
Vasculitis

HAIR
Hair – alopecia

OTHER
Anaphylactoid reaction
Gynecomastia
Paresthesias
Xanthopsia
Xerostomia

*Grinspan's syndrome: the triad of oral lichen planus, diabetes mellitus, and hypertension.

BENZTHIAZIDE

Trade name: Exna (Robins)
Other common trade names: Diurin; Fovane; Regulon
Category: Thiazide diuretic; antihypertensive
Clinically important, potentially serious interactions with: digitalis, lithium

REACTIONS

SKIN
Allergic reactions (sic) (<1%)
Photosensitivity
Purpura
Rash (sic)
Urticaria
Vasculitis

OTHER
Dysgeusia
Paresthesias (<1%)
Xanthopsia

BENZTROPINE

Trade name: Cogentin (Merck)
Other common trade names: Akitan; Apo-Benzthioprine; Cogentine; Cogentinol; Phatropine
Category: Antidyskinetic & anticholinergic
Clinically important, potentially serious interactions with: anticholinergics, antipsychotics, quinidine, tricyclic antidepressants

REACTIONS

SKIN
Exanthems
Pruritus
Rash (sic) (<1%)
Urticaria
Xerosis (>10%)

OTHER
Glossodynia
Paresthesias
Stomatodynia
Xerostomia (>10%)

BEPRIDIL

Trade name: Vascor (McNeil)
Other common trade names: Bepricol; Cordium; Cruor
Category: Calcium channel blocker; antianginal
Clinically important, potentially serious interactions with: beta-blockers, carbamazepine, cyclosporine, digitalis, quinidine, ritonavir

REACTIONS

SKIN
- Hyperhidrosis (<1%)
- Irritation (sic)
- Peripheral edema (<1%)
- Rash (sic) (1–10%)

OTHER
- Dysgeusia (<1%)
- Myalgia (<1%)
- Paresthesias (2.5%)
- Xerostomia (1–10%)

BETA-CAROTENE

Trade name: Solatene (Merck)
Other common trade names: Betavin; B-Tene; Carotaben; Solvin
Category: Fat-soluble vitamin supplement; photosensitivity reaction suppressant
Clinically important, potentially serious interactions with: vitamin A

REACTIONS

SKIN
- Carotenemia (>10%)
- Dermatitis (sic)
- Ecchymoses (<1%)

BETAXOLOL

Trade names: Betoptic (ophthalmic) (Alcon); Kerlone (Searle)
Other common trade names: Betoptic S; Betoptima; Kerlon; Optipres
Category: Beta-adrenergic blocking agent
Clinically important, potentially serious interactions with: calcium channel blockers, clonidine, flecainide, nifedipine, oral contraceptives, verapamil

REACTIONS

SKIN
- Acne
- Allergy (sic) (<2%)
- Angioedema
- Contact dermatitis
- Edema (1.3%)
- Erythema (1–10%)
- Exanthems
- Exfoliative dermatitis
- Facial edema
- Flushing (<2%)
- Hyperhidrosis (<2%)
- Lupus erythematosus
- Photosensitivity
- Pigmentation (palms)
- Pruritus (1–10%)
- Psoriasis
- Purpura
- Rash (sic) (1.2%)
- Raynaud's phenomenon
- Toxic epidermal necrolysis
- Urticaria
- Xerosis

HAIR
- Hair – alopecia (after topical use) (<2%)
- Hair – hypertrichosis (<2%)

NAILS
- Nails – pigmentation (bluish)

OTHER
- Ageusia (<2%)
- Anaphylactoid reaction
- Dysgeusia (<2%)
- Glossitis (after topical use)
- Mastodynia (<2%)
- Myalgia (3.2%)

Myasthenia gravis
Oral ulceration (<2%)
Paresthesias (1.9%)
Peyronie's disease (<2%)
Sialorrhea (<2%)
Xerostomia (<2%)

BETHANECHOL

Trade name: Urecholine (Merck)
Other common trade names: Muscaran; Myocholine-Glenwood; Myotonine Chloride; Urocarb
Category: Urinary tract cholinergic stimulant
Clinically important, potentially serious interactions with: cholinergic & anticholinesterase agents, ganglionic blockers

REACTIONS

SKIN
Flushing (<1%)
Hyperhidrosis (1–10%)
Miliaria

OTHER
Sialorrhea (<1%)

BICALUTAMIDE

Trade name: Casodex (Zeneca)
Category: Antiandrogen antineoplastic
Clinically important, potentially serious interactions with: warfarin

REACTIONS

SKIN
Edema (2–5%)
Exanthems (<1%)
Hot flushes (49%)
Hyperhidrosis (6%)
Peripheral edema (8%)
Paresthesias (6%)
Rash (sic) (6%)

HAIR
Hair – alopecia (2–5%)

OTHER
Gynecomastia (5%)
Injection-site reaction (2–5%)
Mastodynia
Myalgia (2–5%)
Xerostomia (2–5%)

BIPERIDEN

Trade name: Akineton (Knoll)
Other common trade names: Biperen; Bipiden; Dekinet; Desiperiden; Dyskinon
Category: Anticholinergic
Clinically important, potentially serious interactions with: anticholinergics, meperidine, phenothiazines, quinidine, tricyclic antidepressants

REACTIONS

SKIN
Contact dermatitis
Exanthems
Flushing
Rash (sic)
Urticaria

OTHER
Glossodynia
Paresthesias
Stomatodynia
Xerostomia

BISACODYL

Trade names: Dulcolax (Boehringer; Ciba); Fleet Laxative (Fleet)
Category: Irritant/stimulant laxative
Clinically important, potentially serious interactions with: none

REACTIONS

SKIN
- Exanthems
- Fixed eruption
- Urticaria

BISOPROLOL

Trade names: Zebeta (Lederle); Ziac (Lederle)
Other common trade names: Concor; Cordalin; Detensiel; Emcor; Fondril; Monocor; Soprol
Category: Beta-adrenergic blocking agent
Clinically important, potentially serious interactions with: flecainide, nifedipine, salicylates

Ziac is bisoprolol & hydrochlorothiazide

REACTIONS

SKIN
- Acne
- Angioedema
- Ankle edema (1–10%)
- Eczema (sic)
- Edema (3%)
- Exanthems
- Exfoliative dermatitis
- Facial edema
- Flushing
- Hyperhidrosis (1%)
- Lupus erythematosus
- Photosensitivity
- Pigmentation
- Pruritus
- Psoriasis
- Purpura
- Rash (sic)
- Raynaud's phenomenon (1–10%)
- Urticaria
- Xerosis

HAIR
- Hair – alopecia

NAILS
- Nails – bluish

OTHER
- Anaphylactoid reaction
- Dysgeusia
- Hypesthesia (1.5%)
- Myalgia (1–10%)
- Paresthesias
- Peyronie's disease
- Xerostomia (1.3%)

BLEOMYCIN

Trade name: Blenoxane (Mead Johnson)
Other common trade names: Bleocin; Bleomycin; Bleomycine; Bleomycinum
Category: Antineoplastic antibiotic
Clinically important, potentially serious interactions with: CCNU, cisplatin, digoxin, phenytoin

REACTIONS

SKIN
- Acral erythema
- Acral gangrene
- Acral sclerosis
- Angioedema
- Bullous eruption (1–5%)
- Dermatitis (sic)
- Digital necrosis
- Exanthems
- Flagellate erythema
- Flagellate pigmentation
- Gangrene (digital)

Hyperkeratosis (palms & soles)
Ichthyosis
Intertrigo
Linear streaking (sic)
Lymphangitis
Neutrophilic eccrine hidradenitis
Nodular eruption
Painful erythema (elbows, knees, palms)
Palmar nodules
Palmar-plantar erythema
Pigmentation (30 percent)
Pruritus (>5%)
Radiation recall
Raynaud's phenomenon (>10%)
Scleroderma
Stevens-Johnson syndrome
Urticaria
Xerosis

HAIR
Hair – alopecia (>10%)
Hair – gray

NAILS
Nails – Beau's lines (transverse ridging)
Nails – dystrophy
Nails – growth reduced
Nails – loss
Nails – onychodystrophy
Nails – onycholysis
Nails – pigmentation (banding)
Nails – shedding

OTHER
Acrocyanosis
Anaphylactoid reaction (<1%)
Calcinosis
Glossitis
Hypersensitivity (1–10%)
Oral papillomatosus
Oral ulceration
Stomatitis (>10%)
Tongue erosions

BROMFENAC

Trade name: Duract (Wyeth-Ayerst)
Category: Non steroidal anti-inflammatory agent (NSAID)
Clinically important, potentially serious interactions with: anticoagulants, cimetidine, lithium, phenytoin

REACTIONS

SKIN
Ecchymoses (<1%)
Exanthems (<1%)
Facial edema (<1%)
Generalized edema (<1%)
Hyperhidrosis (<1%)
Pruritus (<1%)
Rash (sic) (<1%)
Seborrhea (<1%)
Ulceration (<1%)
Urticaria (<1%)

HAIR
Hair – alopecia (<1%)

OTHER
Anaphylactoid reaction
Dysgeusia (<1%)
Mastodynia (<1%)
Myalgia (<1%)
Paresthesias (<1%)
Phlebitis (<1%)
Stomatitis (<1%)
Xerostomia (<1%)

BROMOCRIPTINE

Trade name: Parlodel (Novartis)
Other common trade names: Apo-Bromocriptine; Bromed; Kripton; Parilac; Pravidel
Category: Dopamine agonist; antihyperprolactinemic; infertility therapy adjunct; lactation inhibitor; antidyskinetic; growth hormone suppressant; ergot alkaloid; anti-parkinsonian
Clinically important, potentially serious interactions with: ergot alkaloids, sympathomimetics

REACTIONS

SKIN
- Exanthems
- Flushing
- Livedo reticularis
- Morphea
- Purpura
- Raynaud's phenomenon (1–10%)
- Scleroderma
- Urticaria (rare)
- Vasculitis

HAIR
- Hair – alopecia

OTHER
- Anaphylactoid reaction
- Erythromelalgia
- Paresthesias
- Stomatopyrosis
- Xerostomia

BROMPHENIRAMINE

Trade name: Dimetane (Robins)
Other common trade names: Bromine; Brommine; Dimegan; Ilvin; Kinmedon; Neo-Meton
Category: Antihistamine
Clinically important, potentially serious interactions with: alcohol, CNS depressants, MAO inhibitors, tricyclic antidepressants

REACTIONS

SKIN
- Angioedema (<1%)
- Exanthems (<1%)
- Photosensitivity (<1%)
- Rash (sic) (<1%)

OTHER
- Myalgia (<1%)
- Paresthesias (<1%)
- Xerostomia (1–10%)

BUCLIZINE

Trade name: Bucladin-S (Stuart)
Other common trade names: Aphilan; Buclixin; Longifene; Odetin; Postafeno; Vibazina
Category: Antiemetic
Clinically important, potentially serious interactions with: CNS depressants, MAO inhibitors, tricyclic antidepressants

REACTIONS

OTHER
- Xerostomia

BUMETANIDE

Trade name: Bumex (Roche)
Other common trade names: Burinex; Fondiuran; Fontego; Lunetoron; Miccil; Primex
Category: Sulfonamide loop diuretic; antihypertensive
Clinically important, potentially serious interactions with: aminoglycosides, digitalis, indomethacin, lithium

REACTIONS

SKIN
- Allergic reactions (sic)
- Bullous eruption
- Bullous pemphigoid
- Contact dermatitis
- Cutaneous side effects (sic) (1.1%)
- Edema (periorbital)
- Erythema multiforme (<1%)
- Exanthems
- Exfoliative dermatitis
- Hyperhidrosis (0.1%)
- Photosensitivity
- Pruritus (<1%)
- Purpura
- Rash (sic) (rare) (0.2%)
- Urticaria (0.2%)
- Vasculitis

OTHER
- Nipple tenderness (0.1%)
- Pseudoporphyria
- Xerostomia (0.1%)

BUPROPION

Trade names: Wellbutrin (Glaxo Wellcome); Zyban (Glaxo Wellcome)
Category: Heterocyclic antidepressant; aid to smoking cessation
Clinically important, potentially serious interactions with: carbamazepine, ritonavir

REACTIONS

SKIN
- Acne (<1%)
- Angioedema
- Ecchymoses (<0.1%)
- Edema (>1%)
- Exanthems (<0.1%)
- Exfoliative dermatitis
- Flushing (4%)
- Hyperhidrosis (5%)
- Lupus panniculitis
- Photosensitivity (<0.1%)
- Pruritus (4%)
- Rash (sic) (4%)
- Stevens-Johnson syndrome
- Urticaria (2%)
- Xerosis (<1%)

HAIR
- Hair – alopecia (<1%)
- Hair – color change (sic) (<1%)
- Hair – hirsutism (<1%)

OTHER
- Bromhidrosis
- Bruxism (<0.1%)
- Dysgeusia (4%)
- Gingivitis
- Glossitis
- Gynecomastia (<1%)
- Hypesthesia (<0.1%)
- Myalgia (6%)
- Oral edema (<1%)
- Paresthesias (2%)
- Priapism
- Sialorrhea
- Stomatitis (>1%)
- Tongue edema (0.1%)
- Twitching (2%)
- Vaginitis
- Xerostomia (up to 64%)

BUSPIRONE

Trade name: Buspar (Bristol-Myers Squibb)
Other common trade names: Ansail; Bespar; Biron; Busirone; Kallmiren; Narol; Neurosine
Category: Nonbenzodiazepine anxiolytic tranquilizer; serotonin antagonist
Clinically important, potentially serious interactions with: MAO inhibitors

REACTIONS

SKIN
- Acne (<0.1%)
- Bullous eruption (<1%)
- Ecchymoses
- Edema
- Exanthems
- Facial edema (1%)
- Flushing
- Hyperhidrosis
- Pruritus (1%)
- Purpura (1%)
- Radiation recall
- Rash (sic) (<1%)
- Seborrheic dermatitis
- Sicca syndrome
- Urticaria (<1%)
- Xerosis (1%)

HAIR
- Hair – alopecia (1%)

NAILS
- Nails – thinning (<0.1%)

OTHER
- Dysgeusia (<1%)
- Galactorrhea (<0.1%)
- Glossodynia (rare)
- Glossopyrosis
- Paresthesias (1%)
- Parosmia (1%)
- Sialorrhea
- Xerostomia (3%)

BUSULFAN

Trade name: Myleran (Glaxo Wellcome)
Other common trade names: Citosulfan; Leukosulfan; Mablin; Misulban
Category: Antineoplastic
Clinically important, potentially serious interactions with: thioguanine

REACTIONS

SKIN
- Bullous eruption
- Cheilitis
- Eccrine squamous syringometaplasia
- Erythema (macular) (sic) (1–10%)
- Erythema multiforme (<1%)
- Erythema nodosum (<1%)
- Exanthems
- Kaposi's sarcoma
- Pigmentation (5–10%)
- Purpura
- Urticaria (1–10%)
- Vasculitis
- Xerosis

HAIR
- Hair – alopecia (1–10%)

NAILS
- Nails – pigmentation

OTHER
- Anhidrosis
- Dysgeusia
- Gynecomastia (<1%)
- Oral mucosal pigmentation
- Porphyria cutanea tarda
- Stomatitis

BUTABARBITAL

Trade name: Butisol (Wallace)
Other common trade names: Butisol; Day-Barb
Category: Sedative-hypnotic barbiturate
Clinically important, potentially serious interactions with: benzodiazepines, chloramphenicol, CNS depressants, methylphenidate, propoxyphene, valproic acid

REACTIONS

SKIN
- Angioedema (<1%)
- Bullous eruption
- Erythema multiforme
- Exanthems
- Exfoliative dermatitis (<1%)
- Fixed eruption
- Herpes simplex
- Lupus erythematosus
- Necrosis
- Photosensitivity
- Pruritus
- Purpura
- Rash (sic) (<1%)
- Stevens-Johnson syndrome (<1%)
- Toxic epidermal necrolysis
- Urticaria
- Vasculitis

OTHER
- Oral ulceration
- Porphyria variegata
- Thrombophlebitis (<1%)

BUTALBITAL

Trade name: Fiorinal (Novartis)
Category: Sedative & analgesic barbiturate
Clinically important, potentially serious interactions with: benzodiazepines, chloramphenicol, CNS depressants, methylphenidate, propoxyphene, valproic acid

REACTIONS

SKIN
- Bullous eruption
- Erythema multiforme
- Exanthems
- Exfoliative dermatitis (<1%)
- Fixed eruption
- Herpes simplex
- Lupus erythematosus
- Necrosis
- Photosensitivity
- Pruritus
- Purpura
- Rash (sic) (1–10%)
- Stevens-Johnson syndrome (<1%)
- Toxic epidermal necrolysis
- Urticaria
- Vasculitis

OTHER
- Anaphylactoid reaction (1–10%)
- Oral erythema multiforme
- Oral ulceration
- Porphyria variegata

BUTORPHANOL

Trade name: Stadol (Bristol-Myers Squibb; Mead Johnson)
Other common trade names: Biforal; Busphen; Stadol NS
Category: Opioid analgesic
Clinically important, potentially serious interactions with: CNS depressants, cimetidine, ranitidine, ritonavir

REACTIONS

SKIN
- Edema (<1%)
- Exanthems
- Flushing (1–10%)
- Hyperhidrosis (1–10%)
- Pruritus
- Rash (sic) (<1%)
- Urticaria (<1%)

OTHER
- Dysgeusia (3–9%)
- Injection-site reactions
- Paresthesias
- Xerostomia (3–9%)

CABERGOLINE

Trade name: Dostinex (Pharmacia & Upjohn)
Category: Dopamine receptor agonist
Clinically important, potentially serious interactions with: butyrophenones, metoclopramide, phenothiazines, thioxanthines

REACTIONS

SKIN
- Acne (1%)
- Ankle edema (1%)
- Facial edema (1%)
- Fixed eruption
- Hot flashes (3%)
- Periorbital edema (1%)
- Peripheral edema (1%)
- Pruritus (1%)

OTHER
- Mastodynia (2%)
- Paresthesias (5%)
- Xerostomia (2%)

CALCITONIN (HUMAN & SALMON)

Trade names: Calcimar (Rhône-Poulenc Rorer); Cibacalcin (Ciba); Miacalcin (Novartis); Osteocalcin (Arcola)
Other common trade names: Cibacalcine; Clasynar; Miacalcic
Category: Osteoporosis therapy adjunct; bone resorption inhibitor
Clinically important, potentially serious interactions with: no data

REACTIONS

SKIN
- Exanthems
- Flushing (>10%)
- Granuloma annulare
- Pruritus
- Rash (sic) (<1%)
- Urticaria (<1%)

OTHER
- Anaphylactoid reaction
- Dysgeusia
- Injection-site inflammation (>10%)
- Injection-site pain
- Paresthesias (<1%)

CAPTOPRIL

Trade names: Capoten (Bristol-Myers Squibb); Capozide (Bristol-Myers Squibb)
Other common trade names: Acenorm; Acepril; Adocor; Captolane; Captoril; Lopirin; Lopril
Category: Angiotensin-converting enzyme (ACE) inhibitor; antihypertensive & vasodilator
Clinically important, potentially serious interactions with: diuretics, lithium

Capozide is captopril & hydrochlorothiazide

REACTIONS

SKIN
- Angioedema (<1%)
- Aphthous stomatitis (<2%)
- Bullous eruption
- Bullous pemphigoid
- Contact dermatitis
- Erythema multiforme
- Erythroderma
- Exanthems (4–7%)
- Exfoliative dermatitis (<2%)
- Flushing (<1%)
- Kaposi's sarcoma
- Lichenoid eruption
- Lichen planus (pemphigoides)
- Linear IgA bullous dermatosis
- Lupus erythematosus
- Mycosis fungoides
- Palmar-plantar pustulosis
- Pemphigus (<2%)
- Penile ulcers
- Photosensitivity
- Phototoxic reaction (<2%)
- Pigmentation
- Pityriasis rosea (<2%)
- Pruritus (4–7%)
- Psoriasis
- Purpura
- Rash (sic) (4–7%)
- Stevens-Johnson syndrome
- Toxic epidermal necrolysis
- Urticaria
- Vasculitis
- Xerosis

HAIR
- Hair – alopecia (<2%)

NAILS
- Nails – dystrophy
- Nails – onycholysis

OTHER
- Ageusia (2–4%)
- Anaphylactoid reaction (during hemodialysis)
- Dysgeusia (metallic or salty taste) (2–4%)
- Glossitis
- Glossopyrosis
- Gynecomastia
- Lymphadenopathy
- Myalgia
- Oral mucosal eruption
- Oral ulceration
- Paresthesias (<2%)
- Scalded mouth (sic)
- Tongue ulceration
- Xerostomia (<2%)

CARBAMAZEPINE

Trade names: Carbatrol (Shire Richwood); Epitol (Teva); Tegretol (Novartis)
Other common trade names: Foxsalepsin; Kodapan; Lexin; Mazepine; Sirtal; Teril; Timonil
Category: Anticonvulsant, antineuralgic, antimanic, antidiuretic & antipsychotic
Clinically important, potentially serious interactions with: cimetidine, danazol, diltiazem, erythromycin, felodipine, isoniazid, propoxyphene, troleandomycin, verapamil

REACTIONS

SKIN
- Acne keloid
- Acute generalized exanthematous pustulosis (AGEP)
- Allergic reactions (sic)
- Angioedema (<1%)
- Ankle edema
- Bullous eruption (<1%)
- Collagen disease (sic)
- Contact dermatitis

Cutaneous side effects (sic)
Dermatitis (sic)
Diaphoresis (1–10%)
Eczematous eruption (sic)
Edema
Eosinophilic pustular folliculitis (Ofuji's disease)
Epidermolysis bullosa
Erythema multiforme
Erythema nodosum (<1%)
Erythroderma
Exanthems (>5%)
Exfoliative dermatitis
Facial edema
Fixed eruption (<1%)
Kawasaki syndrome
Lichenoid eruption
Lupus erythematosus
Mycosis fungoides
Pellagra
Petechiae
Photosensitivity
Pruritus (<1%)
Psoriasis
Purpura
Pustular eruption
Rash (sic) (>10%)
Schamberg's disease
Sheet-like erythema
Stevens-Johnson syndrome (1–10%)
Toxic epidermal necrolysis (1–10%)
Toxicoderma (sic)
Toxic pustuloderma (sic)
Urticaria
Vasculitis

HAIR
Hair – alopecia

NAILS
Nails – discoloration (bluish-black)
Nails – hypoplasia
Nails – lichen planus
Nails – loss (sic)
Nails – onychomadesis

OTHER
Acute intermittent porphyria
Dysgeusia
Glossitis
Hypersensitivity
Lymphoproliferative disease
Mucocutaneous eruption
Oral lichenoid eruption
Oral mucosal eruption
Porphyria cutanea tarda
Pseudolymphoma
Stomatitis
Tongue ulceration
Xerostomia

CARBENICILLIN

Trade name: Geocillin (Roerig)
Other common trade names: Carbecin; Carbelin
Category: Penicillinase-sensitive penicillin
Clinically important, potentially serious interactions with: probenecid

REACTIONS

SKIN
Allergic reactions (sic)
Angioedema
Ecchymoses
Erythema multiforme
Exanthems
Exfoliative dermatitis
Hematomas
Jarisch-Herxheimer reaction
Pruritus
Purpura
Rash (sic) (<1%)
Stevens-Johnson syndrome
Toxic epidermal necrolysis
Urticaria (<1%)

OTHER
Anaphylactoid reaction
Black tongue
Dysgeusia (1–10%)
Glossitis (1–10%)
Glossodynia
Injection-site pain
Oral candidiasis
Serum sickness
Stomatitis
Stomatodynia
Thrombophlebitis (<1%)
Vaginitis (<1%)
Xerostomia

CARBIDOPA

Trade name: Sinemet (Dupont)
Category: Anti-parkinsonian
Clinically important, potentially serious interactions with: MAO inhibitors, tricyclic antidepressants

Sinemet is carbidopa & levodopa

REACTIONS

SKIN
- Ankle edema
- Dermatomyositis
- Edema
- Exanthems
- Exfoliative dermatitis
- Flushing
- Hyperhidrosis
- Melanoma
- Pigmentation
- Pruritus
- Purpura
- Scleroderma
- Urticaria

HAIR
- Hair – alopecia

OTHER
- Black cartilage
- Bromhidrosis
- Chromhidrosis (1–10%)
- Dysgeusia
- Glossopyrosis
- Xerostomia (1–10%)

CARBOPLATIN

Trade name: Paraplatin (Mead Johnson)
Other common trade names: Carboplat; Carbosin; Ercar; Oncocarbin; Paraplatine
Category: Antineoplastic
Clinically important, potentially serious interactions with: aldesleukin, phenytoin

REACTIONS

SKIN
- Depigmentation
- Erosion of body folds
- Erythema (2%)
- Exanthems
- Facial edema
- Pigmentation
- Pruritus (2%)
- Rash (sic) (2%)
- Urticaria (2%)

HAIR
- Hair – alopecia (3%)

OTHER
- Hypersensitivity (2%)
- Injection-site pain (>10%)
- Oral mucosal lesions
- Stomatitis (<1%)

CARISOPRODOL

Trade names: Rela (Schering); Soma (Wallace)
Other common trade names: Artifar; Carisoma; Myolax; Sanoma; Somadril
Category: Skeletal muscle relaxant
Clinically important, potentially serious interactions with: alcohol, CNS depressants, clindamycin, MAO inhibitors, phenothiazines

REACTIONS

SKIN
- Angioedema (1–10%)
- Edema
- Erythema multiforme (<1%)
- Exanthems
- Fixed eruption (<1%)
- Flushing (1–10%)
- Hyperhidrosis
- Photosensitivity
- Pruritus (<1%)
- Rash (sic) (<1%)
- Urticaria (<1%)

OTHER
- Anaphylactoid reaction
- Paresthesias
- Pseudoporphyria
- Xerostomia

CARMUSTINE

Trade name: Bicnu (Bristol-Myers Squibb)
Other common trade names: Bcnu; Becenun; BiCNU; Carmubris; Nitrumon
Category: Antineoplastic
Clinically important, potentially serious interactions with: cimetidine, etoposide

REACTIONS

SKIN
- Contact dermatitis
- Eccrine squamous syringometaplasia
- Erythema
- Exanthems
- Flushing (1–10%)
- Pigmentation (on accidental contact)
- Skin tenderness (sic)
- Telangiectases

HAIR
- Hair – alopecia (1–10%)

OTHER
- Injection-site burning (>10%)
- Injection-site necrosis
- Stomatitis (1–10%)

CARTEOLOL

Trade names: Cartrol (Abbott); Ocupress (ophthalmic) (Otsuka)
Other common trade names: Arteolol; Arteoptic; Calte; Carteol; Endak; Mikelan; Teoptic
Category: Beta-adrenergic blocking agent
Clinically important, potentially serious interactions with: calcium channel blockers, clonidine, flecainide, nifedipine, oral contraceptives, verapamil

REACTIONS

SKIN
- Acne
- Angioedema
- Ankle edema (<1%)
- Dermatitis (sic)
- Exanthems
- Exfoliative dermatitis
- Facial edema
- Flushing
- Hyperhidrosis (<1%)
- Lupus erythematosus
- Peripheral edema (1.7%)
- Photosensitivity
- Pigmentation
- Pruritus
- Psoriasis

Purpura (<1%)
Rash (sic) (2.5%)
Raynaud's phenomenon (<1%)
Vesiculobullous eruption
Xerosis

HAIR
Hair – alopecia

NAILS
Nails – discoloration (bluish)

OTHER
Anaphylactoid reaction
Dysgeusia (from topical application)
Paresthesias (2%)
Peyronie's disease
Xerostomia

CARVEDILOL

Trade name: Coreg (SmithKline Beecham)
Other common trade names: Dibloc; Dilatrend; Dimitone; Kredex; Querto
Category: Beta-adrenergic blocking agent
Clinically important, potentially serious interactions with: antidiabetics, calcium channel blockers, clonidine, flecainide, nifedipine, oral contraceptives, tacrine

REACTIONS

SKIN
Allergy (sic) (<1%)
Angioedema
Edema (1–10%)
Exanthems (<1%)
Hyperhidrosis (<1%)
Peripheral edema (1.4%)
Pruritus (<1%)
Psoriasis (<1%)
Rash (sic) (<1%)
Stevens-Johnson syndrome

HAIR
Hair – alopecia (<0.1%)

OTHER
Hypesthesia (<1%)
Myalgia (<1%)
Paresthesias (<1%)
Xerostomia (<1%)

CEFACLOR

Trade name: Ceclor (Lilly)
Other common trade names: Alfatil; CEC 500; Cefabiocin; Distaclor; Kefolor; Panoral
Category: Second-generation cephalosporin
Clinically important, potentially serious interactions with: anticoagulants, cimetidine, heparin

REACTIONS

SKIN
Acute generalized exanthematous pustulosis (AGEP)
Angioedema
Dermatitis (sic)
Edema
Erythema multiforme
Exanthems
Flushing
Pruritus (<1%)
Purpura
Pustular eruption
Rash (sic) (<1%)
Stevens-Johnson syndrome (<1%)
Toxic epidermal necrolysis
Urticaria (<1%)

OTHER
Anaphylactoid reaction
Candidiasis (vaginal)
Dysgeusia
Glossitis
Hypersensitivity
Paresthesias
Serum sickness
Vaginitis

CEFADROXIL

Trade names: Duricef (Bristol-Myers Squibb); Ultracef (Mead Johnson)
Other common trade names: Baxan; Bidocef; Cedrox; Duracef; Moxacef; Oracefal; Sumacef
Category: First-generation cephalosporin antibiotic
Clinically important, potentially serious interactions with: anticoagulants, cimetidine, heparin

REACTIONS

SKIN
- Angioedema
- Candidiasis
- Erythema
- Erythema multiforme
- Exanthems (<1%)
- Pemphigus
- Pruritus
- Rash (sic)
- Stevens-Johnson syndrome
- Toxic epidermal necrolysis
- Urticaria

OTHER
- Anaphylactoid reaction
- Glossitis
- Oral mucosal eruption
- Oral ulceration
- Serum sickness
- Vaginitis

CEFAMANDOLE

Trade name: Mandol (Lilly)
Other common trade names: Cedol; Cefadol; Kefadol; Kefdole; Mancef; Mandokef
Category: Second generation cephalosporin
Clinically important, potentially serious interactions with: aminoglycosides, anticoagulants, cimetidine, furosemide, heparin

REACTIONS

SKIN
- Acne
- Diaper rash
- Edema
- Erythema multiforme
- Exanthems
- Flushing
- Hyperhidrosis
- Linear IgA bullous dermatosis
- Pruritus
- Purpura
- Rash (sic) (<1%)
- Stevens-Johnson syndrome
- Toxic epidermal necrolysis
- Toxic erythema
- Urticaria (<1%)

OTHER
- Anaphylactoid reaction
- Dysgeusia
- Glossitis
- Injection-site burning
- Injection-site cellulitis
- Injection-site edema
- Injection-site inflammation
- Injection-site pain (<1%)
- Injection-site thrombophlebitis
- Oral candidiasis
- Paresthesias
- Serum sickness
- Vaginal candidiasis
- Vaginitis

CEFAZOLIN

Trade names: Ancef (SmithKline Beecham); Kefzol (Lilly); Zolicef (Mead Johnson)
Other common trade names: Basocef; Cefacidal; Elzogram; Gramaxin; Kefarin; Totacef; Zolin
Category: Second-generation cephalosporin antibiotic
Clinically important, potentially serious interactions with: aminoglycosides, anticoagulants, cimetidine, heparin

REACTIONS

SKIN
- Acute generalized exanthematous pustulosis (AGEP)
- Allergic reactions (sic)
- Erythema multiforme
- Exanthems
- Fixed eruption (linear)
- Pemphigus
- Photo recall phenomenon (sic)
- Photosensitivity
- Pruritus
- Pruritus ani
- Pustular eruption
- Rash (sic) (<1%)
- Stevens-Johnson syndrome
- Toxic epidermal necrolysis
- Urticaria (<1%)

OTHER
- Anaphylactoid reaction
- Injection-site induration
- Injection-site pain
- Injection-site phlebitis
- Serum sickness
- Vaginitis

CEFDINIR

Trade name: Omnicef (Parke-Davis)
Category: Cephalosporin
Clinically important, potentially serious interactions with: aminoglycosides, antacids, anticoagulants, cimetidine, cyclosporine, famotidine, heparin, iron, nizatidine, omeprazole, probenecid, ranitidine

REACTIONS

SKIN
- Candidiasis (1%)
- Erythema multiforme
- Erythema nodosum
- Exanthems (0.2%)
- Exfoliative dermatitis
- Facial edema
- Pruritus (0.2%)
- Purpura
- Rash (sic) (3%)
- Stevens-Johnson syndrome
- Toxic epidermal necrolysis
- Vasculitis

OTHER
- Anaphylactoid reaction
- Stomatitis
- Vaginal candidiasis (5%)
- Vaginitis (1%)

CEFEPIME

Trade name: Maxipime (Bristol-Myers Squibb)
Other common trade name: Maxcef
Category: Fourth-generation cephalosporin
Clinically important, potentially serious interactions with: aminoglycosides, anticoagulants, cimetidine, heparin

REACTIONS

SKIN
- Candidiasis (<1%)
- Erythema multiforme
- Exanthems (<1%)
- Pruritus (<1%)
- Rash (sic) (51%)
- Stevens-Johnson syndrome
- Toxic epidermal necrolysis
- Urticaria (<1%)

OTHER
- Injection-site inflammation (0.6%)
- Injection-site pain (0.6%)
- Injection-site phlebitis (1.3%)
- Injection-site rash (1.1%)
- Vaginitis (<1%)

CEFIXIME

Trade name: Suprax (Lederle)
Other common trade names: Cefspan; Cephoral; Fixime; Oroken; Supran; Uro-cephoral
Category: Third-generation cephalosporin antibiotic
Clinically important, potentially serious interactions with: anticoagulants, cimetidine, heparin

REACTIONS

SKIN
- Erythema multiforme (<2%)
- Pruritus (<2%)
- Rash (sic) (<2%)
- Stevens-Johnson syndrome (<2%)
- Urticaria (<2%)

OTHER
- Anaphylactoid reaction
- Pseudolymphoma
- Serum sickness (<2%)
- Vaginitis (<2%)
- Xerostomia

CEFOTAXIME

Trade name: Claforan (Hoechst Marion Roussel)
Other common trade names: Cefotax; Molelant; Oritaxim; Primafen; Spirosine; Zariviz
Category: Third generation, broad-spectrum, cephalosporin
Clinically important, potentially serious interactions with: aminoglycosides, anticoagulants, cimetidine, furosemide, heparin,tobramycin

REACTIONS

SKIN
- Erythema multiforme
- Exanthems
- Pruritus (2.4%)
- Rash: (sic) (2.4%)
- Urticaria (2.4%)

OTHER
- Anaphylactoid reaction (2.4%)
- Injection-site inflammation (4.3%)
- Injection-site pain (1–10%)
- Phlebitis (<1%)
- Vaginitis (<1%)

CEFOXITIN

Trade name: Mefoxin (Merck)
Other common trade names: Cefmore; Cefoxin; Lephocin; Mefoxil; Mefoxitin
Category: Second generation, broad-spectrum cephalosporin
Clinically important, potentially serious interactions with: aminoglycosides, anticoagulants, cimetidine, furosemide, heparin

REACTIONS

SKIN
- Angioedema
- Exanthems
- Exfoliative dermatitis (<1%)
- Flushing
- Pruritus
- Purpura
- Pustular eruption
- Rash (sic) (<1%)
- Toxic epidermal necrolysis
- Urticaria

OTHER
- Anaphylactoid reaction
- Injection-site induration
- Injection-site pain
- Injection-site tenderness
- Serum sickness

CEFPODOXIME

Trade name: Vantin (Pharmacia & Upjohn)
Other common trade names: Cefodox; Celance; Orelox; Podomexef
Category: Third generation cephalosporin
Clinically important, potentially serious interactions with: anticoagulants, cimetidine, heparin, probenecid

REACTIONS

SKIN
- Acne
- Diaper rash (<1%)
- Edema
- Erythema multiforme
- Flushing (<1%)
- Hyperhidrosis
- Pruritus (<1%)
- Rash (sic)
- Skin peeling (sic) (<1%)
- Stevens-Johnson syndrome
- Toxic epidermal necrolysis

OTHER
- Anaphylactoid reaction (<1%)
- Dysgeusia (<1%)
- Glossitis
- Injection-site burning
- Injection-site cellulitis
- Injection-site edema
- Injection-site inflammation
- Injection-site thrombophlebitis
- Oral candidiasis
- Paresthesias
- Serum sickness
- Sialopenia (<1%)
- Vaginal candidiasis (<1%)
- Vaginitis

CEFTAZIDIME

Trade names: Ceptaz (Glaxo Wellcome); Fortaz (Glaxo Wellcome); Tazicef (SmithKline Beecham); Tazidime (Lilly)
Category: Third-generation cephalosporin
Clinically important, potentially serious interactions with: aminoglycosides, anticoagulants, cimetidine, furosemide, heparin

REACTIONS

SKIN
- Acne
- Allergic reactions (sic)
- Angioedema (2%)
- Diaper rash
- Edema
- Erythema multiforme (2%)
- Exanthems
- Flushing
- Hyperhidrosis
- Pemphigus erythematosus (sic)
- Photosensitivity
- Pruritus (2%)
- Rash (sic) (2%)
- Stevens-Johnson syndrome (2%)
- Toxic epidermal necrolysis (2%)
- Toxic erythema
- Toxic pustuloderma
- Urticaria

OTHER
- Anaphylactoid reaction (2%)
- Dysgeusia
- Glossitis
- Injection-site burning
- Injection-site cellulitis
- Injection-site edema
- Injection-site inflammation (2%)
- Injection-site pain (1–10%)
- Injection-site thrombophlebitis (2%)
- Oral candidiasis
- Paresthesias (<1%)
- Serum sickness
- Vaginal candidiasis
- Vaginitis (1%)

CEFTIBUTEN

Trade name: Cedax (Schering)
Other common trade names: Ceten; Cilecef; Keimax; Seftem
Category: Third-generation cephalosporin
Clinically important, potentially serious interactions with: aminoglycosides, anticoagulants, cimetidine, heparin

REACTIONS

SKIN
- Candidiasis (<1%)
- Pruritus (0.3%)
- Rash (sic) (0.3%)
- Toxic epidermal necrolysis
- Urticaria (<1%)

OTHER
- Dysgeusia (<1%)
- Paresthesias (<1%)
- Vaginitis (<1%)
- Xerostomia (<1%)

CEFTRIAXONE

Trade name: Rocephin (Roche)
Other common trade names: Cefaxone; Rocefin; Rocephalin; Rocephine; Tacex; Zefone
Category: Third-generation cephalosporin
Clinically important, potentially serious interactions with: aminoglycosides, anticoagulants, cimetidine, heparin, probenecid

REACTIONS

SKIN
- Angioedema
- Candidiasis (5%)
- Cutaneous side effects (sic) (3%)
- Dermatitis (sic)
- Erythema multiforme
- Exanthems
- Flushing (<1%)
- Hyperhidrosis (0.2%)
- Jarisch-Herxheimer reaction
- Pemphigus
- Pruritus (<1%)
- Purpura
- Rash (sic) (1.7%)
- Stevens-Johnson syndrome
- Urticaria (0.1%)

OTHER
- Anaphylactoid reaction
- Dysgeusia (<1%)
- Glossitis
- Injection-site induration
- Injection-site pain (1–10%)
- Injection-site phlebitis (<1%)
- Oral mucosal eruption
- Serum sickness
- Vaginitis (<1%)

CEFUROXIME

Trade name: Ceftin (Glaxo Wellcome)
Other common trade names: Cefuril; Cepazine; Elobact; Zinat; Zinnat; Zoref
Category: Second-generation cephalosporin
Clinically important, potentially serious interactions with: aminoglycosides, anticoagulants, cimetidine, heparin

REACTIONS

SKIN
- Acute generalized exanthematous pustulosis (AGEP)
- Angioedema
- Erythema multiforme
- Exanthems
- Jarisch-Herxheimer reaction
- Pemphigus
- Perianal thrush
- Pruritus (<1%)
- Purpura
- Pustular eruption
- Rash (sic) (<1%)
- Stevens-Johnson syndrome
- Toxic epidermal necrolysis
- Urticaria (<1%)

OTHER
- Anaphylactoid reaction
- Hypersensitivity
- Injection-site pain (<1%)
- Oral candidiasis
- Serum sickness
- Thrombophlebitis (1–10%)
- Vaginitis (<1%)

CEPHALEXIN

Trade names: Cefanex (Bristol-Myers Squibb); Keflet (Dista); Keflex (Dista)
Other common trade names: Ceforal; Ceporex; Ceporexine; Kefarol; Novolexin; Ospexin
Category: First-generation cephalosporin
Clinically important, potentially serious interactions with: amikacin, aminoglycosides, anticoagulants, cimetidine, gentamicin, heparin

REACTIONS

SKIN
- Acute generalized exanthematous pustulosis (AGEP)
- Angioedema
- Contact dermatitis
- Cutaneous side effects (sic) (2%)
- Erythema multiforme
- Exanthems
- Fixed eruption
- Pemphigus
- Pruritus
- Pruritus ani et vulvae
- Purpura
- Pustular eruption
- Rash (sic) (<1%)
- Stevens-Johnson syndrome
- Toxic epidermal necrolysis
- Urticaria

NAILS
- Nails – paronychia

OTHER
- Anaphylactoid reaction
- Serum sickness
- Vaginitis

CEPHALOTHIN

Trade names: Keflin (Lilly); Kefzol (Lilly)
Other common trade names: Cepovenin; Keflin-N; Keflin Neutral; Keflin Neutro; Practogen
Category: First generation, broad-spectrum cephalosporin
Clinically important, potentially serious interactions with: amphotericin B, anticoagulants, cimetidine, furosemide, gentamicin, heparin

REACTIONS

SKIN
- Allergic reactions (sic)
- Erythema multiforme
- Exanthems (<1%)
- Pruritus
- Purpura
- Rash (sic)
- Toxic epidermal necrolysis
- Urticaria

OTHER
- Anaphylactoid reaction
- Injection-site pain (<1%)
- Serum sickness

CEPHRADINE

Trade name: Velosef (Bristol-Myers Squibb)
Other common trade names: Cefro; Celex; Doncef; Eskacef; Maxisporin; Opebrin; Sefril
Category: First-generation cephalosporin
Clinically important, potentially serious interactions with: anticoagulants, cimetidine, heparin

REACTIONS

SKIN
- Acute generalized exanthematous pustulosis (AGEP)
- Erythema multiforme
- Exanthems
- Pruritus
- Purpura
- Pustular eruption
- Rash (sic) (<1%)
- Stevens-Johnson syndrome

Toxic epidermal necrolysis
Toxic pustuloderma
Urticaria

OTHER
Anaphylactoid reaction
Serum sickness
Vaginitis

CERIVASTATIN

Trade name: Baycol (Bayer)
Category: A statin (HMG-CoA reductase inhibitor); lipid-lowering agent
Clinically important, potentially serious interactions with: erythromycin, kaolin, mibefradil, nefazodone

REACTIONS

SKIN
Angioedema
Dermatomyositis
Erythema multiforme
Flushing
Lupus erythematosus
Nodules (sic)
Peripheral edema (2%)
Photosensitivity
Pigmentation
Pruritus
Purpura
Rash (sic) (3.4%)
Stevens-Johnson syndrome
Toxic epidermal necrolysis
Urticaria
Vasculitis
Xerosis

HAIR
Hair – alopecia
Hair – changes (sic)

NAILS
Nails – changes (sic)

OTHER
Anaphylactoid reaction
Dysgeusia
Gynecomastia
Hypersensitivity
Myalgia (2.7%)
Paresthesias
Xerostomia

CETIRIZINE

Trade name: Zyrtec (Pfizer)
Other common trade names: Alercet; Alerid; Cetrine; Cezin; Triz; Virlix; Zirtin
Category: Antihistamine
Clinically important, potentially serious interactions with: alcohol; CNS depressants

REACTIONS

SKIN
Acne (<2%)
Angioedema (<2%)
Bullous eruption (<2%)
Dermatitis (<2%)
Edema
Exanthems (<2%)
Flushing (<2%)
Furunculosis (<2%)
Hyperhidrosis (<2%)
Hyperkeratosis (<2%)
Photosensitivity (<2%)
Phototoxic reaction (<2%)
Pruritus (<2%)
Purpura (<2%)
Rash (sic) (<2%)
Seborrhea (<2%)
Urticaria (<2%)
Xerosis (<2%)

HAIR
Hair – alopecia (<2%)
Hair – hypertrichosis (<2%)

OTHER
Ageusia (<2%)
Anaphylactoid reaction (<2%)
Dysgeusia (<2%)
Hyperesthesia (<2%)
Hypesthesia (<2%)

Mastodynia (<2%)
Myalgia (<2%)
Paresthesias (<2%)
Parosmia (<2%)
Sialorrhea (<2%)
Stomatitis (<2%)
Tongue discoloration (<2%)
Tongue edema (<2%)
Vaginitis (<2%)
Xerostomia (5%)

CHLORAL HYDRATE

Trade names: Aquachloral (Alcon); Noctec (Bristol-Myers Squibb)
Other common trade names: Chloraldurat; Medianox; Novochlorhydrate; Somnox; Welldorm
Category: Sedative hypnotic
Clinically important, potentially serious interactions with: alcohol, CNS depressants, furosemide, phenytoin, warfarin

REACTIONS

SKIN
Acne
Angioedema
Bullous eruption
Dermatitis
Eczematous eruption (sic)
Erythema
Erythema multiforme
Exanthems
Fixed eruption
Flushing
Lichenoid eruption
Pruritus
Purpura
Rash (sic) (1–10%)
Ulceration
Urticaria (1–10%)

OTHER
Dysgeusia
Oral mucosal lesions
Oral ulceration
Stomatitis

CHLORAMBUCIL

Trade name: Leukeran (Glaxo Wellcome)
Other common trade names: Chloraminophene; Linfolysin
Category: Antineoplastic; immunosuppressant
Clinically important, potentially serious interactions with: azathioprine

REACTIONS

SKIN
Angioedema
Cutaneous necrosis
Cutaneous side effects (sic)
Edema
Erythema multiforme
Exanthems
Exfoliative dermatitis
Facial erythema
Herpes simplex
Herpes zoster
Kaposi's sarcoma
Lupus erythematosus
Pellagra
Periorbital edema
Photosensitivity
Pruritus
Psoriasis (exacerbation)
Purpura
Rash (sic) (1–10%)
Sezary syndrome
Stevens-Johnson syndrome
Toxic epidermal necrolysis
Urticaria

HAIR
Hair – alopecia

OTHER
Acute intermittent porphyria
Hypersensitivity (<1%)
Oral mucosal lesions
Oral ulceration (<1%)
Stomatitis

CHLORAMPHENICOL

Trade names: Ak-Chlor (Alcon); Chloromycetin (Parke-Davis); Chloroptic (Allergan); Ophthochlor (Parke-Davis)
Other common trade names: Aquamycetin; Cebenicol; Kloramfenicol; Oleomycetin
Category: Broad-spectrum antibiotic
Clinically important, potentially serious interactions with: antidiabetics, chlorpropamide, oral anticoagulants, penicillin, phenytoin

REACTIONS

SKIN
- Acute generalized exanthematous pustulosis (AGEP)
- Angioedema (<1%)
- Bullous eruption
- Contact dermatitis
- Eczematous eruption
- Erythema multiforme (<1%)
- Exanthems (1–5%)
- Fixed eruption
- Gray syndrome*
- Leukoderma
- Pellagra
- Pruritus (<1%)
- Purpura
- Pustular eruption
- Rash (sic) (<1%)
- Sensitization (sic)
- Sheet-like erythema (sic)
- Stevens-Johnson syndrome
- Systemic eczematous contact dermatitis
- Toxic epidermal necrolysis (<1%)
- Urticaria
- Vasculitis

HAIR
- Hair – alopecia

NAILS
- Nails – photo-onycholysis

OTHER
- Acute intermittent porphyria
- Anaphylactoid reaction
- Black hairy tongue
- Glossitis
- Hypersensitivity
- Oral mucosal eruption
- Oral ulceration
- Paresthesias
- Porphyria
- Stomatitis (<1%)
- Xerostomia

*Gray syndrome: toxic reactions in premature infants and newborns. Signs and symptoms include: abdominal distension, blue-gray skin color, low body temperature, and uneven breathing.

CHLORDIAZEPOXIDE

Trade names: Libritabs (Roche); Librium (Roche); Limbitrol (Roche); Lipoxide (Major)
Other common trade names: Huberplex; Multum; Novopoxide; Psicofar; Solium; Tropium
Category: Benzodiazepine; antianxiety, sedative-hypnotic, antipanic & antitremor agent
Clinically important, potentially serious interactions with: alcohol, cimetidine, clarithromycin, diltiazem, levodopa, oral anticoagulants, tricyclic antidepressants, verapamil

Limbitrol is amitriptyline & chlordiazepoxide

REACTIONS

SKIN
- Angioedema (<1%)
- Dermatitis (sic) (1–10%)
- Edema (1–10%)
- Erythema multiforme (<1%)
- Erythema nodosum (<1%)
- Exanthems
- Fixed eruption (<1%)
- Hyperhidrosis (>10%)
- Lupus erythematosus
- Photosensitivity
- Pigmented purpuric eruption
- Pruritus
- Purpura
- Rash (sic) (>10%)
- Urticaria

Vasculitis

HAIR
Hair – alopecia

OTHER
Acute intermittent porphyria
Galactorrhea
Gynecomastia
Paresthesias
Porphyria
Sialopenia (>10%)
Sialorrhea (1–10%)
Xerostomia (>10%)

CHLORMEZANONE

Trade name: Trancopal (Sanofi)
Category: Antianxiety agent & muscle relaxant
Clinically important, potentially serious interactions with: none

REACTIONS

SKIN
Ankle edema
Exanthems
Fixed eruption
Flushing
Pruritus
Rash (sic)
Stevens-Johnson syndrome
Toxic epidermal necrolysis
Urticaria

OTHER
Acute intermittent porphyria
Dysgeusia
Xerostomia

CHLOROQUINE

Trade name: Aralen (Sanofi Winthrop)
Other common trade names: Avloclor; Chlorquin; Emquin; Heliopar; Lagaquin; Malarivon
Category: Antiprotozoal & antirheumatic drug; lupus erythematosus suppressant; polymorphous light eruption, & porphyria cutanea tarda
Clinically important, potentially serious interactions with: cimetidine, cyclosporine, digitalis, etretinate, methotrexate, methoxsalen, penicillamine

REACTIONS

SKIN
Acute generalized exanthematous pustulosis (AGEP)
Angioedema (<1%)
Contact dermatitis
Ephelides
Erythema annulare centrifugum
Erythema multiforme (<1%)
Erythroderma
Exanthems (1–5%)
Exfoliative dermatitis
Fixed eruption (<1%)
Lichenoid eruption
Photosensitivity
Pigmentation
Polymorphous light eruption
Pruritus
Psoriasis
Pustular eruption
Pustular psoriasis
Stevens-Johnson syndrome
Toxic epidermal necrolysis (<1%)
Urticaria (rare)
Vasculitis
Vitiligo

HAIR
Hair – alopecia
Hair – pigmentation (<1%)
Hair – poliosis

NAILS
Nails – discoloration
Nails – pigmentation
Nails – shoreline

OTHER
Acute intermittent porphyria
Gingival pigmentation
Myopathy

Oral mucosal pigmentation
Oral mucosal ulceration
Porphyria
Porphyria cutanea tarda
Stomatitis (<1%)
Stomatopyrosis

CHLOROTHIAZIDE

Trade name: Diuril (Merck)
Other common trade names: Azide; Chlothin; Chlotride; Diurazide; Diuret; Saluretil; Saluric
Category: Thiazide diuretic; antihypertensive
Clinically important, potentially serious interactions with: amantadine, digitalis, furosemide, lithium, probenecid

REACTIONS

SKIN
Bullous eruption
Erythema multiforme
Exanthems
Exfoliative dermatitis
Fixed eruption
Lichenoid eruption
Lupus erythematosus
Photoallergic reaction
Photosensitivity (<1%)
Pruritus
Purpura
Rash (sic) (<1%)
Stevens-Johnson syndrome
Toxic epidermal necrolysis
Urticaria
Vasculitis

HAIR
Hair – alopecia

OTHER
Anaphylactoid reaction
Dysgeusia
Oral mucosal lesions
Paresthesias (<1%)
Xanthopsia

CHLOROTRIANISENE

Trade name: Tace (Hoechst Marion Roussel)
Other common trade names: Estregur; Merbentul
Category: Estrogen replacement
Clinically important, potentially serious interactions with: anticoagulants, felbamate, phenytoin

REACTIONS

SKIN
Acne pustulosa
Candidiasis
Chloasma (<1%)
Edema (>10%)
Erythema multiforme
Erythema nodosum
Melasma (<1%)
Rash (sic) (<1%)
Urticaria

HAIR
Hair – alopecia
Hair – hirsutism

OTHER
Gynecomastia (>10%)
Mastodynia (>10%)
Porphyria cutanea tarda
Vaginitis

CHLORPROMAZINE

Trade name: Thorazine (SmithKline Beecham)
Other common trade names: Chloractil; Chlorazin; Esmino; Largactil; Propaphenin; Prozin
Category: Phenothiazine antipsychotic & antiemetic
Clinically important, potentially serious interactions with: ACE-inhibitors, CNS depressants, epinephrine, lithium, MAO inhibitors, piperazines, valproic acid

REACTIONS

SKIN
- Actinic reticuloid
- Angioedema (<1%)
- Bullous eruption (<1%)
- Contact dermatitis
- Erythema multiforme (<1%)
- Exanthems (>5%)
- Exfoliative dermatitis
- Fixed eruption (<1%)
- Hypohidrosis (>10%)
- Lichenoid eruption
- Lupus erythematosus
- Miliaria
- Peripheral edema
- Photocontact dermatitis
- Photosensitivity
- Phototoxic reaction
- Pigmentation (<1%)
- Pruritus (1–10%)
- Purpura
- Pustular eruption
- Rash (sic) (1–10%)
- Seborrheic dermatitis
- Toxic epidermal necrolysis (<1%)
- Urticaria (rare)
- Vasculitis

NAILS
- Nails – photo-onycholysis
- Nails – pigmentation

OTHER
- Anaphylactoid reaction (<1%)
- Aseptic necrosis following injection
- Galactorrhea (<1%)
- Gynecomastia (1–10%)
- Mastodynia (1–10%)
- Oral mucosal eruption
- Oral mucosal pigmentation
- Oral ulceration
- Polyarteritis nodosa
- Priapism (<1%)
- Pseudolymphoma
- Xerostomia (1–10%)

CHLORPROPAMIDE

Trade name: Diabinese (Pfizer)
Other common trade names: Arodoc C; Chlormide; Diabemide; Diabenese; Melormin; Tesmel
Category: First generation sulfonylurea hypoglycemic & antidiuretic
Clinically important, potentially serious interactions with: beta-blockers, hydantoins, MAO inhibitors, phenylbutazone, salicylates, sulfonamides, thiazides

REACTIONS

SKIN
- Angioedema
- Bullous eruption (<1%)
- Contact dermatitis
- Cutaneous side effects (sic)
- Edema (<1%)
- Erythema multiforme (<1%)
- Erythema nodosum (<1%)
- Exanthems (1–5%)
- Exfoliative dermatitis
- Fixed eruption
- Flushing
- Granulomas
- Lichenoid eruption
- Lupus erythematosus
- Photosensitivity (1–10%)
- Pruritus (<3%)
- Purpura
- Rash (sic) (1–10%)
- Stevens-Johnson syndrome
- Toxic epidermal necrolysis
- Urticaria (1–10%)
- Vasculitis

HAIR
Hair – alopecia

OTHER
Acute intermittent porphyria
Oral lichenoid eruption
Porphyria
Porphyria cutanea tarda
Tongue ulceration

CHLORTHALIDONE

Trade names: Combipres (Boehringer Ingelheim); Hygroton (Rhône-Poulenc Rorer); Thalitone (Boehringer Ingelheim)
Other common trade names: Higroton; Hydro-Long; Hypertol; Igroton; Thalidone; Uridon
Category: Thiazide diuretic; antihypertensive
Clinically important, potentially serious interactions with: antidiabetics, bumetanide, digitalis, furosemide, lithium, probenecid

Combipres is chlorthalidone & clonidine

REACTIONS

SKIN
Exanthems
Lupus erythematosus
Necrotizing angiitis
Photosensitivity
Psoriasis
Purpura
Rash (sic)
Toxic epidermal necrolysis
Urticaria
Vasculitis

OTHER
Paresthesias
Pseudoporphyria
Xanthopsia

CHLORZOXAZONE

Trade names: Paraflex (McNeil); Parafon Forte DSC (McNeil)
Other common trade names: Escoflex; Klorzoxazon; Muscol; Prolax; Solaxin
Category: Skeletal muscle relaxant
Clinically important, potentially serious interactions with: alcohol, CNS depressants, disulfiram

REACTIONS

SKIN
Angioedema (1–10%)
Ecchymoses
Erythema multiforme (<1%)
Exanthems
Flushing (1–10%)
Petechiae
Pruritus (rare)
Rash (sic) (<1%)
Urticaria (<1%)

OTHER
Anaphylactoid reaction

CHOLESTYRAMINE

Trade name: Questran (Bristol-Myers Squibb)
Other common trade names: Chol-Less; Colestrol; Lismol; Quantalan; Questran Lite
Category: Antihyperlipidemic; antipruritic (cholestasis); anti-diarrheal
Clinically important, potentially serious interactions with: acetaminophen, anticoagulants, antidiabetics, digitalis, furosemide, thiazides, tricyclic antidepressants, valproic acid

REACTIONS

SKIN
- Ecchymoses
- Edema
- Exanthems
- Rash (sic) (<1%)
- Urticaria

OTHER
- Dysgeusia
- Paresthesias
- Tongue irritation (sic) (<1%)

CIMETIDINE

Trade name: Tagamet (SmithKline Beecham)
Other common trade names: Azucimet; Cimedine; Cimehexal; Ciuk; Dyspamet; Stomedine
Category: Histamine H_2-receptor antagonist
Clinically important, potentially serious interactions with: beta-blockers, carbamazepine, carmustine, cisapride, fentanyl, isoniazid, itraconazole, ketoconazole, midazolam, moclobemide, morphine, pentazocine, phenytoin, theophylline, tricyclic antidepressants

REACTIONS

SKIN
- Angioedema (<1%)
- Cutaneous side effects (sic) (0.4%)
- Erythema annulare centrifugum
- Erythema multiforme (<1%)
- Erythrosis-like lesions (sic)
- Exanthems
- Exfoliative dermatitis
- Fixed eruption
- Ichthyosis
- Id reaction
- Lupus erythematosus
- Pruritus (<1%)
- Psoriasis
- Purpura
- Pustular psoriasis
- Rash (sic) (<2%)
- Seborrheic dermatitis
- Stevens-Johnson syndrome
- Toxic dermatitis
- Toxic epidermal necrolysis (<1%)
- Urticaria
- Vasculitis
- Xerosis

HAIR
- Hair – alopecia

OTHER
- Anaphylactoid reaction
- Galactorrhea
- Gynecomastia (<1%)
- Hypersensitivity
- Myalgia
- Myopathy
- Porphyria
- Pseudolymphoma
- Xerostomia

CIPROFLOXACIN

Trade names: Ciloxan (Alcon); Cipro (Bayer)
Other common trade names: Ciflox; Ciplox; Ciprobay Uro; Cipromycin; Ciproxin; Uniflox
Category: Synthetic fluoroquinolone antibiotic
Clinically important, potentially serious interactions with: antacids, bismuth subsalicylate, calcium salts, didanosine, foscarnet, glyburide, iron, magnesium salts, sucralfate, theophylline, zinc

Ciprofloxacin is chemically related to nalidixic acid

REACTIONS

SKIN
- Acne
- Angioedema (<1%)
- Bullous eruption
- Candidiasis (<1%)
- Edema (<1%)
- Elastolysis
- Erythema multiforme
- Erythema nodosum (<1%)
- Erythroderma (<1%)
- Exanthems
- Exfoliative dermatitis (<1%)
- Fixed eruption
- Flushing (<1%)
- Hyperhidrosis
- Hyperpigmentation (<1%)
- Lobular panniculitis
- Photosensitivity (<1%)
- Phototoxic reaction
- Pruritus (<1%)
- Purpura
- Rash (sic) (1–10%)
- Stevens-Johnson syndrome (<1%)
- Toxic epidermal necrolysis (<1%)
- Urticaria (<1%)
- Vasculitis (<1%)

OTHER
- Anaphylactoid reaction (<1%)
- Anosmia
- Dysesthesia (<1%)
- Dysgeusia (<1%)
- Gynecomastia (<1%)
- Hypersensitivity
- Injection-site pain
- Oral candidiasis
- Oral mucosal lesions
- Panniculitis (lobular)
- Paresthesias
- Serum sickness
- Stomatitis
- Tendon rupture
- Vaginitis (<1%)
- Xerostomia

CISAPRIDE

Trade name: Propulsid (Janssen)
Other common trade names: Acenalin; Alimix; Prepulsid; Propulsin; Risamol; Sepride; Unamol
Category: Antiemetic; cholinergic enhancer; gastrointestinal emptying adjunct
Clinically important, potentially serious interactions with: cimetidine, clarithromycin, CNS depressants, diazepam, erythromycin, fluconazole, indinavir, itraconazole, ketoconazole, miconazole, nefazodone, ranitidine, ritonavir, troleandomycin

REACTIONS

SKIN
- Edema (>1%)
- Exanthems
- Pruritus (1.2%)
- Rash (sic) (>5%)
- Urticaria

OTHER
- Myalgia (>1%)
- Vaginitis (1.2%)
- Xerostomia (>5%)

CISPLATIN

Trade name: Platinol (Mead Johnson)
Other common trade names: Cisplatyl; Platiblastin; Platinex; Platinol-AQ; Platistil; Plasticin
Category: Antineoplastic
Clinically important, potentially serious interactions with: bleomycin, bumetanide, furosemide, phenytoin

REACTIONS

SKIN
- Angioedema
- Contact dermatitis
- Erythema
- Exanthems
- Exfoliative dermatitis
- Facial edema
- Flushing
- Hyperhidrosis
- Necrosis
- Pigmentation
- Pruritus
- Pyoderma (verrucous)
- Rash (sic)
- Raynaud's phenomenon
- Stevens-Johnson syndrome
- Urticaria

HAIR
- Hair – alopecia (>10%)

NAILS
- Nails – Beau's lines (transverse nail ridging)
- Nails – hypomelanosis

OTHER
- Ageusia
- Anaphylactoid reaction (<1%)
- Gingival pigmentation
- Injection-site cellulitis
- Oral mucosal lesions (<1%)
- Porphyria

CLADRIBINE

Trade name: Leustatin (Ortho)
Category: Antineoplastic
Clinically important, potentially serious interactions with: none

REACTIONS

SKIN
- Allergic cutaneous reactions (sic)
- Diaphoresis (1–10%)
- Edema (6%)
- Erythema (6%)
- Exanthems
- Halogenoderma (sic)
- Petechiae (8%)
- Pruritus (6%)
- Purpura (10%)
- Rash (sic) (27%)
- Toxic epidermal necrolysis
- Transient acantholytic dermatosis (sic)

OTHER
- Injection-site edema (9%)
- Injection-site erythema (9%)
- Injection-site pain (9%)
- Injection-site phlebitis (2%)
- Injection-site thrombosis (2%)
- Myalgia (7%)

CLARITHROMYCIN

Trade name: Biaxin (Abbott)
Other common trade names: Biaxin HP; Clacine; Clarith; Klacid; Macladin; Veclam
Category: Macrolide antibiotic
Clinically important, potentially serious interactions with: astemizole, benzodiazepines, carbamazepine, cisapride, cyclosporine, digoxin, ergot alkaloids, fluconazole, pimozide, terfenadine, theophylline

REACTIONS

SKIN
- Exanthems
- Fixed eruption
- Pruritus
- Psoriasis
- Pustular eruption
- Rash (sic) (3%)
- Stevens-Johnson syndrome
- Urticaria
- Vasculitis

OTHER
- Anaphylactoid reaction
- Black tongue
- Dysgeusia (3%)
- Glossitis
- Hypersensitivity
- Oral candidiasis
- Parosmia
- Pseudolymphoma
- Stomatitis

CLEMASTINE

Trade name: Tavist (Novartis)
Other common trade names: Aller-Eze; Clema; Darvine; Tavegil; Tavegyl
Category: H_1-receptor antihistamine
Clinically important, potentially serious interactions with: CNS depressants, MAO inhibitors, phenothiazines, tricyclic antidepressants

REACTIONS

SKIN
- Angioedema (<1%)
- Edema (<1%)
- Exanthems
- Flushing
- Hyperhidrosis
- Photosensitivity (<1%)
- Purpura
- Rash (sic) (<1%)
- Toxic pustuloderma
- Urticaria

OTHER
- Anaphylactoid reaction
- Myalgia (<1%)
- Paresthesias
- Xerostomia (1–10%)

CLIDINIUM

Trade name: Librax (Roche); Quarzan (Roche)
Other common trade names: Bralix; Diporax; Epirax; Libraxin; Librocol; Nirvaxal; Spasmoten
Category: Anticholinergic
Clinically important, potentially serious interactions with: anticholinergics, atenolol, digitalis

Librax is clidinium & chlordiazepoxide

REACTIONS

SKIN
- Hypohidrosis
- Urticaria

OTHER
- Ageusia
- Anaphylactoid reaction
- Dysgeusia
- Xerostomia

CLINDAMYCIN

Trade name: Cleocin (Pharmacia & Upjohn); Cleocin-T (Pharmacia & Upjohn)
Other common trade names: Aclinda; BB; Clindacin; Dalacin; Dalacin C; Dalacine; Sobelin
Category: Lincosamide antibiotic & antiprotozoal
Clinically important, potentially serious interactions with: antacids, erythromycin, saquinavir

REACTIONS

SKIN
- Allergic reactions (sic)
- Contact dermatitis
- Eczematous eruption (sic)
- Erythema multiforme (<1%)
- Exanthems
- Leukocytoclastic angiitis
- Pruritus (<1%)
- Pruritus ani
- Purpura
- Rash (sic) (1–10%)
- Rosacea
- Stevens-Johnson syndrome (<1%)
- Toxic epidermal necrolysis
- Urticaria (<1%)
- Vasculitis

OTHER
- Anaphylactoid reaction
- Dysgeusia
- Injection-site phlebitis
- Lip edema
- Lymphadenitis

CLOFAZIMINE

Trade name: Lamprene (Novartis)
Other common trade names: Clofozine; Hansepran; Lampren; Lapren
Category: Antileprotic
Clinically important, potentially serious interactions with: none

REACTIONS

SKIN
- Acne (<1%)
- Acute febrile neutrophilic dermatosis (Sweet's syndrome)
- Ankle edema (<1%)
- Cheilitis (candidal) (<1%)
- Discoloration (sic)
- Erythroderma (<1%)
- Exanthems
- Exfoliative dermatitis
- Ichthyosis (8–28%)
- Pedal edema
- Photosensitivity (<1%)
- Pigmentation (pink to brownish-black) (75–100%)
- Pruritus (1–5%)
- Rash (sic) (1–5%)
- Urticaria
- Vitiligo
- Xerosis (8–28%)

NAILS
- Nails – discoloration
- Nails – onycholysis
- Nails – subungual hyperkeratosis

OTHER
- Chromhidrosis (red sweat) (1–10%)
- Dysgeusia (<1%)

CLOFIBRATE

Trade name: Atromid-S (Ayerst)
Other common trade names: Claripex; Col; Lipavlon; Novofibrate; Regelan N; Skleromexe
Category: Antihyperlipidemic
Clinically important, potentially serious interactions with: furosemide, insulin, probenecid, sulfonylureas, warfarin

REACTIONS

SKIN
- Dermatitis (sic)
- Erythema multiforme
- Exanthems
- Exfoliative dermatitis
- Facial dermatitis
- Hyperhidrosis
- Lupus erythematosus
- Photosensitivity
- Pruritus (<1%)
- Purpura
- Rash (sic) (<1%)
- Sarcoidosis
- Stevens-Johnson syndrome
- Toxic epidermal necrolysis
- Urticaria (<1%)
- Vesiculobullous eruption
- Xerosis

HAIR
- Hair – alopecia (<1%)
- Hair – dry (<1%)

OTHER
- Dysgeusia
- Gynecomastia
- Hypogeusia
- Myalgia
- Myopathy (<1%)
- Oral ulceration
- Stomatitis

CLOMIPHENE

Trade names: Clomid (Hoechst Marion Roussel); Serophene (Serono)
Other common trade names: Clom 50; Clomifen; Dyneric; Omifin; Pergotime; Phenate
Category: Infertility therapy adjunct; ovulation stimulator
Clinically important, potentially serious interactions with: no data

REACTIONS

SKIN
- Acne
- Allergic reactions (sic)
- Dermatitis (<1%)
- Edema
- Erythema
- Erythema multiforme
- Erythema nodosum
- Exanthems
- Flushing (10%)
- Hyperhidrosis
- Melanoma
- Pruritus
- Purpura (palpable)
- Rash (<1%)
- Urticaria

HAIR
- Hair – alopecia (<1%)
- Hair – hypertrichosis

OTHER
- Gynecomastia (1–10%)
- Myalgia

CLOMIPRAMINE

Trade name: Anafranil (Novartis)
Other common trade names: Anafranil Retard; Clofranil; Clopress; Placil
Category: Tricyclic antidepressant
Clinically important, potentially serious interactions with: CNS depressants, clonidine, epinephrine, guanethidine, MAO inhibitors, tricyclic antidepressants

REACTIONS

SKIN
- Acne (2%)
- Allergic reactions (sic) (<3%)
- Cellulitis (2%)
- Chloasma
- Contact dermatitis
- Dermatitis (sic) (2%)
- Edema (2%)
- Exanthems
- Flushing (8%)
- Folliculitis
- Hyperhidrosis (29%)
- Photosensitivity (<1%)
- Pigmentation (pseudocyanotic)
- Pruritus (6%)
- Psoriasis
- Purpura (3%)
- Pustular eruption
- Rash (sic) (8%)
- Seborrhea (rare)
- Urticaria (1%)
- Vasculitis
- Xerosis (2%)

HAIR
- Hair – alopecia (<1%)
- Hair – alopecia areata
- Hair – hypertrichosis

OTHER
- Ageusia
- Black tongue
- Cheilitis
- Dysgeusia (8%)
- Galactorrhea (<1%)
- Gingival bleeding
- Gingivitis
- Glossitis
- Gynecomastia (2%)
- Mastodynia (1%)
- Myalgia (13%)
- Paresthesias
- Sialorrhea
- Stomatitis
- Tongue ulceration
- Vaginitis (2%)
- Xerostomia (84%)

CLONAZEPAM

Trade name: Klonopin (Roche)
Other common trade names: Clonex; Iktorivil; Landsen; Lonazep; Rivortil
Category: Benzodiazepine anticonvulsant & antipanic
Clinically important, potentially serious interactions with: CNS depressants, clarithromycin, diltiazem, verapamil

REACTIONS

SKIN
- Angioedema
- Ankle edema
- Dermatitis (sic) (1–10%)
- Exanthems
- Facial edema
- Hyperhidrosis (>10%)
- Hypermelanosis
- Pruritus
- Pseudo-mycosis fungoides
- Purpura
- Rash (sic) (>10%)
- Urticaria

HAIR
- Hair – alopecia
- Hair – hirsutism

OTHER
- Gingivitis
- Oral mucosal eruption
- Oral ulceration
- Paresthesias
- Pseudolymphoma

Sialopenia (>10%)
Sialorrhea (1–10%)
Xerostomia (>10%)

CLONIDINE

Trade names: Catapres (Boehringer Ingelheim); Combipres (Boehringer Ingelheim)
Other common trade names: Barclyd; Catapres; Catapresan; Daipres; Haemiton; Sulmidine
Category: Alpha$_2$-adrenergic agonist antihypertensive
Clinically important, potentially serious interactions with: beta-adrenergic blocking agents, tricyclic antidepressants, verapamil

Combipres is clonidine & chlorthalidone

REACTIONS

SKIN
- Angioedema (<1%)
- Contact dermatitis (20%)
- Depigmentation
- Eczematous eruption (sic)
- Edema
- Erythema
- Exanthems
- Herpes simplex
- Hyperhidrosis
- Hyperpigmentation (to the patch)
- Lupus erythematosus
- Pemphigoid (anogenital & cicatricial)
- Pityriasis rosea
- Pruritus (>5%)
- Psoriasis
- Rash (sic) (1–10%)
- Raynaud's phenomenon (<1%)
- Urticaria (<1%)

HAIR
- Hair – alopecia (<1%)

OTHER
- Acute intermittent porphyria
- Dysgeusia (to the patch)
- Gynecomastia (<1%)
- Immune complex disease
- Vesiculation at site of application
- Xerostomia (40%)

CLOPIDOGREL

Trade name: Plavix (Bristol-Myers Squibb)
Category: Antiplatelet
Clinically important, potentially serious interactions with: anticoagulants, fluvastatin, heparin, naproxen, NSAIDs, phenytoin, tamoxifen, tolbutamide, torsemide, warfarin

REACTIONS

SKIN
- Allergic reaction (sic) (1–2.5%)
- Bullous eruption (1–2.5%)
- Eczema (1–2.5%)
- Edema
- Exanthems (1–2.5%)
- Pruritus (3.3%)
- Purpura (5.3%)
- Rash (sic) (4.2%)
- Ulceration (1–2.5%)
- Urticaria (1–2.5%)

OTHER
- Hypesthesia (1–2.5%)
- Paresthesias (1–2.5%)

CLORAZEPATE

Trade name: Tranxene (Abbott)
Other common trade names: Novoclopate; Transene; Tranxal; Tranxen; Tranxilen; Tranxilium
Category: Benzodiazepine anxiolytic & sedative-hypnotic; anticonvulsant
Clinically important, potentially serious interactions with: alcohol, cimetidine, clarithromycin, CNS depressants, diltiazem, fluconazole, itraconazole, ketoconazole, miconazole, verapamil

REACTIONS

SKIN
- Blistering (sic)
- Dermatitis (sic) (1–10%)
- Exanthems
- Hyperhidrosis (>10%)
- Photosensitivity
- Pruritus
- Purpura
- Rash (sic) (>10%)
- Urticaria
- Vasculitis

NAILS
- Nails – photo-onycholysis

OTHER
- Oral ulceration
- Paresthesias
- Sialopenia (>10%)
- Sialorrhea (1–10%)
- Xerostomia (>10%)

CLOXACILLIN

Trade names: Cloxapen (SmithKline Beecham); Tegopen (Mead Johnson)
Other common trade names: Alclox; Apo-Cloxi; Ekvacillin; Loxavit; Orbenin; Orbenine
Category: Penicillinase-resistant penicillin antibiotic
Clinically important, potentially serious interactions with: anticoagulants, cyclosporine, disulfiram, heparin, probenecid

REACTIONS

SKIN
- Angioedema
- Contact dermatitis
- Ecchymoses
- Erythema multiforme
- Exanthems
- Exfoliative dermatitis
- Hematomas
- Jarisch-Herxheimer reaction
- Pruritus
- Rash (sic) (<1%)
- Stevens-Johnson syndrome
- Urticaria

NAILS
- Nails – onycholysis (rare)
- Nails – shedding

OTHER
- Anaphylactoid reaction
- Black tongue
- Glossitis
- Glossodynia
- Injection-site pain
- Oral candidiasis
- Serum sickness (<1%)
- Stomatitis
- Vaginitis

CLOZAPINE

Trade name: Clozaril (Novartis)
Other common trade names: Entumin; Entumine; Leponex; Lozapin; Sizopin
Category: Tricyclic antipsychotic
Clinically important, potentially serious interactions with: cimetidine, MAO inhibitors, neuroleptics, phenytoin, ritonavir, tricyclic antidepressants

REACTIONS

SKIN
- Dermatitis (sic) (<1%)
- Eczematous eruption (sic) (<1%)
- Edema (<1%)
- Erythema (<1%)
- Erythema multiforme (<1%)
- Exanthems
- Facial erosions
- Hyperhidrosis (6%)
- Lupus erythematosus
- Periorbital edema (<1%)
- Petechiae (<1%)
- Photosensitivity
- Pruritus (<1%)
- Purpura (<1%)
- Rash (sic) (2%)
- Stevens-Johnson syndrome (<1%)
- Urticaria (<1%)
- Vasculitis (<1%)

OTHER
- Dysgeusia (<1%)
- Glossodynia (1%)
- Mastodynia (<1%)
- Priapism
- Sialorrhea
- Xerostomia (6%)

COCAINE

Trade name: Cocaine
Category: Topical anesthetic; substance abuse drug
Clinically important, potentially serious interactions with: beta-blockers, MAO inhibitors

REACTIONS

SKIN
- Bullous eruption
- Cutaneous nodules
- Granulomas (foreign body)
- Hyperkeratosis (fingers & palms)
- Necrosis
- Scleroderma (reversible)
- Thrombophlebitis
- Warts (snorters' warts)

OTHER
- Ageusia (>10%)
- Anosmia (>10%)
- Injection-site scarring
- Nasal septal perforation
- Porphyria

CODEINE

Trade names: Calcidrine; Cheracol; Guaituss AC; Halotussin; Novahistine DH; Nucofed; Robitussin AC; Tussar-2; Tussi-Organidin; & those preparations that include "with Codeine". (Various pharmaceutical companies.)
Other common trade names: Actacode; Codicept; Codiforton; Paveral; Solcodein; Tricodein
Category: Opioid (narcotic) analgesic
Clinically important, potentially serious interactions with: alcohol, barbiturates, cimetidine, CNS depressants, guanabenz, MAO inhibitors, phenothiazines, ranitidine, tricyclic antidepressants

REACTIONS

SKIN
- Acute generalized exanthematous pustulosis (AGEP)
- Angioedema
- Bullous eruption
- Contact dermatitis
- Erythema multiforme (<1%)
- Erythema nodosum (<1%)
- Exanthems
- Exfoliative dermatitis
- Facial edema
- Fixed eruption (<1%)
- Flushing
- Hyperhidrosis
- Pityriasis rosea
- Pruritus (<1%)
- Radiation recall (sunlight & electronic beam)
- Rash (sic) (1–10%)
- Toxic epidermal necrolysis (<1%)
- Urticaria (1–10%)

NAILS
- Nails – shoreline

OTHER
- Anaphylactoid reaction
- Dysgeusia
- Injection-site pain (1–10%)
- Oral ulceration
- Paresthesias
- Xerostomia (1–10%)

COLCHICINE

Trade name: Colbenemid (Merck)
Other common trade names: Colchineos; Colgout; Goutnil; Konicine; Kolkicin
Category: Uricosuric, antigout anti-inflammatory
Clinically important, potentially serious interactions with: CNS depressants, cyclosporine, erythromycin

Colbenemid is colchicine & probenecid

REACTIONS

SKIN
- Bullous eruption (<1%)
- Cutaneous side effects (sic) (14%)
- Erythroderma
- Exanthems
- Fixed eruption
- Flushing
- Lichenoid eruption
- Photocontact dermatitis
- Pruritus (<1%)
- Purpura
- Pyoderma
- Rash (sic) (<1%)
- Staphylococcal scalded skin syndrome
- Toxic epidermal necrolysis
- Urticaria
- Vasculitis
- Vesicular eruption (palms)

HAIR
- Hair – alopecia (1–10%)

OTHER
- Anaphylactoid reaction
- Injection-site thrombophlebitis
- Myopathy (<1%)
- Porphyria cutanea tarda (very rare)

COLESTIPOL

Trade name: Colestid (Pharmacia & Upjohn)
Other common trade names: Cholestabyl; Lestid
Category: Antilipidemic
Clinically important, potentially serious interactions with: acetaminophen, anticoagulants, diclofenac, digitalis, furosemide, lovastatin, pravastatin, simvastatin

REACTIONS

SKIN
- Dermatitis (sic) (<1%)
- Exanthems (<1%)
- Urticaria (<1%)

CORTICOSTEROIDS

Generic names:

Betamethasone
Trade name: Celestone
Cortisone
Trade name: Cortone
Dexamethasone
Trade names: Decadron; Dexameth; Hexadrol
Hydrocortisone
Trade names: Cortef; Solu-Cortef
Methylprednisolone
Trade names: Medrol; Depo-Medrol; Solu-Medrol
Prednisolone
Trade names: Delta-Cortef; Hydeltrasol
Prednisone
Trade names: Deltasone; Meticorten; Orasone
Triamcinolone:
Trade names: Aristocort; Aristospan; Kenalog

Category: Anti-inflammatory

REACTIONS

SKIN
- Acanthosis nigricans
- Acne
- Angioedema
- Atrophy
- Bacterial infection
- Calcification
- Contact dermatitis
- Depigmentation
- Dermal thinning
- Dermatofibromas
- Ecchymoses
- Eczematous eruption (sic)
- Erythema
- Exanthems
- Facial edema
- Fungal infection
- Herpes simplex
- Herpes zoster
- Hyperpigmentation
- Kaposi's sarcoma
- Leucoderma acquisitum
- Linear atrophy
- Linear hypopigmentation
- Lupus erythematosus
- Mycotic infection
- Necrosis
- Perioral dermatitis
- Pigmentation (sic)
- Pityriasis rosea
- Porokeratosis
- Pruritus
- Pseudoxanthoma elasticum
- Purpura
- Pustular psoriasis
- Redness of the face
- Striae
- Telangiectases
- Urticaria
- Vasculitis
- Viral infection

HAIR
- Hair – hirsutism
- Hair – hypertrichosis

OTHER
- Anaphylactoid reaction

Black hairy tongue
Buffalo hump
Impaired wound healing
Injection-site aseptic necrosis
Injection-site lipoatrophy
Moon face
Myopathy
Panniculitis

CORTISONE

Trade name: Cortone (Merck)
Other common trade names: Adreson; Cortate; Cortelan; Cortisone; Cortistab; Scheroson
Category: Short-acting glucocorticoid; anti-inflammatory
Clinically important, potentially serious interactions with: anticoagulants, diuretics, estrogens, NSAIDs, phenytoin, rifabutin, rifampin, salicylates

REACTIONS

SKIN
Acanthosis nigricans
Acne (<1%)
Angioedema
Atrophy (<1%)
Depigmentation (localized)
Ecchymoses
Erythema
Exanthems
Fixed eruption (<1%)
Hyperhidrosis
Hyperpigmentation (<1%)
Kaposi's sarcoma
Lupus erythematosus
Mycotic infection
Pityriasis rosea
Porokeratosis
Pseudoxanthoma elasticum
Purpura (<1%)
Striae
Urticaria
Vasculitis
Viral infection

HAIR
Hair – hypertrichosis (1–10%)

OTHER
Anaphylactoid reaction
Black hairy tongue
Hypersensitivity (<1%)
Impaired wound healing
Injection-site lipoatrophy
Myopathy
Pseudotumor cerebri (<1%)

COTRIMOXAZOLE

Trade names: Bactrim (Roche); Cotrim (Teva); Septra (Glaxo Wellcome)
Category: Antibacterial & antiprotozoal
Clinically important, potentially serious interactions with: anticoagulants, cyclosporine, hypoglycemics, MAO inhibitors, methotrexate, phenytoin, sulfones

Cotrimoxazole is sulfamethoxazole & trimethoprim

REACTIONS

SKIN
Acute febrile neutrophilic dermatosis (Sweet's syndrome)
Acute generalized exanthematous pustulosis (AGEP)
Angioedema
Aphthous stomatitis
Bullous eruption
Cutaneous side effects (sic)
Dermatitis (sic)
Erythema multiforme
Erythema nodosum
Erythroderma
Exanthems
Exfoliative dermatitis
Fixed eruption
Flushing
Lichenoid eruption
Lupus erythematosus
Mucocutaneous syndrome
Photosensitivity
Pruritus

Pruritus vulvae
Psoriasis
Purpura
Pustular eruption
Radiation recall
Rash (sic)
Stevens-Johnson syndrome
Toxic epidermal necrolysis
Urticaria
Vasculitis
Vulvovaginitis

OTHER
Anaphylactoid reaction
Black hairy tongue
Dysgeusia
Gingival hyperplasia
Glossitis
Hypersensitivity
Myalgia
Oral mucosal eruption
Oral ulceration
Pseudolymphoma
Serum sickness
Stomatitis
Tongue ulceration

CROMOLYN (SODIUM CROMOGLYCATE)

Trade names: Gastrocrom (Fisons); Nasalcrom (Fisons); Intal (Fisons)
Other common trade names: Colimune; Cromoptic; Fivent; Nalcrom; Opticron; Rynacrom
Category: Mast cell stabilizer
Clinically important, potentially serious interactions with: none

REACTIONS

SKIN
Angioedema (1–10%)
Contact dermatitis
Dermatitis (sic) (generalized)
Eczematous eruption (sic)
Edema
Erythema
Exanthems
Exfoliative dermatitis
Facial dermatitis (sic)
Flushing
Photosensitivity
Pruritus
Rash (sic) (<1%)
Rosacea
Urticaria (<1%)
Vasculitis

OTHER
Anaphylactoid reaction (<1%)
Anosmia
Dysgeusia (>10%)
Hypersensitivity
Myalgia
Myopathy
Paresthesias
Serum sickness
Xerostomia (1–10%)

CYANOCOBALAMIN

Trade names: Cyanoject (Mayrand); Cyomin (Forest); Nascobal (Schwarz); Rubramin (Bristol-Myers Squibb); Vitamin B_{12}
Other common trade names: Ancobin; Betolvex; Cytamen; Dobetin; Lifaton B12; Vicapan N
Category: Water-soluble nutritional supplement & antianemic
Clinically important, potentially serious interactions with: chloramphenicol, omeprazole

REACTIONS

SKIN
Acne
Allergic reactions (sic)
Angioedema
Bullous eruption (<1%)
Cheilitis
Contact dermatitis
Eczematous eruption (sic)
Exanthems
Folliculitis
Pruritus (1–10%)
Systemic eczematous contact dermatitis
Urticaria (<1%)

OTHER
- Anaphylactoid reaction (<1%)
- Aseptic necrosis following injection
- Embolia cutis medicamentosa (Nicolau syndrome)
- Hypersensitivity
- Injection-site pain
- Porphyria cutanea tarda

CYCLAMATE

Trade name: Sucaryl
Category: Sulfonamide sweetener
Clinically important, potentially serious interactions with: none

Cyclamates cross-react with sulfonamides

REACTIONS

SKIN
- Angioedema
- Bullous eruption
- Exanthems
- Photosensitivity
- Pruritus
- Urticaria

OTHER
- Paresthesias

CYCLOBENZAPRINE

Trade name: Flexeril (Merck)
Other common trade names: Benzamin; Cloben; Cyben; Flexiban; Yurelax
Category: Skeletal muscle relaxant
Clinically important, potentially serious interactions with: anticholinergics, clonidine, epinephrine, guanethidine, MAO inhibitors

REACTIONS

SKIN
- Allergic reactions (sic)
- Angioedema (<1%)
- Facial edema (<1%)
- Flushing
- Hyperhidrosis
- Photosensitivity
- Pruritus (<1%)
- Purpura
- Rash (sic) (<1%)
- Urticaria (<1%)

HAIR
- Hair – alopecia

OTHER
- Ageusia (<1%)
- Anaphylactoid reaction (<1%)
- Dysgeusia (3%)
- Galactorrhea
- Gynecomastia
- Paresthesias (<1%)
- Stomatitis
- Tongue pigmentation
- Tongue edema (<1%)
- Xerostomia (27%)

CYCLOPHOSPHAMIDE

Trade names: Cytoxan (Mead Johnson); Neosar (Pharmacia & Upjohn)
Other common trade names: Cycloblastin; Cyclostin; Endoxan; Endoxana; Procytox;
Category: Antineoplastic & immunosuppressant
Clinically important, potentially serious interactions with: allopurinol, azathioprine, chloramphenicol, cimetidine, digitalis, doxorubicin, phenobarbital, phenytoin, quinolones, thiazides

REACTIONS

SKIN
- Acral erythema
- Angioedema
- Condylomata acuminata
- Contact dermatitis
- Dermatitis herpetiformis
- Dermatofibromas
- Eccrine squamous syringometaplasia
- Erythema multiforme (<1%)
- Erythrodysesthesia syndrome
- Exanthems
- Facial burning
- Flushing (1–10%)
- Hyperhidrosis
- Keratoacanthoma
- Lymphoma
- Myxedema
- Palmar-plantar erythema
- Pigmentation (<1%)
- Polyarteritis nodosa
- Pruritus
- Purpura
- Rash (sic) (1–10%)
- Squamous cell carcinoma
- Stevens-Johnson syndrome
- Toxic epidermal necrolysis (<1%)
- Ultraviolet light recall
- Urticaria
- Vasculitis

HAIR
- Hair – alopecia (universal and severe in one-third)

NAILS
- Nails – Beau's lines (transverse ridging)
- Nails – dystrophy
- Nails – onychodermal band
- Nails – pigmentation (<1%)
- Nails – transverse leukonychia (Muehrcke's lines)

OTHER
- Acute intermittent porphyria
- Anaphylactoid reaction
- Gingival pigmentation
- Hypersensitivity
- Injection-site pain
- Oral mucosal ulceration
- Porphyria cutanea tarda
- Scalp burning
- Stomatitis (1–10%)
- Tooth discoloration

CYCLOSERINE

Trade name: Seromycin (Dura)
Other common trade names: Closerina; Closerin; Cyclomycin; Cyclorine; Cycosin
Category: Tuberculostatic
Clinically important, potentially serious interactions with: alcohol, ethionamide, isoniazid

REACTIONS

SKIN
- Allergic reactions (sic)
- Dermatitis (sic)
- Exanthems
- Lichenoid eruption
- Pruritus
- Rash (sic) (<1%)
- Stevens-Johnson syndrome
- Urticaria

OTHER
- Oral mucosal lesions
- Paresthesias

CYCLOSPORINE

Trade names: Neoral (Novartis); Sandimmune (Novartis)
Other common trade names: Ciclosporin; Consupren; Implanta; Sandimmun
Category: Immunosuppressant
Clinically important, potentially serious interactions with: androgens, clarithromycin, danazol, doxorubicin, erythromycin, etoposide, fluconazole, foscarnet, itraconazole, ketoconazole, lovastatin, penicillamine, penicillins, pravastatin, rifampin, simvastatin

REACTIONS

SKIN
- Acne (6%)
- Angioedema
- Ankle edema
- Aphthous stomatitis
- Basal cell carcinoma
- Bullous eruption (1%)
- Buschke-Lowenstein penile carcinoma
- Cutaneous neoplasms (sic)
- Eccrine squamous syringometaplasia
- Edema
- Epidermal cysts
- Exanthems
- Facial edema
- Flushing (>3%)
- Folliculitis
- Herpes simplex
- Herpes zoster
- Hidradenitis
- Hyperpigmentation
- Hyperkeratosis
- Hypohidrosis
- Ichthyosis
- Kaposi's sarcoma
- Keratoses
- Keratosis pilaris
- Lichenoid eruption
- Lupus erythematosus
- Lymphocytic infiltration
- Lymphoma
- Melanoma
- Mycosis fungoides
- Nodular cutaneous T-lymphocyte infiltrate
- Papillomas (facial)
- Papulovesicular lesions (sic)
- Poikiloderma
- Porokeratosis (superficial actinic)
- Pruritus (<2%)
- Pseudofolliculitis barbae
- Psoriasis
- Purpura (3%)
- Pustular psoriasis
- Rash (sic) (10%)
- Raynaud's phenomenon
- Sebaceous hyperplasia
- Squamous cell carcinoma
- Striae
- Toxic epidermal necrolysis
- Ulceration (1%)
- Urticaria
- Vasculitis
- Vitiligo

HAIR
- Hair – alopecia (3%)
- Hair – alopecia areata
- Hair – breakage
- Hair – growth
- Hair – hypertrichosis (19%)

NAILS
- Nails – abnormal growth
- Nails – brittle (<2%)
- Nails – disorder (sic)
- Nails – ingrown
- Nails – leukonychia
- Nails – periungual granulation tissue

OTHER
- Acromegaloid features
- Anaphylactoid reaction (<1%)
- Breast lumps (sic)
- Dysesthesia
- Gingival hyperplasia (>10%)
- Gingivitis (4%)
- Glossitis (atrophic)
- Gynecomastia (>3%)
- Hyperesthesia
- Lingual fungiform papillae hypertrophy (sic)
- Lymphoproliferative disease
- Myalgia
- Myopathy
- Oral ulceration
- Paresthesias (>8%)
- Pseudolymphoma
- Stomatitis (7%)

CYCLOTHIAZIDE

Trade name: Anhydron (Lilly)
Other common trade names: Doburil; Valmiran
Category: Thiazide diuretic
Clinically important, potentially serious interactions with: antidiabetics, bumetanide, cyclophosphamide, digitalis, lithium, methotrexate

REACTIONS

SKIN
- Exanthems (<1%)
- Photosensitivity
- Purpura
- Rash (sic)
- Urticaria
- Vasculitis

OTHER
- Paresthesias

CYPROHEPTADINE

Trade name: Periactin (Merck)
Other common trade names: Ciplactin; Ciproral; Nuran; Periactine, Periactinol, Peritol
Category: H_1-receptor antihistamine & appetite stimulant
Clinically important, potentially serious interactions with: fluoxetine, MAO inhibitors, phenelzine

REACTIONS

SKIN
- Allergic reactions (sic) (<1%)
- Angioedema (<1%)
- Contact dermatitis
- Dermatitis (sic)
- Edema (<1%)
- Erythema
- Exanthems
- Flushing
- Hyperhidrosis
- Lichenoid eruption
- Lupus erythematosus
- Peripheral edema
- Photosensitivity
- Purpura
- Rash (sic)
- Urticaria
- Vasculitis

OTHER
- Anaphylactoid reaction
- Dysgeusia
- Myalgia (<1%)
- Paresthesias (<1%)
- Xerostomia (1–10%)

CYTARABINE

Trade names: Cytosar-U (Pharmacia & Upjohn); Tarabine (Pharmacia & Upjohn)
Other common trade names: Alexan; Arabitin; Arace; Aracytine; Cytarbel; Cytosar; Uducil
Category: Antineoplastic
Clinically important, potentially serious interactions with: digitalis, methotrexate, quinolones

REACTIONS

SKIN
- Acral erythema
- Acral erythrodysesthesia syndrome
- Actinic keratoses
- Acute febrile neutrophilic dermatosis (Sweet's syndrome)
- Allergic edema (sic)
- Bullous eruption
- Desquamation
- Erythema
- Erythema & swelling of ears
- Erythroderma (generalized)
- Exanthems
- Exfoliative dermatitis

Freckles (1–10%)
Herpes zoster
Neutrophilic eccrine hidradenitis
Pruritus (1–10%)
Rash (sic) (>10%)
Seborrheic keratoses (Leser-Trélat syndrome) (in patients with acute leukemia)
Syringosquamous metaplasia (sic)
Toxic epidermal necrolysis
Ulceration
Urticaria
Vasculitis*

HAIR
Hair – alopecia (1–10%)

NAILS
Nails – Mees' lines
Nails – transverse leukonychia

OTHER
Anal ulceration (>10%)
Anaphylactoid reaction
Hypersensitivity
Injection-site cellulitis (1–10%)
Myalgia (1–10%)
Oral mucosal lesions
Oral ulceration (>10%)
Stomatitis

*Vasculitis, a part of the cytarabine syndrome, consists of fever, malaise, myalgia, conjunctivitis, arthralgia and a diffuse erythematous maculopapular eruption that occurs from 6 to 12 hours following the administration of the drug.

DACARBAZINE

Trade name: DTIC (Dome)
Other common trade names: Dacatic; D.T.I.C.; Deticene; Detimedac
Category: Antineoplastic
Clinically important, potentially serious interactions with: aldesleukin

REACTIONS

SKIN
Angioedema
Erythema
Exanthems
Fixed eruption
Flushing (1–10%)
Photosensitivity (<1%)
Rash (sic) (1–10%)
Urticaria

HAIR
Hair – alopecia (<1%)

NAILS
Nails – pigmentation

OTHER
Anaphylactoid reaction (1–10%)
Dysgeusia (metallic taste) (1–10%)
Hypersensitivity
Injection-site burning (>10%)
Injection-site cellulitis
Injection-site dermatitis
Injection-site necrosis (>10%)
Injection-site pain (>10%)
Injection-site phlebitis
Myalgia (1–10%)
Paresthesias (facial)
Stomatitis (<1%)

DACTINOMYCIN (ACTINOMYCIN-D)

Trade name: Cosmegen (Merck)
Other common trade names: Ac-De; Cosmegen Lyovac; Lyovac
Category: Antineoplastic antibiotic
Clinically important, potentially serious interactions with: aldesleukin

REACTIONS

SKIN
- Acne (>10%)
- Bullous pemphigoid
- Cellulitis
- Cheilitis
- Dermatitis (sic)
- Erythema
- Erythema, brawny localized
- Erythema multiforme
- Exanthems
- Folliculitis
- Keratoses (reactivation of)
- Pigmentation
- Pruritus
- Pustular eruption
- Radiation recall (>10%)
- Toxic epidermal necrolysis
- Urticaria

HAIR
- Hair – alopecia (>10%)

OTHER
- Anaphylactoid reaction (<1%)
- Injection-site extravasation
- Injection-site necrosis (>10%)
- Injection-site phlebitis (>10%)
- Myalgia
- Oral mucosal lesions
- Phlebitis
- Stomatitis (ulcerative) (>5%)

DALTEPARIN

Trade name: Fragmin (Pharmacia & Upjohn)
Other common trade name: Fragmine
Category: Anticoagulant
Clinically important, potentially serious interactions with: anticoagulants, aspirin, ketorolac

REACTIONS

SKIN
- Allergic reactions (sic) (1–10%)
- Bullous eruption (1–10%)
- Exanthems (<1%)
- Pruritus (1–10%)
- Rash (sic) (1–10%)

OTHER
- Anaphylactoid reaction (1–10%)
- Injection-site hematoma (1–10%)
- Injection-site pain (1–10%)
- Necrosis

DANAZOL

Trade name: Danocrine (Sanofi-Winthrop)
Other common trade names: Azol; Bonzol; Cyclomen; D-Zol; Danol; Winobanin
Category: Synthetic pituitary gonadotropin inhibitor
Clinically important, potentially serious interactions with: anticoagulants, carbamazepine, cyclosporine, lovastatin, oral contraceptives, retinoids

REACTIONS

SKIN
- Acne (>10%)
- Angioedema
- Edema (>10%)
- Erythema multiforme
- Exanthems
- Flushing
- Guillain-Barré syndrome

Hyperhidrosis (3%)
Lupus erythematosus
Lymphomatoid papulosis
Petechiae
Photosensitivity (<1%)
Pruritus
Purpura
Rash (sic) (3%)
Seborrhea
Stevens-Johnson syndrome
Urticaria

HAIR
Hair – alopecia
Hair – hirsutism (>10%)

OTHER
Acute intermittent porphyria
Bleeding gums
Breast changes (sic)
Paresthesias
Vaginal dryness (sic)
Vaginitis (<1%)

DANTROLENE

Trade name: Dantrium (Procter-Gamble)
Other common trade names: Dantamacrin; Dantrolen
Category: Muscle relaxant
Clinically important, potentially serious interactions with: CNS depressants, clindamycin, clofibrate, estrogens, MAO inhibitors, phenothiazines, tolbutamide, verapamil, warfarin

REACTIONS

SKIN
Acne
Dermatitis (sic)
Exanthems
Hyperhidrosis
Pruritus
Rash (sic) (>10%)
Urticaria

HAIR
Hair – abnormal growth

OTHER
Anaphylactoid reaction
Dysgeusia
Malignant lymphoma
Myalgia
Parageusia

DAPSONE

Trade name: Dapsone (Jacobus)
Other common trade names: Avlosulfon; Dapson; Dapson-Fatol; Protogen; Sulfona
Category: Antileprotic & dermatitis herpetiformis suppressant
Clinically important, potentially serious interactions with: didanosine, folic acid antagonists, rifampin, saquinavir, trimethoprim

Note: A hypersensitivity reaction – termed the "sulfone syndrome" or "dapsone syndrome" – may infrequently develop during the first six weeks of treatment. This syndrome consists of exfoliative dermatitis, fever, malaise, nausea, anorexia, hepatitis, jaundice, lymphadenopathy and hemolytic anemia.

REACTIONS

SKIN
Bullous eruption (<1%)
Cyanosis
Dapsone syndrome
Epidermolysis bullosa
Erythema multiforme (<1%)
Erythema nodosum
Erythroderma
Exanthems (1–5%)
Exfoliative dermatitis (<1%)
Fixed eruption
Lichenoid eruption
Lupus erythematosus
Photosensitivity
Pigmentation
Pruritus
Purpura
Rash (sic)
Scleroderma
Stevens-Johnson syndrome

Subcorneal pustular dermatosis
Toxic epidermal necrolysis (<1%)
Toxic erythema (sic)
Urticaria

NAILS
Nails – Beau's lines

OTHER
Acute intermittent porphyria
Hypersensitivity
Nodular panniculitis
Oral mucosal eruption
Oral mucosal fixed eruption
Oral mucosal pigmentation
Porphyria cutanea tarda

DAUNORUBICIN

Trade names: Cerubidine (Bedford); Daunoxome (Nexstar)
Other common trade name: Daunoxome
Category: Antineoplastic
Clinically important, potentially serious interactions with: aldesleukin, quinolones

REACTIONS

SKIN
Angioedema
Contact dermatitis
Exanthems
Folliculitis
Hypopigmentation
Neutrophilic eccrine hidradenitis
Pigmentation
Rash (sic) (<1%)
Urticaria (<1%)

HAIR
Hair – alopecia (>10%)

NAILS
Nails – pigmentation (<1%)

OTHER
Anaphylactoid reaction
Injection-site cellulitis
Injection-site necrosis (1–10%)
Injection-site phlebitis
Injection-site ulceration (1–10%)
Oral mucosal lesions
Stomatitis (>10%)

DEFEROXAMINE

Trade name: Desferal (Novartis)
Other common trade name: Desferin
Category: Chelating agent; antidote
Clinically important, potentially serious interactions with: no data

REACTIONS

SKIN
Acne
Angioedema
Dermatitis (sic)
Erythema (<1%)
Erythema multiforme
Exanthems
Flushing (<1%)
Pigmentation
Pruritus (<1%)
Purpura
Rash (sic) (<1%)
Toxic epidermal necrolysis
Urticaria (<1%)

OTHER
Anaphylactoid reaction (<1%)
Injection-site erythema
Injection-site inflammation (1–10%)
Injection-site pain (1–10%)
Oral mucosal lesions

DELAVIRDINE

Trade name: Rescriptor (Pharmacia & Upjohn)
Category: Reverse transcriptase inhibitor
Clinically important, potentially serious interactions with: amphetamines, antiarrhythmics, anticoagulants, astemizole, calcium channel blockers, carbamazepine, cimetidine, cisapride, ergot, famotidine, phenytoin, quinidine, rifabutin, rifampin, terfenadine

REACTIONS

SKIN
- Allergic reaction (sic) (<2%)
- Angioedema (<2%)
- Aphthous stomatitis (<2%)
- Dermatitis (sic) (<2%)
- Desquamation (<2%)
- Diaphoresis (<2%)
- Ecchymoses (<2%)
- Edema (<2%)
- Epidermal cyst (<2%)
- Erythema (<2%)
- Erythema multiforme (<2%)
- Exanthems (6.6%)
- Folliculitis (<2%)
- Fungal dermatitis (sic) (<2%)
- Lip edema (<2%)
- Nodule (sic) (<2%)
- Peripheral edema (<2%)
- Petechiae (<2%)
- Pruritus (<2%)
- Purpura (<2%)
- Rash (sic) (9.8%)
- Seborrhea (<2%)
- Stevens-Johnson syndrome (<2%)
- Urticaria (<2%)
- Vasculitis (<2%)
- Vesiculobullous eruption (<2%)
- Xerosis (<2%)

HAIR
- Hair – alopecia (<2%)

NAILS
- Nails – disorder (sic) (<2%)

OTHER
- Dysgeusia (<2%)
- Gingivitis (<2%)
- Gynecomastia (<2%)
- Hypesthesia (<2%)
- Hyperesthesia (<2%)
- Myalgia (<2%)
- Oral ulceration (<2%)
- Paresthesias (<2%)
- Sialorrhea (<2%)
- Stomatitis (<2%)
- Tingling (<2%)
- Tongue edema (<2%)
- Vaginal candidiasis (<2%)
- Xerostomia (<2%)

DEMECLOCYCLINE

Trade name: Declomycin (Lederle)
Other common trade names: Ledermicina; Ledermycin; Rynabron
Category: Tetracycline antibiotic & antiprotozoal
Clinically important, potentially serious interactions with: antacids, calcium carbonate, digitalis, penicillins, warfarin

REACTIONS

SKIN
- Acne
- Angioedema
- Bullous eruption
- Exanthems
- Exfoliative dermatitis (<1%)
- Fixed eruption
- Lichenoid eruption
- Lupus erythematosus
- Perianal rash
- Photosensitivity (1–10%)
- Phototoxic reaction
- Pigmentation
- Pruritus (<1%)
- Pruritus ani
- Purpura
- Toxic epidermal necrolysis
- Urticaria

NAILS
- Nails – onycholysis
- Nails – photo-onycholysis
- Nails – pigmentation (<1%)

OTHER
- Anaphylactoid reaction (<1%)
- Glossitis
- Mucous membrane pigmentation
- Oral mucosal eruption
- Paresthesias (<1%)
- Porphyria
- Pseudotumor cerebri
- Tongue pigmentation
- Tooth discoloration

DESIPRAMINE

Trade name: Norpramin (Hoechst Marion Roussel)
Other common trade names: Deprexan; Nebril; Nortimil; Pertofran; Petylyl
Category: Tricyclic antidepressant & antipanic
Clinically important, potentially serious interactions with: alcohol, anticholinergics, cimetidine, clonidine, CNS depressants, diltiazem, epinephrine, guanethidine, MAO inhibitors, phenytoin, verapamil

Reactions

SKIN
- Acne
- Allergic reactions (sic) (<1%)
- Angioedema
- Ecchymoses
- Edema
- Exanthems
- Exfoliative dermatitis
- Flushing
- Hyperhidrosis (1–10%)
- Petechiae
- Photosensitivity (1.4%)
- Pigmentation (blue-gray) (photosensitive)
- Pruritus
- Purpura
- Rash (sic)
- Urticaria

HAIR
- Hair – alopecia (<1%)

OTHER
- Black tongue
- Bromhidrosis
- Dysgeusia (>10%)
- Galactorrhea (<1%)
- Gynecomastia (<1%)
- Mucous membrane desquamation
- Paresthesias
- Pseudolymphoma
- Stomatitis
- Xerostomia (>10%)

DESMOPRESSIN

Trade name: DDAVP (Rhône-Poulenc Rorer)
Other common trade names: Defirin; Desmospray; Minirin; Minurin; Octostim
Category: Antidiuretic; antihemophilic; antihemorrhagic
Clinically important, potentially serious interactions with: chlorpropamide

Reactions

SKIN
- Allergic reactions (sic)
- Flushing (1–10%)
- Hyperhidrosis
- Rash (sic)

OTHER
- Injection-site edema
- Injection-site erythema
- Injection-site pain

DEXFENFLURAMINE

Trade name: Redux (Wyeth)
Other common trade names: Adifax; Dipondal; Glypolix; Isomeride; Obesine; Siran
Category: Anorexiant
Clinically important, potentially serious interactions with: selective serotonin reuptake inhibitors (SSRI), MAO inhibitors

REACTIONS

SKIN
- Allergic reactions (sic) (<1%)
- Angioedema
- Bullous eruption
- Ecchymoses
- Eczema (sic) (<1%)
- Edema (<1%)
- Erythema multiforme
- Exanthems (sic) (<1%)
- Hyperhidrosis (>1%)
- Pityriasis rosea (<1%)
- Pruritus (>1%)
- Psoriasis (<1%)
- Purpura
- Rash (sic) (2.3%)
- Stevens-Johnson syndrome
- Urticaria (>1%)

HAIR
- Hair – alopecia (>1%)
- Hair – hirsutism (<1%)

OTHER
- Digital necrosis
- Dysgeusia (>1%)
- Gynecomastia
- Hyperesthesia (<1%)
- Hypesthesia
- Mastodynia (<1%)
- Myalgia (>1%)
- Myopathy (<1%)
- Oral mucosal lesions
- Oral ulceration (<1%)
- Paresthesias (>1%)
- Tongue disorder (sic)
- Xerostomia (12.5%)

DEXTROAMPHETAMINE

Trade name: Dexedrine (SmithKline Beecham)
Other common trade names: Dexamphetamine; Dexamphetamini
Category: Central nervous system stimulant
Clinically important, potentially serious interactions with: MAO inhibitors, meperidine, norepinephrine, phenobarbital, phenothiazines, phenytoin, propoxyphene, tricyclic antidepressants

REACTIONS

SKIN
- Hyperhidrosis (1–10%)
- Rash (sic) (<1%)
- Toxic epidermal necrolysis
- Urticaria (<1%)

OTHER
- Dysgeusia
- Xerostomia (1–10%)

DEXTROMETHORPHAN

Trade names: Benylin; Cheracol-D; Drixoral; Pertussin; Robitussin; Sucrets; Suppress; Vicks Formula 44; etc. (Various pharmaceutical companies.)
Category: Antitussive
Clinically important, potentially serious interactions with: fluoxetine, fluvoxamine, MAO inhibitors, paroxetine, sertraline

REACTIONS

SKIN
- Bullous eruption
- Fixed eruption

DIAZEPAM

Trade names: Diastat (Athena); Valium (Roche); Vazepam (Major)
Other common trade names: Assival; Dialar; Diapax; Diazemuls; Ducene; Novazam; Solis
Category: Benzodiazepine anxiolytic & sedative-hypnotic; anticonvulsant
Clinically important, potentially serious interactions with: alcohol, antituberculosis agents, cisapride, clarithromycin, CNS antidepressants, diltiazem, levodopa, methadone, phenothiazines, ritonavir, valproic acid, verapamil

REACTIONS

SKIN
- Acne (rare)
- Allergic reactions (sic)
- Angioedema
- Bullous eruption
- Contact dermatitis
- Dermatitis (sic) (1–10%)
- Eczematous eruption (sic)
- Exanthems
- Exfoliative dermatitis
- Fixed eruption (<1%)
- Flushing
- Granuloma disciformis (Miescher)
- Hyperhidrosis
- Melanoma
- Pellagra
- Pigmentation
- Pruritus
- Purpura
- Rash (sic) (>10%)
- Urticaria

NAILS
- Nails – parrot beak nails

OTHER
- Anaphylactoid reaction
- Gynecomastia
- Injection-site phlebitis (>10%)
- Paresthesias
- Porphyria
- Porphyria variegata
- Sialorrhea
- Xerostomia

DIAZOXIDE

Trade name: Hyperstat (Schering)
Other common trade names: Eudimine; Proglicem
Category: Antihypoglycemic
Clinically important, potentially serious interactions with: diuretics, hydralazine, phenytoin, warfarin

REACTIONS

SKIN
- Candidiasis
- Exanthems
- Flushing (<1%)
- Herpes (sic)
- Hyperhidrosis
- Leukomelanoderma (sic)
- Lichenoid eruption
- Photosensitivity
- Pruritus

Purpura
Rash (sic) (<1%)
Urticaria
Xerosis

HAIR
Hair – alopecia
Hair – hypertrichosis (<1%)

OTHER
Ageusia
Cellulitis (<1%)
Dysgeusia
Hypersensitivity
Injection-site pain (<1%)
Injection-site phlebitis
Paresthesias
Sialorrhea
Xerostomia

DICLOFENAC

Trade names: Arthrotec (Searle); Cataflam (Novartis); Voltaren (Novartis)
Other common trade names: Allvoran; Fenac; Monoflam; Remethan; Taks; Voltarene; Voltarol
Category: Nonsteroidal anti-inflammatory (NSAID)
Clinically important, potentially serious interactions with: aminoglycosides, anticoagulants, aspirin, cyclosporine, digoxin, diuretics, insulin, lithium, methotrexate, sulfonylureas, triamterene

Arthrotec is diclofenac & misoprostol

REACTIONS

SKIN
Allergic reactions (sic)
Angioedema (1–3%)
Aphthous stomatitis
Bullous eruption (1–3%)
Contact dermatitis
Dermatitis (sic) (1–3%)
Dermatitis herpetiformis
Dermatomyositis
Eczema (1–3%)
Erythema (sic)
Erythema multiforme (<1%)
Erythema nodosum (<1%)
Exanthems (1–5%)
Exfoliative dermatitis (<1%)
Flushing (<1%)
Hyperhidrosis (<1%)
Linear IgA bullous dermatosis
Lupus erythematosus
Photosensitivity (1–3%)
Pruritus (1–10%)
Pseudoallergic reactions (sic)
Psoriasis
Purpura (1–3%)
Pustular psoriasis
Rash (sic) (1–10%)
Skin reactions (sic)
Stevens-Johnson syndrome (1–3%) (one fatal case report)
Still's disease
Toxic epidermal necrolysis
Urticaria (1–3%)
Vasculitis

HAIR
Hair – alopecia (1–3%)

OTHER
Acute intermittent porphyria
Anaphylactoid reaction (1–3%)
Dysgeusia (1–3%)
Injection-site necrosis
Oral ulceration (rare)
Paresthesias (<1%)
Serum sickness
Stomatitis (<1%)
Tongue edema (1–3%)
Xerostomia (1–3%)

DICLOXACILLIN

Trade names: Dycill (SmithKline Beecham); Dynapen (Mead Johnson)
Other common trade names: Dichlor-Stapenor; Diclo; Diclocil; Diclocillin; Diclox; Novapen
Category: Penicillinase-resistant penicillin
Clinically important, potentially serious interactions with: anticoagulants, cyclosporine, methotrexate

Reactions

SKIN
- Angioedema
- Ecchymoses
- Erythema multiforme
- Erythroderma
- Exanthems
- Exfoliative dermatitis
- Hematomas
- Jarisch-Herxheimer reaction
- Pruritus
- Rash (sic) (<1%)
- Stevens-Johnson syndrome
- Urticaria

NAILS
- Nails – shoreline

OTHER
- Anaphylactoid reaction
- Black tongue
- Dysgeusia
- Glossitis
- Glossodynia
- Injection-site pain
- Myalgia
- Oral candidiasis
- Serum sickness
- Stomatitis
- Stomatodynia
- Vaginitis
- Xerostomia

DICUMAROL

Trade name: Dicumarol (Abbott)
Other common trade name: Embolin
Category: Oral anticoagulant
Clinically important, potentially serious interactions with: several dozen, too numerous to mention here

Reactions

SKIN
- Acral purpura
- Angioedema (<1%)
- Bullous eruption
- Dermatitis (sic)
- Ecchymoses
- Exanthems (rare)
- Hemorrhagic skin infarcts
- Necrosis
- Pigmentation
- Pruritus (<1%)
- Purplish erythema (feet & toes)
- Purpura
- Rash (sic)
- Urticaria
- Vesicular eruption

HAIR
- Hair – alopecia

OTHER
- Hypersensitivity
- Oral ulceration (rare)
- Priapism

DICYCLOMINE

Trade name: Bentyl (Hoechst Marion Roussel)
Other common trade names: Bentylol; Merbentyl; Notensyl; Panakiron; Spasmoban; Swityl
Category: Anticholinergic; antispasmodic
Clinically important, potentially serious interactions with: amantadine, antiarrhythmics, anticholinergics, antihistamines, atenolol, clozapine, digitalis, narcotic analgesics, phenothiazines, tacrine, tricyclic antidepressants

REACTIONS

SKIN
- Exanthems
- Hypohidrosis (>10%)
- Pruritus
- Rash (sic) (<1%)
- Urticaria
- Xerosis (>10%)

OTHER
- Ageusia
- Anaphylactoid reaction
- Injection-site reactions (sic) (>10%)
- Xerostomia (>10%)

DIDANOSINE

Trade name: Videx (Bristol-Myers Squibb)
Category: Antiviral; reverse transcriptase inhibitor
Clinically important, potentially serious interactions with: ganciclovir, indinavir, itraconazole, ketoconazole, pentamidine, sulfones

REACTIONS

SKIN
- Acral erythema
- Erythema multiforme
- Exanthems
- Pruritus (9%)
- Purpura
- Rash (sic) (9%)
- Stevens-Johnson syndrome
- Urticaria
- Vasculitis

HAIR
- Hair – alopecia

OTHER
- Anaphylactoid reaction
- Hypersensitivity (<1%)
- Myalgia
- Myopathy
- Paresthesias
- Xerostomia

DIDEOXYCYTIDINE (ddC) (See ZALCITABINE)

DIETHYLPROPION

Trade name: Tenuate (Hoechst Marion Roussel)
Other common trade names: Anorex; Linea; Prefamone; Regenon; Tenuate Retard
Category: Anorexiant
Clinically important, potentially serious interactions with: barbiturates, CNS depressants, MAO inhibitors, phenothiazines, sympathomimetics

REACTIONS

SKIN
- Ecchymoses
- Erythema (<1%)
- Erythema multiforme
- Exanthems (<1%)
- Flushing (<1%)
- Hyperhidrosis (<1%)
- Pruritus (<1%)
- Purpura (<1%)
- Rash (sic)
- Scleroderma
- Systemic sclerosis

Urticaria

HAIR
Hair – alopecia (<1%)

OTHER
Dysgeusia
Gynecomastia
Myalgia (<1%)
Xerostomia

DIETHYLSTILBESTROL

Trade name: Diethylstilbestrol (Lilly)
Other common trade names: Diethyl Stilbestrol; Distilbene; Stilboestrol
Category: Estrogen; antineoplastic; osteoporosis prophylactic
Clinically important, potentially serious interactions with: anticoagulants, felbamate, fluconazole, itraconazole, ketoconazole, phenytoin, propranolol

REACTIONS

SKIN
Acanthosis nigricans
Angioedema
Bullous eruption
Chloasma (<1%)
Edema
Erythema multiforme
Erythema nodosum
Exanthems
Exfoliative dermatitis
Flushing
Hyperkeratosis of nipples
Lupus erythematosus
Melasma (<1%)
Peripheral edema (>10%)
Pruritus
Purpura
Rash (sic) (<1%)
Urticaria

HAIR
Hair – alopecia
Hair – hirsutism

OTHER
Gynecomastia (>10%)
Mastodynia (>10%)
Periarteritis nodosa
Porphyria cutanea tarda
Vaginal candidiasis

DIFLUNISAL

Trade name: Dolobid (Merck)
Other common trade names: Ansal; Diflonid; Diflusal; Dolobis; Donobid; Fluniget; Flustar
Category: Nonsteroidal anti-inflammatory (NSAID)
Clinically important, potentially serious interactions with: acetaminophen, anticoagulants, digoxin, hydrochlorothiazide, indomethacin, lithium, methotrexate, phenytoin, sulfonamides, sulfonylureas

REACTIONS

SKIN
Angioedema (<1%)
Aphthous stomatitis
Bullous eruption
Edema (<1%)
Erythema multiforme (<1%)
Erythroderma
Exanthems
Exfoliative dermatitis (<1%)
Fixed eruption
Flushing (<1%)
Hyperhidrosis (<1%)
Lichenoid eruption
Photosensitivity (<1%)
Pruritus (1–10%)
Purpura
Rash (sic) (3–9%)
Skin reactions (sic)
Stevens-Johnson syndrome (<1%)
Toxic epidermal necrolysis (<1%)
Urticaria (<1%)
Vasculitis (<1%)

HAIR
Hair – alopecia

NAILS
Nails – onycholysis

OTHER
Anaphylactoid reaction (<1%)
Hypersensitivity (<1%)
Oral lichen planus
Oral ulceration
Paresthesias (<1%)
Pseudoporphyria
Stomatitis (<1%)
Xerostomia

DIGOXIN

Trade names: Lanoxicaps (Glaxo Wellcome); Lanoxin (Glaxo Wellcome)
Other common trade names: Cardigox; Digacin; Digoxine; Eudigox; Lanicor; Lenoxin
Category: Cardiac glycoside; inotropic; antiarrhythmic
Clinically important, potentially serious interactions with: amiodarone, amphotericin B, bumetanide, calcium preparations, clarithromycin, cyclosporine, doxycycline, erythromycin, ethacrynic acid, furosemide, itraconazole, phenytoin, propafenone, quinidine, quinine, reserpine, rifampin, tetracycline, verapamil

REACTIONS

SKIN
Bullous eruption
Diaphoresis
Exanthems
Pruritus
Psoriasis
Purpura
Rash (sic) (rare)
Urticaria (rare)
Vasculitis

OTHER
Gynecomastia

DIHYDROTACHYSTEROL

Trade names: DHT (Roxane); Hytakerol (Sanofi-Winthrop)
Other common trade names: AT 10; Dihydral; Dygratyl; Vitamin D
Category: Fat soluble vitamin
Clinically important, potentially serious interactions with: thiazide diuretics, verapamil

REACTIONS

SKIN
Livedo reticularis

OTHER
Calcification
Ulcerative necrosis

DILTIAZEM

Trade names: Cardizem (Hoechst Marion Roussel); Dilacor XR (Watson); Teczem (Hoechst Marion Roussel); Tiazac (Forest)
Other common trade names: Britiazem; Calcicard; Deltazen; Dilrene; Diltahexal; Tildiem
Category: Calcium channel blocker; antianginal, antiarrhythmic & antihypertensive
Clinically important, potentially serious interactions with: amiodarone, beta-blockers, carbamazepine, cyclosporine, digitalis, fentanyl, nifedipine, quinidine, theophylline

Teczem is diltiazem & enalapril

REACTIONS

SKIN
Acne
Acute generalized exanthematous pustulosis (AGEP)

Angioedema
Ankle edema
Cutaneous side effects (sic)
Edema (1–10%)
Erythema
Erythema multiforme (<1%)
Exanthems
Exfoliative dermatitis (<1%)
Flushing (<1%)
Hyperhidrosis
Hyperkeratosis (feet)
Lichenoid eruption (photosensitive)
Lupus erythematosus
Peeling of palms & soles (sic)
Periorbital edema
Peripheral edema
Petechiae (<1%)
Photosensitivity (<1%)
Pruritus (<1%)
Psoriasis
Purpura (<1%)
Pustular eruption
Pustular psoriasis
Rash (sic) (1.3%)
Skin thickening (sic)
Stevens-Johnson syndrome
Subcorneal pustular dermatosis
Toxic dermatitis (sic)
Toxic epidermal necrolysis
Toxic erythema
Toxic skin eruptions
Ulcerations of legs
Urticaria (<1%)
Vasculitis (<1%)

HAIR
Hair – alopecia (<1%)
Hair – hirsutism

NAILS
Nails – dystrophy

OTHER
Dysgeusia (<1%)
Erythromyalgia
Gingival hyperplasia
Gynecomastia
Hypersensitivity
Lymphadenopathy
Parageusia (<1%)
Paresthesias (<1%)
Pseudolymphoma
Xerostomia (<1%)

DIMENHYDRINATE

Trade names: Calm-X; Dimetabs; Dramamine; Marmine; Nico-Vert; Tega-Cert; Tega-Vert; Triptone; Vertab; Wehamine (Various pharmaceutical companies.)
Other common trade names: Andrumin; Lomarin; Nauseatol; Nausicalm; Vomacur; Vomex A
Category: H_1-receptor antihistamine & antinauseant
Clinically important, potentially serious interactions with: aminoglycoside antibiotics, anticholinergics, CNS depressants, MAO inhibitors, tricyclic antidepressants

REACTIONS

SKIN
Angioedema (<1%)
Eczematous eruption (sic)
Exanthems
Fixed eruption (<1%)
Flushing
Hyperhidrosis
Photosensitivity (<1%)
Rash (sic) (<1%)
Systemic eczematous contact dermatitis
Urticaria

OTHER
Acute intermittent porphyria
Injection-site pain (<1%)
Myalgia (<1%)
Paresthesias (<1%)
Xerostomia (1–10%)

DIPHENHYDRAMINE

Trade names: Allermax; Benadryl (Parke-Davis); Benylin (Warner-Lambert); Compoz; Sominex 2; Valdrene
Other common trade names: Allerdryl; Allermin; Dibrondrin; Dolestan; Nytol; Resmin; Sediat
Category: Antihistamine; antidyskinetic; antiemetic; sedative-hypnotic
Clinically important, potentially serious interactions with: chloral hydrate, CNS depressants, glutethimide, MAO inhibitors

REACTIONS

SKIN
- Allergic reactions (sic)
- Angioedema (<1%)
- Contact dermatitis
- Eczema (sic)
- Edema (<1%)
- Exanthems
- Fixed eruption
- Hyperhidrosis
- Livedo reticularis
- Photosensitivity (<1%)
- Pruritus
- Purpura
- Rash (sic) (<1%)
- Toxic epidermal necrolysis
- Urticaria
- Vasculitis

OTHER
- Anaphylactoid reaction
- Injection-site gangrene
- Injection-site necrosis
- Myalgia (<1%)
- Paresthesias (<1%)
- Xerostomia (1–10%)

DIPHENOXYLATE

Trade name: Lomotil (Searle)
Category: Antidiarrheal
Clinically important, potentially serious interactions with: anticholinergics, CNS depressants, digitalis, MAO inhibitors

Note: Lomotil is diphenoxylate with atropine. The reactions listed below are a result of this combination.

REACTIONS

SKIN
- Angioedema
- Flushing
- Hyperhidrosis (<1%)
- Pruritus (<1%)
- Urticaria (<1%)

OTHER
- Anaphylactoid reaction
- Gingivitis
- Xerostomia (1–10%)

DIPYRIDAMOLE

Trade name: Persantine (Boehringer Dupont)
Other common trade names: Cardoxin; Cleridium; Coronarine; Coroxin; Curantyl N; Persantin
Category: Platelet aggregation inhibitor & coronary vasodilator
Clinically important, potentially serious interactions with: beta-blockers, heparin, indomethacin

REACTIONS

SKIN
- Allergic reactions (sic) (<1%)
- Angioedema
- Diaphoresis (0.4%)
- Edema (0.3%)
- Erythema multiforme

Exanthems
Flushing (3.4%)
Pruritus
Psoriasis
Purpura
Rash (sic) (2.3%)
Stevens-Johnson syndrome
Toxic epidermal necrolysis
Urticaria

OTHER
Anaphylactoid reaction
Dysgeusia (0.1%)
Hypesthesia (0.5%)
Injection-site pain (0.1%)
Injection-site reactions (0.4%)
Mastodynia (0.03%)
Myalgia (0.9%)
Paresthesias (1.3%)
Pseudopolymyalgia rheumatica

DIRITHROMYCIN

Trade name: Dynabac (Bock)
Category: Macrolide antibiotic
Clinically important, potentially serious interactions with: estrogens

REACTIONS

SKIN
Allergic reactions (sic) (<1%)
Bullous eruption
Edema (<1%)
Hyperhidrosis (<1%)
Peripheral edema (<1%)
Pruritus (1.2%)
Rash (sic) (1.4%)
Urticaria (1.2%)

OTHER
Anaphylactoid reaction
Dysgeusia (<1%)
Myalgia (<1%)
Oral ulceration (<1%)
Paresthesias (<1%)
Vaginal candidiasis (<1%)
Vaginitis (<1%)
Xerostomia (<1%)

DISOPYRAMIDE

Trade name: Norpace (Searle)
Other common trade names: Dirythmin SA; Disonorm; Durbis; Isorythm; Rythmodan
Category: Antiarrhythmic
Clinically important, potentially serious interactions with: astemizole, beta-blockers, digoxin, erythromycin, terfenadine

REACTIONS

SKIN
Angioedema
Edema (1–3%)
Erythema nodosum
Exanthems (1–5%)
Lupus erythematosus (<1%)
Photosensitivity
Pruritus (1–3%)
Purpura
Rash (sic) (generalized) (1–3%)
Urticaria

HAIR
Hair – alopecia

OTHER
Gynecomastia (<1%)
Oral mucosal lesions (40%)
Paresthesias (<1%)
Xerostomia (32%)

DISULFIRAM

Trade name: Antabuse (Ayerst)
Other common trade names: Antabus; Busetal; Esperal; Nocbin; Refusal; Tetradin
Category: Deterrent to alcohol consumption
Clinically important, potentially serious interactions with: alcohol, anticoagulants, benzodiazepines, chlorzoxazone, isoniazid, MAO inhibitors, metronidazole, phenytoin, tricyclic antidepressants, warfarin

REACTIONS

SKIN
- Acne
- Allergic dermatitis (sic)
- Bullous eruption
- Contact dermatitis (on exposure to rubber)
- Dermatitis recall (nickel)
- Diaphoresis (<1%) (with alcohol)
- Eczematous eruption (sic)
- Exanthems
- Fixed eruption (<1%)
- Flushing (<1%) (with alcohol)
- Periarteritis nodosa
- Purpura
- Pustular eruption
- Rash (sic) (1–10%)
- Skin reaction (sic) (from beer-containing shampoo)
- Systemic eczematous contact dermatitis (sic)
- Toxic epidermal necrolysis
- Urticaria
- Vasculitis
- Yellow palms

OTHER
- Dysgeusia (metallic or garlic aftertaste) (1–10%)
- Hypogeusia
- Paresthesias
- Periarteritis nodosa

DIVALPROEX

Trade name: Depakote (Abbott)
Other common trade name: Epival
Category: Antimigraine
Clinically important, potentially serious interactions with: aspirin, barbiturates, carbamazepine, cimetidine, clonazepam, clozapine, diazepam, ethosuximide, felbamate, isoniazid, lamotrigine, phenobarbital, phenytoin, primidone, rifampin, salicylates, tolbutamide, warfarin, zidovudine

REACTIONS

SKIN
- Allergic reactions (sic) (<5%)
- Ecchymoses (<5%)
- Erythema multiforme
- Exanthems (<5%)
- Facial edema (<5%)
- Furunculosis (<5%)
- Lupus erythematosus
- Peripheral edema (<5%)
- Petechiae (<5%)
- Photosensitivity
- Pruritus (<5%)
- Rash (sic) (<5%)
- Seborrhea
- Stevens-Johnson syndrome
- Toxic epidermal necrolysis
- Vasculitis
- Xerostomia (<5%)

HAIR
- Hair – alopecia (7%)

OTHER
- Acute intermittent porphyria
- Dysgeusia (<5%)
- Galactorrhea
- Glossitis (<5%)
- Gynecomastia
- Hypesthesia
- Myalgia (<5%)
- Paresthesias (<5%)
- Stomatitis (<5%)
- Vaginitis (<5%)
- Xerostomia (<5%)

DOCETAXEL

Trade name: Taxotere (Rhône-Poulenc Rorer)
Category: Antineoplastic
Clinically important, potentially serious interactions with: cyclosporine, erythromycin, ketoconazole, terfenadine, troleandomycin

REACTIONS

SKIN
Ankle edema
Edema
Erythema (0.9%)
Erythrodysesthesia syndrome
Exanthems
Flushing
Photo-recall phenomenon
Photosensitivity
Pruritus
Rash (sic) (0.9%)
Scleroderma
Urticaria

HAIR
Hair – alopecia (80%)

NAILS
Nails – onycholysis
Nails – pigmentation
Nails – transverse superficial loss of nail plate

OTHER
Dysesthesia (3.9%)
Hypersensitivity (0.9%)
Infusion-site erythema
Infusion-site fixed eruption
Infusion-site hyperpigmentation
Infusion-site inflammation
Paresthesias (3.9%)
Stomatitis (42.3%)

DOCUSATE

Trade names: Colase; Dialose; Doxinate; Modane; Regutol; Sulfalax; Surfak, etc. (Various pharmaceutical companies.)
Other common trade names: Coloxyl; Hisof; Jamylene; Lambanol; Mollax; Regutol; Softon
Category: Laxative; stool softener
Clinically important, potentially serious interactions with: mineral oil, phenolphthalein

REACTIONS

SKIN
Exanthems (1%)

OTHER
Dysgeusia

DOLASETRON

Trade name: Anzemet (Hoechst Marion Roussel)
Category: Antiemetic & antinauseant
Clinically important, potentially serious interactions with: none

REACTIONS

SKIN
Edema
Facial edema
Flushing
Hyperhidrosis
Peripheral edema
Purpura
Rash (sic)
Urticaria

OTHER
Anaphylactoid reaction
Dysgeusia
Myalgia
Paresthesias
Photophobia
Thrombophlebitis
Twitching (sic)

DONEPEZIL

Trade name: Aricept (Roerig)
Category: Reversible acetylcholinesterase inhibitor for Alzheimer's disease
Clinically important, potentially serious interactions with: no data

REACTIONS

SKIN
- Dermatitis (sic) (<1%)
- Diaphoresis (>1%)
- Ecchymoses (4%)
- Erythema (<1%)
- Facial edema (<1%)
- Flushing
- Hyperkeratosis (sic) (<1%)
- Neurodermatitis (sic) (<1%)
- Periorbital edema (<1%)
- Pigmentation (<1%)
- Pruritus (>1%)
- Striae (<1%)
- Ulceration (<1%)
- Urticaria (>1%)

HAIR
- Hair – alopecia (<1%)
- Hair – hirsutism (<1%)

OTHER
- Dysgeusia (<1%)
- Gingivitis (<1%)
- Paresthesias (<1%)
- Tongue edema (<1%)
- Vaginitis (<1%)
- Xerostomia (<1%)

DOPAMINE

Trade name: Intropin
Other common trade names: Cardiosteril; Dopamin; Dopamin AWD; Dynatra; Revimine
Category: Adrenergic agonist; sympathomimetic
Clinically important, potentially serious interactions with: furazolidone, MAO inhibitors, phenytoin

REACTIONS

SKIN
- Exanthems
- Pruritus
- Raynaud's phenomenon (<1%)
- Urticaria

HAIR
- Hair – alopecia

OTHER
- Injection-site extravasation
- Injection-site gangrene
- Injection-site necrosis (<1%)
- Injection-site piloerection & vasoconstriction (sic)
- Peripheral ischemia
- Symmetric peripheral gangrene (sic)

DOXAPRAM

Trade name: Dopram (Robins)
Category: Respiratory stimulant
Clinically important, potentially serious interactions with: MAO inhibitors, sympathomimetics

REACTIONS

SKIN
- Flushing
- Hyperhidrosis (<1%)
- Pruritus

OTHER
- Injection-site erythema
- Injection-site pain
- Injection-site phlebitis (<1%)
- Paresthesias

DOXAZOSIN

Trade name: Cardura (Roerig)
Other common trade names: Alfadil; Cardoxan; Cardular; Dedralen; Diblocin; Supressin
Category: Alpha-adrenergic blocking; antihypertensive
Clinically important, potentially serious interactions with: beta-blockers, nifedipine, verapamil

REACTIONS

SKIN
- Bruising
- Eczema (sic) (<0.5%)
- Edema (4%)
- Exanthems (1.7%)
- Facial edema (1%)
- Flushing (1%)
- Hyperhidrosis (1.4%)
- Lichen planus
- Lupus erythematosus
- Pruritus (1%)
- Purpura (<0.5%)
- Rash (sic) (1%)
- Urticaria
- Xerosis (<0.5%)

HAIR
- Hair – alopecia (<0.5%)
- Hair – growth (sic)

OTHER
- Dysgeusia (<0.5%)
- Myalgia (1%)
- Paresthesias
- Parosmia (<0.05%)
- Xerostomia (2%)

DOXEPIN

Trade names: Sinequan (Roerig); Zonalon (topical) (Medicis)
Other common trade names: Anten; Aponal; Doneurin; Gilex; Mareen; Sinquan; Triadapin
Category: Tricyclic antidepressant, antipanic & antipruritic
Clinically important, potentially serious interactions with: alcohol, clonidine, diltiazem, epinephrine, fluoxetine, guanethidine, MAO inhibitors, selegiline, verapamil

REACTIONS

SKIN
- Ankle edema
- Aphthous stomatitis
- Contact dermatitis (from topical)
- Edema
- Exanthems
- Flushing
- Hyperhidrosis (1–10%)
- Photosensitivity (<1%)
- Pruritus
- Purpura
- Rash (sic)
- Red, dry skin (sic)
- Toxic dermatitis (sic)
- Urticaria

HAIR
- Hair – alopecia (<1%)

OTHER
- Burning at site of application
- Dysgeusia (>10%)
- Edema at site of application
- Galactorrhea (<1%)
- Glossalgia
- Glossitis
- Gynecomastia (<1%)
- Paresthesias
- Pseudolymphoma
- Stomatitis
- Xerostomia (>10%)

DOXORUBICIN

Trade names: Adriamycin (Pharmacia & Upjohn); Rubex (Immunex)
Other common trade names: Adiblastine; Adriablastine; Adriacin; Adriblatina; Farmablastina
Category: Anthracycline antibiotic & antineoplastic
Clinically important, potentially serious interactions with: cyclophosphamide, digitalis, mercaptopurine, quinolones, streptozocin, verapamil

REACTIONS

SKIN
- Acral erythrodysesthesia syndrome
- Allergic reactions (sic) (<1%)
- Angioedema
- Cellulitis
- Contact dermatitis
- Dermatitis herpetiformis
- Erythema of palms & soles (painful)
- Exanthems
- Exfoliative dermatitis
- Flushing (1–10%)
- Hyperpigmentation
- Keratoderma
- Necrosis (local)
- Pigmentation
- Postirradiation erythema
- Pruritus
- Purpura
- Radiation recall (<1%)
- Rash (sic)
- Raynaud's phenomenon
- Toxic epidermal injury (sic)
- Urticaria (<1%)

HAIR
- Hair – alopecia (>10%)

NAILS
- Nails – Beau's lines (transverse ridging)
- Nails – onycholysis
- Nails – pigmentation (1–10%)
- Nails – pigmented bands

OTHER
- Anaphylactoid reaction (<1%)
- Injection-site erythema
- Injection-site extravasation (>10%)
- Injection-site necrosis (>10%)
- Injection-site ulceration (>10%)
- Oral mucosal lesions
- Oral mucosal pigmentation
- Oral ulceration
- Stomatitis (>10%)
- Tongue pigmentation

DOXYCYCLINE

Trade names: Monodox (Oclassen); Vibramycin (Pfizer); Vibra-Tabs (Pfizer)
Other common trade names: Azudoxat; Bactidox; Doximed; Doxylin; Vibramycine; Vibravenos
Category: Tetracycline antibiotic
Clinically important, potentially serious interactions with: antacids, bismuth, digitalis, iron, penicillins, phenytoin, warfarin, zinc

REACTIONS

SKIN
- Acute generalized exanthematous pustulosis (AGEP)
- Allergic reactions (sic) (0.47%)
- Angioedema
- Erythema multiforme
- Exanthems
- Exfoliative dermatitis
- Fixed eruption (<1%)
- Lupus erythematosus
- Painful eruption of hands (sic)
- Photosensitivity (<1%)
- Phototoxic reaction
- Pigmentation
- Pruritus ani
- Psoriasis
- Purpura
- Rash (sic) (<1%)
- Seborrhea (sic)
- Stevens-Johnson syndrome
- Toxic epidermal necrolysis
- Urticaria
- Vasculitis

NAILS
Nails – discoloration (painful)
Nails – onycholysis
Nails – photo-onycholysis

OTHER
Anaphylactoid reaction
Anosmia
Dysgeusia
Glossitis
Injection-site phlebitis (<1%)
Paresthesias
Tongue pigmentation
Tooth discoloration (>10%) (in children)
Vaginitis

DRONABINOL (THC)

Trade name: Marinol (Roxane)
Category: Antiemetic; appetite stimulant
Clinically important, potentially serious interactions with: none

REACTIONS

SKIN
Flushing (<1%)
Hyperhidrosis (<1%)

OTHER
Myalgia (<1%)
Xerostomia (1–10%)

EDROPHONIUM

Trade names: Enlon (Ohmeda); Reversol (Organon); Tensilon (ICN)
Category: Cholinesterase inhibitor; antidote
Clinically important, potentially serious interactions with: corticosteroids, succinylcholine, tacrine

REACTIONS

SKIN
Hyperhidrosis (>10%)

OTHER
Hypersensitivity (<1%)
Sialorrhea (<1%)
Thrombophlebitis (<1%)

ENALAPRIL

Trade names: Lexxel (Astra Merck); Teczem (Hoechst Marion Roussel); Vasotec (Merck)
Other common trade names: Amprace; Enapren; Innovace; Pres; Renitec; Reniten; Xanef
Category: Angiotensin-converting enzyme (ACE) inhibitor; antihypertensive & vasodilator
Clinically important, potentially serious interactions with: allopurinol, bumetanide, lithium, potassium-sparing diuretics, salicylates

Lexxel is enalapril & felodipine; Teczem is enalapril & diltiazem; Vaseretic is enalapril & hydrochlorothiazide

REACTIONS

SKIN
Angioedema (<1%)
Bullous pemphigoid
Erythema
Erythema multiforme (<1%)
Exanthems
Exfoliative dermatitis (<1%)
Flushing (<1%)
Herpes zoster (<1%)
Hyperhidrosis (<1%)
Lichenoid eruption
Lupus erythematosus
Mycosis fungoides
Pemphigus
Pemphigus foliaceus
Pemphigus vegetans
Photodermatitis
Photosensitivity (<1%)
Pruritus (<1%)
Psoriasis

Purpura
Rash (sic) (1.4%)
Stevens-Johnson syndrome (<1%)
Toxic epidermal necrolysis (<1%)
Toxic pustuloderma
Urticaria (<1%)
Vasculitis (<1%)

HAIR
Hair – alopecia (<1%)

NAILS
Nails – dystrophy

OTHER
Ageusia
Anaphylactoid reaction (<1%)
Anosmia (<1%)
Dysesthesia (<1%)
Dysgeusia (1–10%)
Glossitis (<1%)
Glossopyrosis
Gynecomastia
Myalgia (<1%)
Oral bleeding (sic)
Oral mucosal lesions
Oral mucosal lichenoid eruption
Oral ulceration
Paresthesias (<1%)
Pseudopolymyalgia
Scalded mouth (sic)
Stomatitis (<1%)
Tongue edema
Xerostomia (<1%)

ENOXACIN

Trade name: Penetrex (Rhône-Poulenc Rorer)
Other common trade names: Bactidan; Comprecin; Enoxacine; Enoxen; Enoxor; Gyramid
Category: Quinolone antibacterial
Clinically important, potentially serious interactions with: caffeine, cimetidine, cyclosporine, digoxin, famotidine, metoprolol, nizatidine, propranolol, ranitidine, warfarin

REACTIONS

SKIN
Erythema multiforme (<1%)
Erythema nodosum
Exanthems
Hyperhidrosis (<1%)
Hyperpigmentation
Photoallergic reaction
Photosensitivity (<1%)
Phototoxic reaction
Purpura (<1%)
Rash (sic) (<1%)
Stevens-Johnson syndrome (<1%)
Toxic epidermal necrolysis (<1%)
Urticaria (<1%)

OTHER
Hypersensitivity
Injection-site phlebitis
Myalgia (<1%)
Paresthesias (<1%)
Stomatitis (<1%)
Vaginal candidiasis (<1%)
Vaginitis (<1%)

ENOXAPARIN

Trade name: Lovenox (Rhône-Poulenc Rorer)
Other common trade names: Clexan; Clexane 40; Klexane
Category: Anticoagulant (heparin, low weight)
Clinically important, potentially serious interactions with: ketorolac, oral anticoagulants, platelet inhibitors

REACTIONS

SKIN
Cutaneous side effects (sic) (0.2%)
Ecchymoses (2%)
Edema (3%)
Erythema (1–10%)
Peripheral edema (3%)
Urticaria

OTHER
Hypersensitivity

Injection-site erythema
Injection-site necrosis
Injection-site pain

EPHEDRINE

Trade names: Ectasule; Efedron; Ephedsol; Vicks Vatronol, etc.
Category: Adrenergic agonist, sympathomimetic bronchodilator
Clinically important, potentially serious interactions with: atropine, guanethidine, isocarboxazid, MAO inhibitors, methyldopa, phenylpropanolamine, selegiline, theophylline, tranylcypromine

REACTIONS

SKIN
Contact dermatitis (after topical application)
Bullous eruption
Dermatitis
Exanthems
Exfoliative dermatitis
Fixed eruption
Hyperhidrosis (1–10%)
Purpura
Urticaria
Vasculitis

OTHER
Xerostomia (1–10%)

EPINEPHRINE

Trade names: Adrenalin (Parke-Davis); Epifrin (Allergan); Epipen (CTR Labs); Sus-Phrine (Forest)
Other common trade names: Adrenaline; Eppy; Eppystabil; Isopto-Epinal; Simplene
Category: Adrenergic agonist, sympathomimetic bronchodilator
Clinically important, potentially serious interactions with: albuterol, atenolol, digitalis, ergotamine, imipramine, MAO inhibitors, metoprolol, propranolol, tranylcypromine, tricyclic antidepressants, vasopressors

REACTIONS

SKIN
Contact dermatitis
Exanthems
Fixed eruption
Flushing (1–10%)
Hyperhidrosis (1–10%)
Necrosis
Pemphigoid (cicatricial)
Urticaria

HAIR
Hair – alopecia

OTHER
Injection-site necrosis
Injection-site pain
Injection-site urticaria
Xerostomia (<1%)

EPOETIN ALFA

Trade names: Epogen (Amgen); Erythropoietin; Procrit (Ortho)
Other common trade names: Epoxitin; Erypo
Category: Colony stimulating factor; growth factor
Clinically important, potentially serious interactions with: none

REACTIONS

SKIN
Acne
Angioedema (1–5%)
Contact dermatitis
Edema (17%)
Exanthems
Lichenoid eruption
Photosensitivity
Pruritus
Rash (sic) (1–10%)
Urticaria

HAIR
Hair – hypertrichosis

OTHER
Anaphylactoid reaction
Hypersensitivity (<1%)
Injection-site pain
Injection-site reactions (sic) (7%)
Injection-site ulceration
Myalgia
Paresthesias (11%)
Porphyria cutanea tarda

ERGOCALCIFEROL

Trade names: Calciferol (Schwarz); Deltalin (Lilly); Drisdol (Sanofi); Vitamin D
Other common trade names: Kalciferol; Radiostol Forte; Sterogyl-5; Vigantol; Vitaminol
Category: Fat-soluble nutritional supplement, antihypocalcemic & antihypoparathyroid
Clinically important, potentially serious interactions with: thiazide diuretics, verapamil

REACTIONS

SKIN
Granulomas (perforating)
Pruritus (1–10%)

OTHER
Dysgeusia (metallic taste) (1–10%)
Xerostomia

ERYTHROMYCIN

Trade names: E.E.S; E-Mycin; Eryc; Erypar; Ery-Ped; Ery-Tab; Erythrocin; Eryzole; Ilosone; Ilotycin; PCE; Pediazole; Robimycin; Wintrocin (Various pharmaceutical companies.)
Other common trade names: Too numerous to list
Category: Bacteriostatic macrolide antibiotic
Clinically important, potentially serious interactions with: astemizole, bromocriptine, carbamazepine, cisapride, clindamycin, colchicine, cyclosporine, digitalis, dihydroergotamine, ergotamine, lovastatin, methadone, midazolam, pimozide, terfenadine, theophylline, triazolam, warfarin

REACTIONS

SKIN
Acne
Acute generalized exanthematous pustulosis (AGEP)
Allergic reactions (sic) (<1%)
Contact dermatitis (systemic)
Eczema (sic)
Erythema multiforme
Exanthems (1–5%)
Fixed eruption
Pruritus
Pustular eruption
Rash (sic) (<1%)
Red neck syndrome
Stevens-Johnson syndrome
Toxic epidermal necrolysis
Urticaria
Vasculitis

OTHER
Anaphylactoid reaction
Enamel hypoplasia (teeth)
Gingival hyperplasia
Glossodynia
Hypersensitivity (1–10%)
Injection-site phlebitis (1–10%)
Oral candidiasis (1–10%)
Oral ulceration
Stomatodynia
Tooth discoloration

ESMOLOL

Trade name: Brevibloc (Ohmeda)
Category: Beta-adrenergic blocker; antiarrhythmic
Clinically important, potentially serious interactions with: antidiabetics, calcium channel blockers, clonidine, digoxin, flecainide, morphine, nifedipine, oral contraceptives, verapamil

REACTIONS

SKIN
- Diaphoresis (>10%)
- Edema (<1%)
- Erythema (<1%)
- Flushing (<1%)
- Pigmentation (<1%)

OTHER
- Dysgeusia
- Infusion-site reactions (1–10%)
- Injection-site inflammation
- Paresthesias (<1%)
- Thrombophlebitis (<1%)
- Xerostomia (<1%)

ESTAZOLAM

Trade name: Prosom (Abbott)
Other common trade names: Domnamid; Esilgan; Eurodin; Kainever; Nuctalon; Tasedan
Category: Benzodiazepine sedative-hypnotic
Clinically important, potentially serious interactions with: CNS depressants, clarithromycin, diltiazem, fluconazole, itraconazole, ketoconazole, levodopa, miconazole, verapamil

REACTIONS

SKIN
- Acne (<1%)
- Allergic reactions (sic) (<1%)
- Dermatitis (sic) (<1%)
- Edema (<1%)
- Flushing (<1%)
- Hyperhidrosis (>10%)
- Photosensitivity
- Pruritus (1%)
- Purpura (<1%)
- Rash (sic) (>10%)
- Urticaria (<1%)
- Vaginal pruritus
- Xerosis (<1%)

OTHER
- Dysgeusia (<1%)
- Glossitis
- Gynecomastia (<1%)
- Myalgia (<1%)
- Oral ulceration (<1%)
- Paresthesias (<1%)
- Sialopenia (>10%)
- Sialorrhea (<1%)
- Xerostomia (>10%)

ESTRAMUSTINE

Trade name: Emcyt (Pharmacia & Upjohn)
Other common trade name: Cellmusin
Category: Antineoplastic
Clinically important, potentially serious interactions with: aldesleukin

REACTIONS

SKIN
- Allergic reactions (sic)
- Edema (>10%)
- Exanthems
- Flushing (1%)
- Pigmentary changes (sic) (<1%)
- Pruritus (2%)
- Purpura (3%)
- Rash (sic) (1%)
- Urticaria
- Xerosis (2%)

HAIR
Hair – alopecia (<1%)

OTHER
Gynecomastia (>10%)
Injection-site thrombophlebitis (1–10%)
Mastodynia (66%)
Thrombophlebitis (3%)

ETHACRYNIC ACID

Trade name: Edecrin (Merck)
Other common trade names: Edecril; Edecrina; Hydromedin; Reomax
Category: Loop diuretic
Clinically important, potentially serious interactions with: ACE-inhibitors, aminoglycosides, digoxin, lithium, thiazides, warfarin

REACTIONS

SKIN
Exanthems
Photosensitivity
Purpura (rare)
Rash (sic) (<1%)
Urticaria
Vasculitis

OTHER
Injection-site pain

ETHAMBUTOL

Trade name: Myambutol (Lederle)
Other common trade names: Apo-Ethambutol; Dexambutol; EMB; Etapiam; Etibi; Stambutol
Category: Antimycobacterial
Clinically important, potentially serious interactions with: antacids, kaolin

REACTIONS

SKIN
Acne
Angioedema
Bullous eruption
Contact dermatitis
Erythema multiforme
Dermatitis (sic)
Exanthems
Exfoliative dermatitis
Hyperhidrosis
Lichenoid eruption
Lupus erythematosus
Photosensitivity
Pruritus (<1%)
Purpura
Rash (sic) (<1%)
Stevens-Johnson syndrome
Toxic epidermal necrolysis
Urticaria

HAIR
Hair – alopecia

OTHER
Anaphylactoid reaction (<1%)
Hypersensitivity
Paresthesias

ETHANOLAMINE

Trade name: Ethamolin (Reed & Carnrick)
Other common trade name: Ethanolamine Oleate
Category: Sclerosing agent
Clinically important, potentially serious interactions with: none

REACTIONS

SKIN
Contact dermatitis

OTHER
Anaphylactoid reaction (<1%)

ETHCHLORVYNOL

Trade name: Placidyl (Abbott)
Other common trade names: Arvynol; Nostel
Category: Sedative-hypnotic
Clinically important, potentially serious interactions with: alcohol, anticoagulants, CNS depressants, MAO inhibitors, tricyclic antidepressants

REACTIONS

SKIN
- Allergic reactions (sic)
- Bullous eruption (from overdose)
- Fixed eruption
- Hyperhidrosis
- Pruritus
- Purpura
- Rash (sic) (1–10%)
- Urticaria

OTHER
- Acute intermittent porphyria
- Dysgeusia (>10%)
- Paresthesias
- Pressure necrosis

ETHIONAMIDE

Trade name: Trecator-SC (Wyeth)
Other common trade names: Ethatyl; Etiocidan; Myobid-50; Tubermin
Category: Tuberculostatic
Clinically important, potentially serious interactions with: none

REACTIONS

SKIN
- Acne
- Allergic reactions (sic)
- Butterfly eruptions on the face (sic)
- Eczema (sic)
- Exanthems
- Ichthyosis
- Lupus erythematosus
- Pellagra
- Photosensitivity
- Purpura
- Rash (sic) (<1%)
- Seborrheic dermatitis
- Urticaria (1–5%)

HAIR
- Hair – alopecia

OTHER
- Dysgeusia (metallic taste) (1–10%)
- Gynecomastia (<1%)
- Oral ulceration
- Sialorrhea
- Stomatitis (<1%)
- Stomatodynia
- Xerostomia

ETHOSUXIMIDE

Trade name: Zarontin (Parke-Davis)
Other common trade names: Emeside; Petinimid; Petnidan; Pyknolepsinum; Suxinutin
Category: Succinimide anticonvulsant
Clinically important, potentially serious interactions with: isoniazid, phenytoin, valproic acid

REACTIONS

SKIN
- Cutaneous side effects (sic) (3.4%)
- Erythema multiforme (<1%)
- Exanthems (1–5%)
- Exfoliative dermatitis (<1%)
- Lupus erythematosus (>10%)
- Periorbital edema
- Pruritus
- Purpura
- Rash (sic) (<1%)

Raynaud's phenomenon
Stevens-Johnson syndrome (>10%)
Urticaria (1–5%)

HAIR
Hair – alopecia
Hair – hirsutism

OTHER
Acute intermittent porphyria
Gingival hyperplasia
Oral ulceration
Tongue edema

ETHOTOIN

Trade name: Peganone (Abbott)
Other common trade name: Accenon
Category: Hydantoin anticonvulsant
Clinically important, potentially serious interactions with: chloramphenicol, cyclosporine, disulfiram, dopamine, isoniazid, itraconazole

REACTIONS

SKIN
Bullous eruption
Fixed eruption
Lupus erythematosus
Purpura
Rash (sic)

OTHER
Gingival hyperplasia

ETIDRONATE

Trade name: Didronel (Procter Gamble)
Other common trade names: Didronate; Difosfen; Dinol; Diphos; Osteum
Category: Bone resorption inhibitor; antihypercalcemic
Clinically important, potentially serious interactions with: none

REACTIONS

SKIN
Angioedema (<1%)
Exanthems
Pruritus
Rash (sic) (<1%)
Stevens-Johnson syndrome
Toxic epidermal necrolysis
Urticaria

HAIR
Hair – alopecia

OTHER
Dysgeusia (<1%)
Glossitis
Hypersensitivity (<1%)
Paresthesias

ETODOLAC

Trade name: Lodine (Ayerst)
Other common trade names: Antilak; Ecridoxan; Edolan; Elderin; Lonine; Tedolan; Zedolac
Category: Nonsteroidal anti-inflammatory (NSAID)
Clinically important, potentially serious interactions with: aminoglycosides, aspirin, cyclosporine, digoxin, lithium, methotrexate, probenecid, warfarin

REACTIONS

SKIN
Angioedema (<1%)
Dermatitis (sic)
Ecchymoses
Edema
Erythema multiforme (<1%)
Exanthems
Exfoliative dermatitis
Facial edema
Fixed eruption

Flushing
Furunculosis
Hyperhidrosis
Hyperpigmentation
Peeling skin (sic)
Peripheral edema
Photosensitivity
Pruritus (1–10%)
Purpura
Rash (sic) (>10%)
Stevens-Johnson syndrome (<1%)
Toxic epidermal necrolysis (<1%)
Urticaria (<1%)
Vasculitis
Vesiculobullous eruption

HAIR
Hair – alopecia

OTHER
Gingival ulceration
Glossitis
Gynecomastia
Parageusia
Paresthesias
Sialorrhea
Stomatitis
Ulcerative stomatitis
Xerostomia

ETOPOSIDE

Trade names: Toposar (Pharmacia & Upjohn); VePesid (Mead Johnson)
Other common trade names: Aside; Etopos; Etosid; Lastet; Serozide; Vepeside; VP-TEC
Category: Antineoplastic
Clinically important, potentially serious interactions with: calcium antagonists, carmustine, cyclosporine, methotrexate, warfarin

REACTIONS

SKIN
Allergic reactions (sic) (1–2%)
Diaphoresis
Ecchymoses
Eccrine squamous syringometaplasia
Erythema
Erythema multiforme
Exanthems
Facial edema
Flushing (<1%)
Pigmentation
Pruritus
Purpura
Radiation recall
Rash (sic)
Stevens-Johnson syndrome
Urticaria

HAIR
Hair – alopecia (8–66%)

NAILS
Nails – Beau's lines (transverse ridging)
Nails – onycholysis

OTHER
Anaphylactoid reaction (<2%)
Dysgeusia
Hypersensitivity (<1%)
Injection-site pain
Oral mucosal lesions
Paresthesias
Stomatitis (1–10%)
Tongue edema

FAMCICLOVIR

Trade name: Famvir (SmithKline Beecham)
Category: Antiviral
Clinically important, potentially serious interactions with: cimetidine, digoxin, probenecid

REACTIONS

SKIN
Dermatitis
Pruritus (3.7%)

OTHER
Paresthesias (2.6%)

FAMOTIDINE

Trade name: Pepcid (Merck)
Other common trade names: Amfamox; Famodil; Ganor; Gastro; Motiax; Pepcidine; Pepdul
Category: Histamine H_2-receptor antagonist & anti-ulcer
Clinically important, potentially serious interactions with: cephalosporins, ketoconazole, nifedipine, nisoldipine

REACTIONS

SKIN
- Acne (<1%)
- Allergic reactions (sic) (<1%)
- Angioedema
- Contact dermatitis
- Cutaneous side effects (sic)
- Dermographism
- Exanthems
- Facial edema
- Flushing
- Periorbital edema
- Pruritus (<1%)
- Purpura
- Rash (sic)
- Toxic epidermal necrolysis
- Urticaria (<1%)
- Vasculitis
- Xerosis (<1%)

HAIR
- Hair – alopecia

OTHER
- Dysgeusia
- Gynecomastia
- Oral mucosal lesions
- Paresthesias (<1%)
- Xerostomia

FELBAMATE

Trade name: Felbatol (Wallace)
Other common trade names: Felbamyl; Taloxa
Category: Antiepileptic
Clinically important, potentially serious interactions with: barbiturates, carbamazepine, estrogens, phenytoin, valproic acid

REACTIONS

SKIN
- Acne (3.4%)
- Bullous eruption (<1%)
- Diaphoresis
- Edema
- Facial edema (3.4%)
- Flushing
- Lichen planus
- Livedo reticularis
- Lupus erythematosus
- Photosensitivity (<0.01%)
- Pruritus (>1%)
- Purpura
- Pustular eruption
- Rash (sic) (3.5%)
- Stevens-Johnson syndrome (<0.01%)
- Toxic epidermal necrolysis
- Urticaria (<1%)

HAIR
- Hair – alopecia

OTHER
- Anaphylactoid reaction (<0.01%)
- Dysgeusia (6.1%)
- Foetor ex ore (halitosis)
- Gingival bleeding
- Glossitis
- Myalgia (2.6%)
- Oral mucosal edema (>1%)
- Paresthesias (3.5%)
- Thrombophlebitis
- Xerostomia (2.6%)

FELODIPINE

Trade names: Lexxel (Astra Merck); Plendil (Astra Merck)
Other common trade names: AGON SR; Hydac; Modip; Munobal; Penedil; Renedil; Splendil
Category: Calcium channel blocker
Clinically important, potentially serious interactions with: barbiturates, beta-blockers, carbamazepine, cimetidine, cyclosporine, digitalis, metoprolol, phenytoin, prazosin, quinidine, theophylline. Also grapefruit

Lexxel is enalapril & felodipine

REACTIONS

SKIN
- Ankle edema
- Edema
- Erythema (1.5%)
- Exanthems
- Facial edema (1.5%)
- Flushing (3.9–6.9%)
- Hyperhidrosis
- Peripheral edema (2–17.4%)
- Pruritus
- Purpura
- Rash (sic) (1.5%)
- Telangiectases (truncal)
- Urticaria (1.5%)

NAILS
- Nails – brittle

OTHER
- Gingival hyperplasia (<1%)
- Myalgia (1.5%)
- Paresthesias (2.5%)
- Xerostomia (<1%)

FENFLURAMINE

Trade name: Pondimin (Robins)
Other common trade names: Dima-Fen; Pesos; Ponderal; Ponderax; Ponflural; Wate Down
Category: Anorexiant
Clinically important, potentially serious interactions with: antidiabetics, furazolidone, guanethidine, insulin, MAO inhibitors, phenothiazines

REACTIONS

SKIN
- Burning (sic)
- Exanthems
- Hyperhidrosis (<1%)
- Pruritus
- Rash (sic)
- Urticaria

HAIR
- Hair – alopecia (<1%)

OTHER
- Dysgeusia
- Myalgia (<1%)
- Xerostomia

FENOFIBRATE

Trade name: Tricor (Abbott)
Category: Fibric acid cholesterol-lowering
Clinically important, potentially serious interactions with: anticoagulants, cyclosporine, statins

REACTIONS

SKIN
- Exanthems
- Photoallergic reaction
- Photosensitivity
- Phototoxic reaction
- Pruritus
- Rash (sic)
- Skin reactions (sic)

Urticaria

HAIR
Hair – alopecia

OTHER
Polymyositis
Muscle tenderness
Muscle toxicity (sic)
Myopathy

FENOPROFEN

Trade name: Nalfon (Dista)
Other common trade names: Fenoprex; Fenopron; Fepron; Feprona; Nalgesic; Progesic
Category: Nonsteroidal anti-inflammatory (NSAID)
Clinically important, potentially serious interactions with: anticoagulants, cyclosporine, methotrexate, phenytoin, salicylates, sulfonamides, sulfonylureas

REACTIONS

SKIN
Acne
Angioedema (<1%)
Aphthous stomatitis (<1%)
Bruising (<1%)
Erythema multiforme (<1%)
Exanthems
Exfoliative dermatitis (<1%)
Hyperhidrosis (<0.5%)
Peripheral edema (<1%)
Pruritus (>5%)
Purpura (<1%)
Rash (sic) (>10%)
Stevens-Johnson syndrome (<1%)
Toxic epidermal necrolysis (<1%)
Urticaria (<1%)
Vesiculobullous eruption

HAIR
Hair – alopecia (<1%)

OTHER
Anaphylactoid reaction
Dysgeusia (metallic taste) (<1%)
Glossopyrosis (<1%)
Mastodynia (<1%)
Oral ulceration (rare)
Stomatitis (rare)
Xerostomia (>1%)

FENTANYL

Trade name: Duragesic (Janssen)
Other common trade names: Beatryl; Durogesic; Fentanest; Leptanal
Category: Narcotic agonist analgesic
Clinically important, potentially serious interactions with: amiodarone, cimetidine, ranitidine, ritonavir

REACTIONS

SKIN
Edema
Erythema (at application site) (<1%)
Exanthems
Exfoliative dermatitis
Flushing (3–10%)
Hyperhidrosis (>10%)
Papular eruption (sic) (>1%)
Pruritus (3–10%)
Pustules (sic) (<1%)
Rash (sic) (>1%)
Urticaria (<1%)

OTHER
Anaphylactoid reaction
Dysgeusia (<1%)
Paresthesias (<1%)
Xerostomia (>10%)

FEXOFENADINE

Trade name: Allegra (Hoechst Marion Roussel)
Category: H_1-receptor antagonist; antihistamine
Clinically important, potentially serious interactions with: no data

REACTIONS

SKIN
Acne

FINASTERIDE

Trade names: Propecia (Merck); Proscar (Merck)
Other common trade names: Pro-Cure; Proscar 5
Category: Androgen hormone inhibitor; antineoplastic; hair growth stimulant
Clinically important, potentially serious interactions with: none

REACTIONS

SKIN
Exanthems
Rash (sic)
Urticaria

HAIR
Hair – hypotrichosis (sic)
Hair – patchy hair loss of beard (sic)

OTHER
Gynecomastia
Lip swelling

FLAVOXATE

Trade name: Urispas (Beecham)
Other common trade names: Bladderon; Genurin; Harnin; Patricin; Spasuret; Urispadol; Uronid
Category: Antispasmodic
Clinically important, potentially serious interactions with: amantadine, anticholinergics, atenolol, clozapine, digitalis, haloperidol, phenothiazines, tacrine, tricyclic antidepressants

REACTIONS

SKIN
Exanthems
Rash (sic) (<1%)
Urticaria

OTHER
Hypersensitivity
Oral ulceration
Xerostomia (>10%)

FLECAINIDE

Trade name: Tambocor (3M)
Other common trade names: Almarytm; Apocard; Corflene; Flecaine; Tabco
Category: Antiarrhythmic
Clinically important, potentially serious interactions with: amiodarone, beta-blockers, digoxin, disopyramide, ritonavir, verapamil

REACTIONS

SKIN
Edema (3.5%)
Exanthems
Exfoliative dermatitis (<1%)
Flushing (<3%)
Hyperhidrosis (<3%)
Pruritus (<1%)
Psoriasis

Rash (sic) (<3%)
Urticaria (<1%)

HAIR
Hair – alopecia (<1%)

OTHER
Dysgeusia
Hypesthesia (<1%)
Myalgia (<1%)
Oral edema
Paresthesias (<1%)
Tongue edema (<1%)
Xerostomia (<1%)

FLUCONAZOLE

Trade name: Diflucan (Roerig)
Other common trade names: Biozolene; Flucazol; Flukezol; Fluzone; Fungata; Triflucan
Category: Broad-spectrum bis-triazole antifungal
Clinically important, potentially serious interactions with: alprazolam, anticoagulants, astemizole, cimetidine, cisapride, cyclosporine, midazolam, phenytoin, terfenadine, triazolam, warfarin

REACTIONS

SKIN
Acne
Angioedema
Bullous eruption
Erythema multiforme
Exanthems (1.8%) (in AIDS patients)
Exfoliative dermatitis (rare)
Fixed eruption
Petechiae
Pruritus
Purpura
Rash (sic) (1.8%)
Skin hypertrophy (sic)
Stevens-Johnson syndrome
Toxic epidermal necrolysis
Urticaria

HAIR
Hair – alopecia

NAILS
Nail – disorder (sic)

OTHER
Anaphylactoid reaction (in patients with AIDS)
Dysgeusia
Hypersensitivity
Oral ulceration
Paresthesias
Xerostomia

FLUCYTOSINE

Trade name: Ancobon (Roche)
Other common trade names: Alcobon; Ancotil
Category: Antifungal
Clinically important, potentially serious interactions with: amphotericin B

REACTIONS

SKIN
Exanthems
Photosensitivity (<1%)
Pruritus
Purpura
Rash (sic) (1–10%)
Urticaria

OTHER
Anaphylactoid reaction
Paresthesias (<1%)
Xerostomia

FLUMAZENIL

Trade name: Romazicon (Roche)
Other common trade names: Anexate; Lanexat
Category: Benzodiazepine receptor antagonist
Clinically important, potentially serious interactions with: cyclic antidepressants

REACTIONS

SKIN
- Flushing
- Hyperhidrosis (3–9%)
- Rash (sic)

OTHER
- Hypesthesia
- Injection-site pain (3–9%)
- Injection-site reactions (sic)
- Paresthesias
- Thick tongue (sic) (<1%)
- Thrombophlebitis
- Xerostomia (1–10%)

FLUOROURACIL

Trade names: Adrucil (Pharmacia & Upjohn); Efudex (Roche); Fluoroplex (Allergan)
Other common trade names: Efudix; Efurix
Category: Antineoplastic antimetabolite
Clinically important, potentially serious interactions with: aldesleukin, allopurinol, anticoagulants, cimetidine, methotrexate, metronidazole, thiazides

REACTIONS

SKIN
- Acral erythema
- Angioedema
- Bullous eruption
- Contact dermatitis
- Dermatitis (sic) (>10%)
- Eczematous eruption (sic)
- Erythema
- Erythema multiforme
- Exanthems
- Fissuring
- Hand-foot syndrome
- Palmar-plantar erythrodysesthesia syndrome
- Pellagra
- Photosensitivity
- Phototoxic reaction
- Pigmentation (<1%)
- Pruritus
- Radiation recall
- Reactivation phenomenon (sic)
- Seborrheic dermatitis
- Urticaria
- Xerosis (1–10%)

HAIR
- Hair – alopecia (>10%)

NAILS
- Nails – onycholysis
- Nails – pigmentation (<1%)

OTHER
- Anaphylactoid reaction
- Dysgeusia
- Ectropion
- Injection-site burning
- Injection-site desquamation
- Injection-site edema
- Injection-site erythema
- Injection-site necrosis
- Injection-site pain
- Injection-site ulceration
- Paresthesias (<1%)
- Stomatitis (>10%)

FLUOXETINE

Trade name: Prozac (Dista)
Other common trade names: Adofen; Fluctin; Fludac; Fluctine; Fluoxeren; Fluxil; Fontex
Category: Selective serotonin reuptake inhibitor (SSRI); antidepressant & antiobsessional
Clinically important, potentially serious interactions with: alprazolam, diazepam, haloperidol, isocarboxazid, lithium, MAO inhibitors, metoprolol, phenelzine, phenothiazines, phenytoin, pimozide, selegiline, sotalol, terfenadine, tranylcypromine, trazodone, tricyclic antidepressants, tryptophan

REACTIONS

SKIN
- Acne (<1%)
- Angioedema
- Aphthous stomatitis (<1%)
- Bruising
- Bullous eruption (<1%)
- Candidiasis (rare)
- Cellulitis (rare)
- Contact dermatitis (<1%)
- Cutaneous reaction (sic)
- Eczema (sic) (<1%)
- Erythema multiforme (rare)
- Erythema nodosum
- Exanthems (4%)
- Exfoliative dermatitis
- Facial edema (<1%)
- Flushing
- Furunculosis (<1%)
- Herpes simplex (reactivation)
- Herpes zoster (rare)
- Hyperhidrosis (8.4%)
- Lichenoid eruption
- Lupus erythematosus (discoid)
- Mycosis fungoides (exacerbation)
- Peripheral edema (<1%)
- Petechiae (<1%)
- Phototoxic reaction (<1%)
- Pigmentation (<1%)
- Pruritus (2.4%)
- Pseudo-mycosis fungoides (sic)
- Psoriasis (<1%)
- Purpura (<1%)
- Pustular eruption (<1%)
- Rash (sic) (6%)
- Seborrhea (<1%)
- Stevens-Johnson syndrome
- Subcutaneous nodule (sic)
- Toxic epidermal necrolysis
- Ulcers (<1%)
- Urticaria (4%)
- Vasculitis
- Xerosis

HAIR
- Hair – alopecia (<1%)
- Hair – hirsutism (<1%)

OTHER
- Ageusia (<1%)
- Anaphylactoid reaction (<1%)
- Dysgeusia (1.8%)
- Gingivitis (<1%)
- Glossitis (<1%)
- Glossodynia
- Gynecomastia (<1%)
- Hyperesthesia (<1%)
- Hypersensitivity
- Hypesthesia (<1%)
- Mastodynia (<1%)
- Myopathy (<1%)
- Oral ulceration (<1%)
- Paresthesias
- Parosmia (<1%)
- Priapism (<1%)
- Pseudolymphoma
- Serum sickness
- Sialorrhea (<1%)
- Stomatitis (<1%)
- Thrombophlebitis (<1%)
- Tongue edema (<1%)
- Tongue pigmentation (<1%)
- Vaginal anesthesia
- Xerostomia (12%)

FLUOXYMESTERONE

Trade names: Android-F; Halotensin (Pharmacia & Upjohn)
Other common trade names: Stenox; Vewon
Category: Androgen; antineoplastic; antianemic
Clinically important, potentially serious interactions with: anticoagulants, cyclosporine

REACTIONS

SKIN
- Acne (>10%)
- Contact dermatitis
- Edema (1–10%)
- Exanthems
- Flushing (1–5%)
- Furunculosis
- Lichenoid eruption
- Lupus erythematosus
- Pruritus
- Psoriasis
- Purpura
- Seborrhea
- Seborrheic dermatitis
- Striae
- Urticaria

HAIR
- Hair – alopecia
- Hair – hirsutism (1–10%)

OTHER
- Anaphylactoid reaction
- Gynecomastia (<1%)
- Hypersensitivity (<1%)
- Injection-site pain
- Mastodynia (>10%)
- Paresthesias
- Priapism (>10%)
- Stomatitis

FLUPHENAZINE

Trade names: Permitil (Schering); Prolixin (Bristol-Myers Squibb)
Other common trade names: Anatensol; Dapotum D; Dapatum D25; Fludecate; Modecate
Category: Phenothiazine antipsychotic
Clinically important, potentially serious interactions with: ACE-inhibitors, alcohol, barbiturates, levodopa, lithium, meperidine, piperazine, tricyclic antidepressants, valproic acid

REACTIONS

SKIN
- Angioedema (<1%)
- Eczema (sic)
- Erythema
- Exanthems
- Exfoliative dermatitis
- Hyperhidrosis
- Hypohidrosis (>10%)
- Lupus erythematosus
- Peripheral edema
- Photosensitivity
- Pigmentation (<1%) (blue-gray)
- Pruritus (<1%)
- Purpura
- Rash (sic) (1–10%)
- Seborrhea
- Toxic epidermal necrolysis
- Urticaria
- Vitiligo

OTHER
- Anaphylactoid reaction
- Galactorrhea (1–10%)
- Gynecomastia (1–10%)
- Mastodynia (1–10%)
- Priapism (<1%)
- Sialorrhea
- Xerostomia (<1%)

FLURAZEPAM

Trade name: Dalmane (Roche)
Other common trade names: Benozil; Dalmadorm; Flunox; Nergart; Novoflupam; Valdorm
Category: Benzodiazepine hypnotic sedative
Clinically important, potentially serious interactions with: CNS depressants, cimetidine, clarithromycin, diltiazem, fluconazole, itraconazole, ketoconazole, miconazole, verapamil

REACTIONS

SKIN
- Dermatitis (sic) (1–10%)
- Exanthems
- Flushing
- Hyperhidrosis (>10%)
- Pruritus
- Purpura
- Rash (sic) (>10%)
- Urticaria

OTHER
- Acute intermittent porphyria
- Dysgeusia (metallic taste) (3.4%)
- Oral mucosal lesions
- Paresthesias
- Sialopenia (>10%)
- Sialorrhea (1–10%)
- Xerostomia (>10%)

FLURBIPROFEN

Trade name: Ansaid (Pharmacia & Upjohn)
Other common trade names: Apo-Flurbiprofen; Cebutid; Flurofen; Flurozin; Froben; Lapole
Category: Nonsteroidal anti-inflammatory (NSAID)
Clinically important, potentially serious interactions with: aminoglycosides, anticoagulants, methotrexate

REACTIONS

SKIN
- Angioedema (<1%)
- Aphthous stomatitis (rare)
- Cutaneous side effects (sic) (6%)
- Dermatitis herpetiformis
- Discoloration (sic)
- Eczema (sic) (3–9%)
- Edema (3–9%)
- Erythema multiforme (<1%)
- Exanthems
- Exfoliative dermatitis (<1%)
- Fixed eruption
- Flushing
- Furunculosis
- Herpes simplex
- Herpes zoster
- Hyperhidrosis
- Photosensitivity (<1%)
- Pruritus (1–5%)
- Pseudoallergic reactions (sic)
- Purpura (rare)
- Rash (sic) (1–3%)
- Seborrhea
- Stevens-Johnson syndrome (<1%)
- Toxic epidermal necrolysis (<1%)
- Ulceration
- Urticaria (<1%)
- Vasculitis
- Xerosis

HAIR
- Hair – alopecia (<1%)

NAILS
- Nails – disorder (sic) (<1%)
- Nails – pigmentation

OTHER
- Anaphylactoid reaction (<1%)
- Dysgeusia (<1%)
- Hypersensitivity
- Oral lichenoid eruption
- Paresthesias (<1%)
- Parosmia (<1%)
- Vulvovaginitis
- Xerostomia (<1%)

FLUTAMIDE

Trade name: Eulexin (Schering)
Other common trade names: Drogenil; Euflex; Eulexine; Flucinom; Fluken; Flulem; Fugerel
Category: Antineoplastic (prostate carcinoma); antiandrogen
Clinically important, potentially serious interactions with: none

REACTIONS

SKIN
- Bullous eruption
- Edema (4%)
- Erythema
- Exanthems
- Hot flashes (61%)
- Hyperhidrosis
- Lupus erythematosus
- Photosensitivity
- Rash (sic) (3%)
- Toxic epidermal necrolysis
- Urticaria

OTHER
- Gynecomastia (9%)
- Injection-site irritation (3%)
- Paresthesias
- Pseudoporphyria

FLUVASTATIN

Trade name: Lescol (Novartis)
Other common trade names: Cranoc; Locol
Category: Antihyperlipidemic; HMG-CoA reductase inhibitor
Clinically important, potentially serious interactions with: anticoagulants, gemfibrozil, warfarin

REACTIONS

SKIN
- Allergic reactions (sic) (2.6%)
- Angioedema
- Discoloration (sic)
- Erythema multiforme
- Flushing
- Lupus erythematosus
- Photosensitivity
- Pruritus
- Purpura
- Rash (sic) (2.7%)
- Stevens-Johnson syndrome
- Toxic epidermal necrolysis
- Urticaria
- Vasculitis
- Xerosis

HAIR
- Hair – alopecia
- Hair – changes (sic)

NAILS
- Nails – changes (sic)

OTHER
- Anaphylactoid reaction
- Dysgeusia
- Gynecomastia
- Paresthesias

FLUVOXAMINE

Trade name: Luvox (Solvay)
Other common trade names: Dumirox; Dumyrox; Faverin; Favoxil; Fevarin; Maveral
Category: Selective serotonin reuptake inhibitor (SSRI); antidepressant
Clinically important, potentially serious interactions with: alprazolam, anticoagulants, astemizole, beta-blockers, carbamazepine, cimetidine, diltiazem, lithium, MAO inhibitors, methadone, metoprolol, terfenadine, trazodone, triazolam, tricyclic antidepressants

REACTIONS

SKIN
- Acne (<1%)
- Allergic reaction (sic) (<1%)
- Angioedema
- Bullous eruption
- Cutaneous reaction (sic)
- Ecchymoses (<1%)
- Edema (<1%)
- Exanthems
- Exfoliative dermatitis (<1%)
- Furunculosis (<1%)
- Hyperhidrosis (7%)
- Photosensitivity (<1%)
- Pigmentation (<1%)
- Pruritus
- Purpura (<1%)
- Rash (sic)
- Seborrhea (<1%)
- Stevens-Johnson syndrome
- Toxic epidermal necrolysis (<1%)
- Urticaria (<1%)
- Xerosis

HAIR
- Hair – alopecia (<1%)
- Hair – alopecia areata

OTHER
- Ageusia (<1%)
- Anaphylactoid reaction
- Dysgeusia (3%)
- Gingivitis (<1%)
- Glossitis (<1%)
- Mastodynia (<1%)
- Myalgia
- Myopathy (<1%)
- Oral mucosal lesions
- Paresthesias
- Parosmia (<1%)
- Priapism
- Sialorrhea
- Stomatitis (<1%)
- Vaginitis (<1%)
- Xerostomia (14%)

FOLIC ACID

Trade name: Folvite (Lederle)
Other common trade names: Acfol; Apo-Folic; Folacin; Folina; Folinsyre; Folsan; Lexpec
Category: Nutritional supplement; water-soluble vitamin
Clinically important, potentially serious interactions with: phenytoin, pyrimethamine

REACTIONS

SKIN
- Acne
- Allergic reactions (sic) (<1%)
- Dermatitis (sic)
- Erythema
- Exanthems
- Flushing (<1%)
- Pruritus (<1%)
- Rash (sic) (<1%)
- Urticaria

OTHER
- Anaphylactoid reaction

FOSCARNET

Trade name: Foscavir (Astra)
Other common trade name: Foscovir
Category: Antiviral; inhibits various viral DNA & RNA polymerases
Clinically important, potentially serious interactions with: ciprofloxacin, cyclosporine, pentamidine, quinolones

REACTIONS

SKIN
- Acne
- Dermatitis (<1%)
- Edema (<1%)
- Exanthems (>5%)
- Facial edema (>5%)
- Fixed eruption
- Flushing (1–5%)
- Herpes simplex (<1%)
- Hyperhidrosis (>5%)
- Leg edema (<1%)
- Penile ulcers
- Periorbital edema
- Peripheral edema
- Pigmentation (>5%)
- Pruritus (>5%)
- Pruritus ani (<1%)
- Psoriasis (<1%)
- Rash (sic) (generalized) (>5%)
- Seborrhea (>5%)
- Toxic epidermal necrolysis
- Ulceration (>5%)
- Urticaria (<1%)
- Vulvar ulceration
- Warts (<1%)
- Xerosis (<1%)

HAIR
- Hair – alopecia (<1%)

OTHER
- Dysgeusia (>5%)
- Hyperesthesia (<1%)
- Gynecomastia (<1%)
- Injection-site pain (1–10%)
- Injection-site thrombophlebitis
- Myalgia (>5%)
- Oral leukoplakia
- Oral ulceration
- Paresthesias (1–10%)
- Stomatitis (<1%)
- Thrombophlebitis (<1%)
- Tongue ulceration (<1%)
- Ulcerative stomatitis (>5%)

FOSFOMYCIN

Trade name: Monurol (Forest)
Category: Antibiotic (acute cystitis)
Clinically important, potentially serious interactions with: metoclopramide

REACTIONS

SKIN
- Angioedema
- Exanthems (<1%)
- Pruritus (<1%)
- Rash (sic) (1.4%)

OTHER
- Myalgia (<1%)
- Paresthesias (<1%)
- Vaginitis (7.6%)
- Xerostomia (<1%)

FOSINOPRIL

Trade name: Monopril (Bristol-Myers Squibb)
Other common trade names: Acenor-M; Dynacil; Fosinorm; Fozitec; Staril; Vasopril
Category: Angiotensin-converting enzyme (ACE) inhibitor
Clinically important, potentially serious interactions with: allopurinol, amiloride, bumetanide, digitalis, diuretics, furosemide, indomethacin, lithium, phenothiazines, salicylates, spironolactone, torsemide

REACTIONS

SKIN
- Angioedema (<1%)
- Bullous pemphigoid
- Edema (<1%)
- Exfoliative dermatitis
- Flushing
- Hyperhidrosis (<1%)
- Photosensitivity (<1%)
- Pruritus (<1%)
- Rash (sic) (<1%)
- Urticaria (<1%)
- Vasculitis

OTHER
- Ageusia (<1%)
- Anaphylactoid reaction
- Dysgeusia (<1%)
- Myalgia (<1%)
- Paresthesias (<1%)
- Xerostomia (<1%)

FURAZOLIDONE

Trade name: Furoxone (Roberts)
Other common trade names: Furion; Furoxona
Category: Nitrofuran antibiotic; antidiarrheal; antiprotozoal
Clinically important, potentially serious interactions with: anorexiants, antidepressants, dextromethorphan, dopamine, ephedrine, epinephrine, fluoxetine, MAO inhibitors, meperidine, paroxetine, phenylephrine, sertraline, sympathomimetics, trazodone. Also tyramine-containing foods

REACTIONS

SKIN
- Contact dermatitis
- Erythema multiforme
- Exanthems (<1%)
- Flushing (with alcohol) (<1%)
- Photosensitivity
- Pruritus
- Rash (sic) (<1%)
- Urticaria (<1%)

OTHER
- Serum sickness

FUROSEMIDE

Trade name: Lasix (Hoechst Marion Roussel)
Other common trade names: Discoid; Dryptal; Frusid; Furorese; Fusid; Lasilix; Urex; Uritol
Category: Sulfonamide loop diuretic; antihypertensive
Clinically important, potentially serious interactions with: ACE-inhibitors, aminoglycoside antibiotics, digitalis, lithium

REACTIONS

SKIN
- Acute febrile neutrophilic dermatosis (Sweet's syndrome)
- Acute generalized exanthematous pustulosis (AGEP)
- Bullous eruption (<1%)
- Bullous pemphigoid
- Cutaneous side effects (sic)
- Epidermolysis bullosa
- Erythema multiforme (<1%)
- Erythema nodosum
- Exanthems

Exfoliative dermatitis
Flushing
Grinspan's syndrome*
Lichenoid eruption
Lupus erythematosus
Periorbital edema
Photosensitivity (1–10%)
Phototoxic reaction
Pruritus (<1%)
Purpura
Pustular eruption
Rash (sic) (<1%)
Stevens-Johnson syndrome
Urticaria
Vasculitis

OTHER
Acute intermittent porphyria
Anaphylactoid reaction
Injection-site erythema (<1%)
Injection-site pain
Paresthesias
Porphyria
Porphyria cutanea tarda
Pseudolymphoma
Thrombophlebitis
Ulcerative stomatitis
Xanthopsia
Xerostomia

*Grinspan's syndrome is the triad of oral lichen planus, diabetes mellitus, and hypertension.

GABAPENTIN

Trade name: Neurontin (Parke-Davis)
Category: Anticonvulsant
Clinically important, potentially serious interactions with: cimetidine

REACTIONS

SKIN
Acne (>1%)
Exanthems
Facial edema (<1%)
Peripheral edema (1.7%)
Pruritus (1.3%)
Purpura (<1%)
Rash (sic) (>1%)
Urticaria

HAIR
Hair – alopecia

OTHER
Gingivitis (<1%)
Glossitis
Myalgia (2%)
Paresthesias (<1%)
Sialorrhea
Stomatitis
Tooth discoloration
Xerostomia (1.7%)

GANCICLOVIR

Trade name: Cytovene (Syntex)
Other common trade names: Cymevan; Cymeven; Cymevene
Category: Antiviral
Clinically important, potentially serious interactions with: didanosine, probenecid, zidovudine

REACTIONS

SKIN
Acne (<1%)
Bullous eruption (<1%)
Diaphoresis
Edema (<1%)
Exanthems (<1%)
Exfoliative dermatitis
Facial edema (<1%)
Fixed eruption (<1%)
Photosensitivity (<1%)
Pigmentation (<1%)
Pruritus (<1%)
Psoriasis
Purpura

Rash (sic) (1–10%)
Stevens-Johnson syndrome
Urticaria (<1%)

HAIR
Hair – alopecia (<1%)

OTHER
Anaphylactoid reaction
Anosmia
Dysgeusia (<1%)
Gingival hypertrophy
Hypesthesia (<1%)
Injection-site edema (<1%)
Injection-site inflammation (2%)
Injection-site pain
Mastodynia (<1%)
Myalgia (<1%)
Oral ulceration (<1%)
Paresthesias (<1%)
Phlebitis (2%)
Tongue disorder (sic) (<1%)
Xerostomia (<1%)

GEMCITABINE

Trade name: Gemzar (Lilly)
Category: Antineoplastic nucleoside analogue
Clinically important, potentially serious interactions with: aldesleukin

REACTIONS

SKIN
Edema (13%)
Exanthems
Hyperhidrosis
Infections (sic) (16%)
Peripheral edema (20%)
Pruritus (13%)
Petechiae (16%)
Rash (sic) (30%)

HAIR
Hair – alopecia (15%)

OTHER
Anaphylactoid reaction
Injection-site reactions (4%)
Myalgia
Paresthesias (10%)
Stomatitis (11%)

GEMFIBROZIL

Trade name: Lopid (Parke-Davis)
Other common trade names: Bolutol; Decrelip; Fibrocit; Gemlipid; Gevilon Uno; Jezil; Lipur
Category: Antihyperlipidemic
Clinically important, potentially serious interactions with: anticoagulants, fluvastatin, lovastatin, pravastatin, simvastatin, warfarin

REACTIONS

SKIN
Abscesses
Acanthosis nigricans
Angioedema
Basal cell carcinoma
Dermatitis (sic) (0.4%)
Eczema (sic) (1.9%)
Erythema multiforme
Exanthems
Exfoliative dermatitis
Ichthyosis
Lichen planus
Lupus erythematosus
Melanoma
Petechiae
Pruritus (0.8%)
Psoriasis
Rash (sic) (1–10%)
Raynaud's phenomenon
Seborrhea
Skin thickening (sic)
Urticaria (0.1%)
Vasculitis
Xerosis

HAIR
Hair – alopecia
Hair – hirsutism

NAILS
Nails – discoloration
Nails – increased growth (sic)

OTHER
Anaphylactoid reaction
Dysgeusia
Hyperesthesia (<1%)
Myalgia
Myopathy
Myositis
Paresthesias (<1%)
Polymyositis
Pseudolymphoma

GENTAMICIN

Trade name: Garamycin (Schering)
Other common trade names: Alcomicin; Cidomycin; Gentalline; Gentalol; Refobacin; Sedanazin
Category: Aminoglycoside antibiotic
Clinically important, potentially serious interactions with: aminoglycosides, amphotericin B, bumetanide, cephalosporins, ethacrynic acid, furosemide, loop diuretics, penicillins, torsemide

REACTIONS

SKIN
Contact dermatitis
Eczematous eruption (sic)
Edema (1–10%)
Erythema (1–10%)
Exanthems
Exfoliative dermatitis
Photosensitivity (<1%)
Pruritus (1–10%)
Purpura
Rash (sic)
Urticaria
Toxic epidermal necrolysis
Vasculitis

HAIR
Hair – alopecia

OTHER
Anaphylactoid reaction
Injection-site erythema
Injection-site necrosis
Injection-site pain (<1%)
Paresthesias
Pseudotumor cerebri (<1%)
Sialorrhea (<1%)
Stomatitis

GLIMEPIRIDE

Trade name: Amaryl (Hoechst Marion Roussel)
Category: Second generation sulfonylurea antidiabetic
Clinically important, potentially serious interactions with: androgens, anticoagulants, beta-blockers, cimetidine, digitalis, fluconazole, gemfibrozil, MAO inhibitors, methyldopa, phenylbutazone, probenecid, salicylates, sulfonamides, tricyclic antidepressants

REACTIONS

SKIN
Allergic reactions (sic) (<1%)
Edema (<1%)
Erythema (<1%)
Exanthems (<1%)
Photosensitivity (<1%)
Pruritus (<1%)
Psoriasis
Rash (sic) (<1%)
Urticaria (<1%)

OTHER
Porphyria cutanea tarda

GLIPIZIDE

Trade name: Glucotrol (Roerig)
Other common trade names: Glibenese; Glipid; Glyde; Melizide; Mindiab; Minidiab; Minodiab
Category: Second generation sulfonylurea antidiabetic
Clinically important, potentially serious interactions with: androgens, anticoagulants, cimetidine, digitalis, fluconazole, gemfibrozil, MAO inhibitors, methyldopa, phenylbutazone, probenecid, salicylates, sulfonamides, tricyclic antidepressants

REACTIONS

SKIN
- Eczema (sic)
- Edema (<1%)
- Erythema (<1%)
- Exanthems (<1%)
- Flushing (<1%)
- Grinspan's syndrome*
- Lichenoid eruption
- Photosensitivity (1–10%)
- Pruritus (<3%)
- Psoriasis (induced)
- Purpura
- Rash (sic) (1–10%)
- Urticaria (1–10%)

OTHER
- Hypesthesia (<3%)
- Myalgia (<3%)
- Oral lichen planus
- Paresthesias (<3%)
- Porphyria (coproporphyria-like)
- Porphyria cutanea tarda

*Grinspan's syndrome: the triad of oral lichen planus, diabetes mellitus, and hypertension.

GLUCAGON

Trade name: Glucagon Emergency Kit (Lilly)
Category: Antihypoglycemic; antispasmodic; antidote
Clinically important, potentially serious interactions with: beta-blockers, oral anticoagulants

REACTIONS

SKIN
- Acute febrile neutrophilic dermatosis (Sweet's syndrome)
- Angioedema
- Epidermolysis bullosa acquisita
- Erythema multiforme
- Erythema nodosum
- Exanthems
- Folliculitis
- Glucagonoma syndrome (necrolytic migratory erythema)
- Pyoderma gangrenosum
- Rash (sic)
- Urticaria (1–10%)
- Vasculitis

OTHER
- Injection-site cutaneous reaction

GLYBURIDE

Trade names: Diabeta (Hoechst Marion Roussel); Glynase (Pharmacia & Upjohn); Micronase (Pharmacia & Upjohn)
Other common trade names: Daonil; Euglucan; Euglucon; Glimel; Hemi-Daonil; Miglucan
Category: Second generation sulfonylurea antidiabetic
Clinically important, potentially serious interactions with: alcohol, beta-blockers, hydantoins, NSAIDs, oral anticoagulants, phenylbutazone, salicylates, sulfonamides, thiazides

REACTIONS

SKIN
- Allergic reaction (sic) (0.21%)
- Angioedema
- Bullous eruption
- Erythema (1–5%)
- Exanthems (1–5%)
- Eyelid edema
- Flushing
- Linear IgA bullous dermatosis
- Pellagra
- Pemphigus
- Photosensitivity (1–10%)
- Pruritus (1–10%)
- Psoriasis
- Purpura
- Rash (sic) (1–10%)
- Urticaria (1–5%)
- Vasculitis
- Vesiculobullous eruption

OTHER
- Hypersensitivity (generalized)
- Myalgia
- Paresthesias (<1%)
- Porphyria cutanea tarda

GOLD & GOLD COMPOUNDS

Generic names:
- Auranofin
  - Trade name: Ridaura (SmithKline Beecham)
- Aurothioglucose
  - Trade name: Solganal (Schering)
- Gold sodium thiomalate (sodium aurothiomalate)
  - Trade name: Myochrysine (Merck)

Other common trade names: Aureotan; Aurothio; Miocrin; Myocrisine; Shiosol; Tauredon
Category: Antiarthritic
Clinically important, potentially serious interactions with: antimalarials, cytotoxic agents, hydroxychloroquine, immunosuppressants, penicillamine

REACTIONS

SKIN
- Acne
- Angioedema (<1%)
- Angiofibromatosis
- Aphthous stomatitis
- Bullous eruption
- Bullous pemphigoid
- Cheilitis
- Contact dermatitis
- Dermatitis (sic)
- Eczematous eruption (sic)
- Erythema annulare centrifugum
- Erythema multiforme
- Erythema nodosum
- Exanthems (>5%)
- Exfoliative dermatitis
- Fixed eruption
- Granuloma annulare
- Herpes zoster
- Lichenoid eruption
- Lichen planus
- Lichen spinulosus
- Lupus erythematosus
- Lymphocytoma cutis
- Pemphigus
- Photosensitivity
- Pigmentation (chrysiasis)
- Pityriasis rosea
- Pruritus (>10%)
- Psoriasis
- Purpura
- Pyoderma gangrenosum

Radiation keratosis
Rash (sic) (>10%)
Seborrheic dermatitis
Squamous cell carcinoma
Toxic dermatitis (sic)
Toxic epidermal necrolysis
Urticaria (1–10%)
Vasculitis
Vitiligo
Xerosis

HAIR
Hair – alopecia (1–10%)
Hair – pigmentation

NAILS
Nails – dystrophy
Nails – exfoliation
Nails – lichen planus
Nails – onycholysis
Nails – pigmentation

OTHER
Acute intermittent porphyria
Burning mouth syndrome
Dysgeusia
Gingivitis (>10%)
Gingivostomatitis
Glossitis (>10%)
Hypersensitivity
Injection-site pain
Mucocutaneous reactions
Oral lichenoid eruption
Oral lichen planus
Oral mucosal eruption
Oral mucosal pigmentation
Oral ulceration
Pseudolymphoma
Stomatitis (>10%)
Vaginitis

GRANISETRON

Trade name: Kytril (SmithKline Beecham)
Other common trade name: Kevatril
Category: Antiemetic & antinauseant
Clinically important, potentially serious interactions with: none

REACTIONS

SKIN
Allergic reaction (sic)
Exanthems
Rash (sic)
Urticaria

HAIR
Hair – alopecia (3%)

OTHER
Anaphylactoid reaction
Hypersensitivity
Dysgeusia (2%)

GRANULOCYTE COLONY-STIMULATING FACTOR (GCSF)

Generic names:
Filgrastim (rG-CSF)
Trade name: Neupogen (Amgen)
Sargramostin (rGM-CSF)
Trade names: Leukine (Immunex); Prokine
Other common trade names: Grasin; Leucogen; Neupogen 30
Category: Hematopoietic growth factor; neutrophil stimulator
Clinically important, potentially serious interactions with: corticosteroids, lithium

REACTIONS

SKIN
Acne
Acute febrile neutrophilic dermatosis (Sweet's syndrome)
Erythema
Erythema nodosum
Exanthems
Exfoliative dermatitis
Flushing (>10%)
Folliculitis
Peripheral edema (1–10%)
Pruritus

Psoriasis
Pyoderma gangrenosum
Rash (sic)
Urticaria
Vasculitis

HAIR
Hair – alopecia (>10%)

OTHER
Anaphylactoid reaction (<1%)
Injection-site bullous eruption
Injection-site erythema
Injection-site nodules
Injection-site pain (1–10%)
Injection-site pruritus
Injection-site urticaria
Lymphoproliferative disease
Myalgia (>10%)
Oral mucosal lesions
Stomatitis (>10%)

GREPAFLOXACIN

Trade name: Raxar (Glaxo Wellcome)
Category: Fluoroquinolone antibiotic
Clinically important, potentially serious interactions with: antacids, antidiabetics, caffeine, cimetidine, cisapride, cyclophosphamide, cyclosporine, iron, loop diuretics, NSAIDs, omeprazole, propranolol, tacrine, theophylline, warfarin

REACTIONS

SKIN
Acne (<1%)
Balanitis (<1%)
Cheilitis (<1%)
Edema (<1%)
Exanthems (<1%)
Exfoliative dermatitis (<1%)
Facial edema (<1%)
Fungal dermatitis (sic) (<1%)
Herpes simplex (<1%)
Hyperhidrosis (<1%)
Peripheral edema (<1%)
Photosensitivity
Phototoxic reaction (2%)
Pruritus (<1%)
Rash (sic) (1.9%)
Toxic epidermal necrolysis (<1%)
Urticaria (<1%)
Vesiculobullous eruption (<1%)
Xerosis (<1%)

HAIR
Hair – alopecia (<1%)

OTHER
Ageusia (<1%)
Bromhidrosis (<1%)
Dysgeusia (17%) (metallic taste)
Gingivitis (<1%)
Glossitis (<1%)
Hypesthesia (<1%)
Myalgia (<1%)
Oral candidiasis (<1%)
Oral ulceration (<1%)
Paresthesias (<1%)
Parosmia (<1%)
Stomatitis (<1%)
Tongue disorder (sic) (<1%)
Tongue edema (<1%)
Tongue pigmentation (<1%)
Vaginitis (3.3%)
Xerostomia (1.1%)

GRISEOFULVIN

Trade names: Fulvicin (Schering); Grifulvin (Ortho); Grisactin (Ayerst); Gris-Peg (Allergan)
Other common trade names: Fulcin; Grisefuline; Griseostatin; Grisovin; Likudin M; Polygris
Category: Antifungal
Clinically important, potentially serious interactions with: alcohol, anticoagulants, barbiturates, cyclosporine, estrogens, salicylates

REACTIONS

SKIN
Allergic reaction (sic) (1–5%)
Angioedema (<1%)
Angular stomatitis

Bullous eruption (<1%)
Candidiasis
Cold urticaria
Erythema multiforme (<1%)
Exanthems
Exfoliative dermatitis
Fixed eruption (<1%)
Flushing
Hemorrhagic eruption (sic)
Herpes zoster
Hypohidrosis
Jarisch-Herxheimer reaction
Kawasaki syndrome
Leprosy (exacerbation)
Lichenoid eruption
Lupus erythematosus
Petechiae
Photosensitivity (1–10%)
Pigmentation
Pityriasis rosea
Pruritus (<1%)
Purpura
Rash (sic) (>10%)
Seborrheic dermatitis
Stevens-Johnson syndrome
Toxic epidermal necrolysis
Urticaria (1–5%)
Vasculitis

NAILS
Nails – yellow
Nails – subungual hemorrhages

OTHER
Acute intermittent porphyria
Anaphylactoid reaction
Black tongue
Dysgeusia
Glossodynia
Gynecomastia
Hypogeusia
Oral thrush (1–10%)
Paresthesias
Porphyria
Porphyria cutanea tarda
Protoporphyria
Serum sickness
Stomatodynia
Xerostomia

GUANABENZ

Trade name: Wytensin (Wyeth)
Other common trade names: Rexitene; Wytens
Category: Alpha$_2$-adrenergic agonist, antihypertensive
Clinically important, potentially serious interactions with: tricyclic antidepressants

REACTIONS

SKIN
Edema (<3%)
Hyperhidrosis
Pruritus (<3%)
Rash (sic) (<3%)

OTHER
Dysgeusia (<3%)
Gynecomastia (<3%)
Sialorrhea
Xerostomia (28%)

GUANADREL

Trade name: Hylorel (Fisons; Medeva)
Category: Adrenergic blocking agent, antihypertensive
Clinically important, potentially serious interactions with: beta-blockers, epinephrine, tricyclic antidepressants, vasodilators

REACTIONS

SKIN
Peripheral edema (28.6%)

OTHER
Glossitis (8.4%)
Paresthesias (25.1%)
Xerostomia (1.7%)

GUANETHIDINE

Trade name: Ismelin (Novartis)
Other common trade names: Apo-Guanethidine; Ismeline
Category: Alpha$_2$-adrenergic agonist, antihypertensive
Clinically important, potentially serious interactions with: epinephrine, MAO inhibitors, minoxidil, phenothiazines, tricyclic antidepressants

REACTIONS

SKIN
- Dermatitis (sic)
- Edema (>10%)
- Exanthems
- Fixed eruption
- Lupus erythematosus
- Purpura
- Urticaria
- Vasculitis

HAIR
- Hair – alopecia

OTHER
- Myalgia
- Paresthesias (>10%)
- Priapism
- Sialorrhea
- Xerostomia (1–10%)

GUANFACINE

Trade name: Tenex (Robins)
Other common trade names: Entulic; Estulic
Category: Alpha$_2$-adrenergic agonist, antihypertensive
Clinically important, potentially serious interactions with: barbiturates, tricyclic antidepressants

REACTIONS

SKIN
- Dermatitis (sic) (<3%)
- Edema
- Exanthems
- Exfoliative dermatitis
- Hyperhidrosis (<3%)
- Peripheral edema
- Pruritus (<3%)
- Purpura (<3%)
- Rash (sic)
- Urticaria

HAIR
- Hair – alopecia

OTHER
- Dysgeusia (<3%)
- Paresthesias (<3%)
- Sialorrhea
- Xerostomia (5–28%)

HALOPERIDOL

Trade name: Haldol (McNeil)
Other common trade names: Dozic; Duraperidol; Haloper; Peridol; Seranace; Serenace
Category: Phenothiazine, antipsychotic & sedative
Clinically important, potentially serious interactions with: CNS depressants, epinephrine, lithium, phenytoin, propranolol

REACTIONS

SKIN
- Acne
- Cellulitis
- Contact dermatitis (<1%)
- Exanthems
- Exfoliative dermatitis
- Flushing
- Hyperhidrosis
- Photosensitivity (<1%)
- Pigmentation (<1%)
- Pruritus (<1%)
- Purpura

Rash (sic) (<1%)
Seborrheic dermatitis
Urticaria

HAIR
Hair – alopecia (<1%)
Hair – alopecia areata
Hair – depigmentation

OTHER
Galactorrhea (<1%)
Gynecomastia (<1%)
Injection-site hypersensitivity
Injection-site pain & itching
Injection-site reactions
Mastodynia
Priapism
Sialorrhea
Xerostomia (<1%)

HALOTHANE

Trade name: Fluothane (Ayerst)
Other common trade names: Halothan; Trothane
Category: Anesthetic
Clinically important, potentially serious interactions with: xanthines

REACTIONS

SKIN
Acne
Angioedema
Exanthems
Sensitivity (sic)
Urticaria

HAIR
Hair – alopecia

HEPARIN

Trade names: Calciparine (DuPont); Hep-Flush; Hep-Lock; Liquaemin; (Organon)
Other common trade names: Calcilean; Calciparin; Caprin; Heparine; Liquemin; Uniparin
Category: Anticoagulant
Clinically important, potentially serious interactions with: anticoagulants, aspirin, dextran, dipyridamole, hydroxychloroquine, salicylates

REACTIONS

SKIN
Allergic reactions (sic) (1–10%)
Angioedema (<1%)
Baboon syndrome
Burning (soles) (sic)
Contact dermatitis
Ecchymoses
Erythema
Exanthems
Fixed eruption
Hemorrhage
Livedo reticularis
Necrosis
Peripheral edema
Petechiae
Pruritus (<1%)
Purpura (>10%)
Rash (sic)
Scleroderma
Skin lesions (sic)
Toxic dermatitis (sic)
Toxic epidermal necrolysis
Urticaria (<1%)
Vasculitis

HAIR
Hair – alopecia

NAILS
Nails – discoloration of lunulae

OTHER
Anaphylactoid reaction
Hypersensitivity
Injection-site eczematous patches (<1%)
Injection-site hematoma
Injection-site induration
Injection-site necrosis (<1%)
Injection-site plaques
Injection-site urticaria
Priapism

HEROIN (DIACETYLMORPHINE)

Trade name: Heroin
Category: A semisynthetic narcotic; substance abuse drug
Clinically important, potentially serious interactions with: no data

REACTIONS

SKIN
- Abscesses
- Acanthosis nigricans
- Acne
- Angioedema
- Blistering (arms)
- Bullous impetigo
- Candidiasis
- Cellulitis
- Contact dermatitis
- Cutaneous side effects (85%)
- Ecthyma
- Ecthyma gangrenosum
- Edema
- Exanthems
- Excoriations
- Fixed eruption
- Folliculitis (candidal)
- Kaposi's sarcoma
- Necrolytic migratory erythema
- Necrosis
- Necrotizing fasciitis
- Pemphigus
- Pemphigus erythematosus
- Perforating collagenosis
- Photosensitivity
- Pigmentation
- Polyarteritis nodosa
- Pruritus
- Purpura
- Pustular eruption
- Toxic epidermal necrolysis
- Ulceration
- Urticaria
- Vasculitis

OTHER
- Hypersensitivity
- Injection-site scarring
- Injection-site ulceration
- Myopathy
- Necrotizing vasculitis (tongue)
- Oral mucosal ulceration (tongue)
- Serum sickness
- Sweat gland necrosis
- Tongue pigmentation (fixed eruption)

HYDRALAZINE

Trade names: Apresazide (Ciba); Apresoline (Novartis); Ser-Ap-Es (Ciba)
Other common trade names: Alphapress; Apdormin; Apresolin; Novo-Hylazin; Solesorin
Category: Vasodilator antihypertensive
Clinically important, potentially serious interactions with: indomethacin, MAO inhibitors, metoprolol, propranolol

Apresazide is hydralazine & hydrochlorothiazide; Ser-Ap-Es is hydralazine, reserpine & hydrochlorothiazide

REACTIONS

SKIN
- Acute febrile neutrophilic dermatosis (Sweet's syndrome)
- Allergic reactions (sic)
- Angioedema (<1%)
- Bullous eruption
- Edema (<1%)
- Erythema nodosum
- Exanthems
- Fixed eruption (<1%)
- Flushing (>10%)
- Lupus erythematosus
- Photosensitivity
- Pruritus
- Purpura
- Pyoderma gangrenosum
- Rash (sic) (<1%)
- Sjøgren's syndrome
- Systemic eczematous contact dermatitis
- Ulceration
- Urticaria
- Vasculitis

OTHER
- Oral ulceration
- Orogenital ulceration
- Paresthesias
- Relapsing polychondritis

HYDROCHLOROTHIAZIDE

Trade names: Aldactazide; Aldoril; Apresazide; Capozide; Dyazide; Esidrix; E-Zide; Hydro-Chlor; Hydro-D; Hydrodiuril; Hydro-Par; Maxzide; Microzide; Oretic; Prinizide; Ser-Ap-Es. (Various pharmaceutical companies.)
Other common trade names: Clothia; Dichlotride; Diu-Melsin; Diuchlor H; Esidrex
Category: Thiazide diuretic; antihypertensive
Clinically important, potentially serious interactions with: antidiabetics, bumetanide, digoxin, lithium, methotrexate, tetracyclines

REACTIONS

SKIN
- Actinic reticuloid
- Bullous eruption (<1%)
- Dermatitis (sic)
- Erythema annulare centrifugum
- Erythema multiforme (<1%)
- Exanthems
- Fixed eruption
- Hyperhidrosis
- Lichenoid eruption
- Lupus erythematosus
- Photoallergic reaction
- Photosensitivity (<1%)
- Phototoxic reaction
- Porokeratosis (Mibelli)
- Pruritus (<1%)
- Purpura
- Rash (sic)
- Systemic eczematous contact dermatitis
- Toxic epidermal necrolysis
- Urticaria
- Vasculitis

OTHER
- Oral lichenoid eruption (erosive)
- Paresthesias
- Pseudoporphyria
- Xerostomia

HYDROFLUMETHIAZIDE

Trade names: Diucardin (Ayerst); Saluron (Mead Johnson)
Other common trade names: Diademil; Hydravern; Hydrenox; Leodrine; Rivosil; Rontyl
Category: Thiazide diuretic; antihypertensive
Clinically important, potentially serious interactions with: antidiabetics, digitalis, furosemide, lithium, loop diuretics

REACTIONS

SKIN
- Photosensitivity (<1%)
- Purpura
- Rash (sic) (<1%)
- Urticaria
- Vasculitis

OTHER
- Dysgeusia
- Paresthesias (<1%)
- Xanthopsia

HYDROMORPHONE

Trade name: Dilaudid (Knoll)
Other common trade names: Dilaudid HP; Palladone
Category: Narcotic analgesic; antitussive
Clinically important, potentially serious interactions with: CNS depressants, cimetidine, phenothiazines, ranitidine, tricyclic antidepressants

REACTIONS

SKIN
- Diaphoresis
- Exanthems
- Flushing (1–10%)
- Pruritus
- Rash (sic) (<1%)
- Urticaria (<1%)

HAIR
- Hair – alopecia

OTHER
- Dysgeusia
- Injection-site reactions
- Paresthesias
- Xerostomia (1–10%)

HYDROXYCHLOROQUINE

Trade name: Plaquenil (Sanofi Winthrop)
Other common trade names: Ercoquin; Oxiklorin; Plaquinol; Quensyl; Toremonil; Yuma
Category: Antimalarial, anti-lupus & antirheumatic
Clinically important, potentially serious interactions with: cyclosporine, digitalis

REACTIONS

SKIN
- Acute generalized exanthematous pustulosis (AGEP)
- Angioedema (<1%)
- Bullous eruption
- Dermatomyositis
- Erythema annulare centrifugum
- Erythema multiforme (<1%)
- Erythroderma
- Exanthems (1–5%)
- Exfoliative dermatitis
- Fixed eruption (<1%)
- Lichenoid eruption
- Photosensitivity
- Pigmentation (1–10%)
- Polymorphous light eruption
- Pruritus (>10%)
- Psoriasis (exacerbation)
- Purpura
- Pustular eruption
- Pustular psoriasis
- Rash (sic) (1–10%)
- Toxic epidermal necrolysis (<1%)
- Urticaria
- Vasculitis

HAIR
- Hair – alopecia
- Hair – pigmentation (bleaching) (1–10%)

NAILS
- Nails – discoloration
- Nails – pigmentation

OTHER
- Dysgeusia
- Gingival pigmentation
- Lymphoproliferative disease
- Myopathy
- Oral mucosal pigmentation
- Oral mucosal ulceration
- Porphyria
- Stomatopyrosis

HYDROXYUREA

Trade name: Hydrea (Bristol-Myers Squibb, Immunex)
Other common trade names: Litalir; Onco-Carbide
Category: Antineoplastic
Clinically important, potentially serious interactions with: fluorouracil

REACTIONS

SKIN
- Acral erythema
- Atrophy
- Cutaneous carcinoma
- Cutaneous side effects (sic)
- Dermatitis (sic) (dry, scaly)
- Dermatomyositis
- Erythema multiforme (<1%)
- Exanthems (1–10%)
- Facial erythema (<1%)
- Fixed eruption (<1%)
- Ichthyosis
- Keratoderma (palmar & plantar)
- Keratoses
- Lichenoid eruption
- Lichen planus
- Lupus erythematosus
- Photosensitivity
- Pigmentation
- Poikiloderma
- Pruritus (<1%)
- Purpura
- Radiation recall (sic)
- Rash (sic)
- Telangiectases
- Tumors
- Ulceration
- Urticaria
- Vasculitis
- Xerosis (1–10%)

HAIR
- Hair – alopecia (1–10%)

NAILS
- Nails – atrophic
- Nails – dystrophy
- Nails – onycholysis
- Nails – pigmentation
- Nails – pigmented bands

OTHER
- Oral mucosal lesions
- Oral ulceration
- Stomatitis (>10%)
- Tongue pigmentation

HYDROXYZINE

Trade names: Atarax (Roerig); Vistaril (Roerig)
Other common trade names: AH3 N; Bobsule; Iremofar; Masmoran; Multipax; Otarex; Paxistil
Category: Antihistamine, anxiolytic & antiemetic
Clinically important, potentially serious interactions with: anticholinergics, CNS depressants

REACTIONS

SKIN
- Angioedema (<1%)
- Edema (<1%)
- Erythema multiforme (<1%)
- Exanthems
- Fixed eruption
- Flushing
- Hyperhidrosis
- Photosensitivity (<1%)
- Purpura
- Rash (sic) (<1%)
- Urticaria

OTHER
- Hypersensitivity
- Injection-site necrosis
- Myalgia (<1%)
- Priapism
- Xerostomia (1–10%)

IBUPROFEN

Trade names: Advil (Wyeth); Medipren; Midol; Motrin (McNeil; Pharmacia & Upjohn); Nuprin; Pamprin; Profen; Rufen; etc.
Other common trade names: Act-3; Anco; Apsifen; Brufen; Ebufac; Lidifen; Proflex; Urem
Category: Nonsteroidal anti-inflammatory (NSAID); antipyretic
Clinically important, potentially serious interactions with: beta-blockers, digoxin, furosemide, lithium, methotrexate, NSAIDs, phenytoin

REACTIONS

SKIN
Angioedema (<1%)
Aphthous stomatitis
Bullous eruption (<1%)
Bullous pemphigoid
Contact dermatitis (<1%)
Dermatitis herpetiformis
Eczematous eruption (sic)
Erythema multiforme (<1%)
Erythema nodosum
Exanthems
Fixed eruption (<1%)
Flushing
Hyperhidrosis
Livedo reticularis
Lupus erythematosus
Pemphigoid
Periorbital edema
Photoallergic reaction
Photosensitivity
Pruritus (1–5%)
Psoriasis (palms)
Purpura
Rash (sic) (>10%)
Stevens-Johnson syndrome (<1%)
Toxic epidermal necrolysis (<1%)
Urticaria (>10%)
Vasculitis
Vesiculobullous eruption

HAIR
Hair – alopecia (<1%)
Hair – disorders (sic)

NAILS
Nails – disorder (sic)
Nails – onycholysis

OTHER
Anaphylactoid reaction (<1%)
Gingival ulceration (<1%)
Gynecomastia (<1%)
Hypersensitivity
Impaired wound healing
Myopathy
Oral lichenoid eruption
Oral mucosal lesions
Oral ulceration
Paresthesias
Pseudoporphyria
Serum sickness
Stomatitis
Xerostomia (<1%)

IDARUBICIN

Trade name: Idamycin (Pharmacia & Upjohn)
Other common trade name: Zavedos
Category: Antineoplastic antibiotic
Clinically important, potentially serious interactions with: aldesleukin

REACTIONS

SKIN
Acral erythema
Bullous eruption (palms & soles)
Exanthems (<1%)
Radiation recall
Rash (sic) (>10%)
Urticaria (>10%)

HAIR
Hair – alopecia (77%)

NAILS
Nails – pigmentary changes

OTHER
- Injection-site urticaria
- Mucositis (50%)
- Necrosis after extravasation (>10%)
- Stomatitis (>10%)

IFOSFAMIDE

Trade name: Ifex (Mead Johnson)
Other common trade names: Holoxan; Ifoxan; Mitoxana; Tronoxal
Category: Antineoplastic; nitrogen mustard
Clinically important, potentially serious interactions with: anticoagulants

REACTIONS

SKIN
- Allergic reactions (sic) (1–10%)
- Dermatitis (sic) (<1%)
- Pigmentation (1–10%)

HAIR
- Hair – alopecia (50–83%)

NAILS
- Nails – ridging (1–10%)

OTHER
- Anaphylactoid reaction
- Oral mucosal lesions
- Phlebitis (2%)
- Sialorrhea (<1%)
- Stomatitis (<1%)

IMIPENEM/CILASTATIN

Trade name: Primaxin (Merck)
Other common trade names: Tenacid; Tienam; Tienam 500; Zienam
Category: Antibiotic
Clinically important, potentially serious interactions with: beta-lactam antibiotics, cyclosporine, probenecid

REACTIONS

SKIN
- Acute generalized exanthematous pustulosis (AGEP)
- Allergic reactions (sic)
- Angioedema (0.2%)
- Candidiasis (0.2%)
- Erythema multiforme (0.2%)
- Exanthems (<1%)
- Flushing (0.2%)
- Hyperhidrosis (0.2%)
- Pruritus (0.3%)
- Pruritus vulvae (0.2%)
- Pustular eruption
- Rash (sic) (4%)
- Toxic epidermal necrolysis (0.2%)
- Urticaria (0.2%)
- Vasculitis

OTHER
- Dysgeusia (0.2%)
- Glossitis (0.2%)
- Hypersensitivity
- Injection-site erythema (0.4%)
- Injection-site pain (0.2%)
- Injection-site phlebitis
- Oral mucosal lesions
- Paresthesias (0.2%)
- Phlebitis (1–10%)
- Sialorrhea (0.2%)

IMIPRAMINE

Trade names: Janimine (Abbott); Tofranil (Novartis)
Other common trade names: Apo-Imipramine; Imidol; Imipramin; Impril; Primonil; Pryleugan
Category: Tricyclic antidepressant
Clinically important, potentially serious interactions with: cimetidine, clonidine, CNS depressants, epinephrine, guanethidine, MAO-inhibitors, sympathomimetics, warfarin

REACTIONS

SKIN
- Angioedema (<1%)
- Ankle edema
- Bullous eruption
- Edema
- Exanthems (1–5%)
- Exfoliative dermatitis
- Fixed eruption (<1%)
- Flushing
- Hyperhidrosis (1–10%)
- Lichen planus
- Lupus erythematosus
- Petechiae
- Photoallergic reaction
- Photosensitivity (<1%)
- Pigmentation
- Pruritus
- Purpura
- Rash (sic)
- Urticaria
- Vasculitis

HAIR
- Hair – alopecia (<1%)
- Hair – alopecia areata

NAILS
- Nails – parrot beak nails

OTHER
- Black tongue
- Dysgeusia (>10%)
- Galactorrhea (<1%)
- Glossitis
- Glossodynia
- Gynecomastia (<1%)
- Hypogeusia
- Mucous membrane desquamation
- Oral mucosal lesions
- Oral ulceration
- Paresthesias
- Stomatitis
- Xerostomia (>10%)

INDAPAMIDE

Trade name: Lozol (Rhône-Poulenc Rorer)
Other common trade names: Dapa-tabs; Fludex; Ipamix; Lozide; Naplin; Natrilix; Pamid
Category: Oral antihypertensive diuretic
Clinically important, potentially serious interactions with: antidiabetics, digoxin, furosemide, lithium, loop diuretics

REACTIONS

SKIN
- Angioedema
- Bullous eruption
- Erythema multiforme
- Exanthems
- Flushing (<5%)
- Hyperhidrosis
- Peripheral edema (<5%)
- Photosensitivity (<1%)
- Pruritus (<5%)
- Purpura
- Rash (sic) (<5%)
- Stevens-Johnson syndrome
- Toxic epidermal necrolysis
- Urticaria (<5%)
- Vasculitis (<5%)

OTHER
- Anaphylactoid reaction
- Paresthesias (<5%)
- Xanthopsia
- Xerostomia (<5%)

INDINAVIR

Trade name: Crixivan (Merck)
Category: Antiviral; protease inhibitor
Clinically important, potentially serious interactions with: astemizole, benzodiazepines, cisapride, ketoconazole, midazolam, rifampin, terfenadine, triazolam. Also grapefruit juice

REACTIONS

SKIN
- Allergic reaction (sic)
- Aphthous stomatitis (<2%)
- Contact dermatitis (<2%)
- Dermatitis (sic) (<2%)
- Eyelid edema (<2%)
- Flushing (<2%)
- Folliculitis (<2%)
- Herpes simplex (<2%)
- Herpes zoster (<2%)
- Hyperhidrosis (<2%)
- Pruritus (<2%)
- Pyogenic granuloma
- Seborrhea (<2%)
- Urticaria (<2%)
- Xerosis (<2%)

HAIR
- Hair – alopecia

NAILS
- Nails – paronychia

OTHER
- Bromhidrosis (<2%)
- Bruxism (<2%)
- Cheilitis (<2%)
- Dysesthesia (<2%)
- Dysgeusia (2.6%)
- Foetor ex ore (<2%)
- Gingivitis (<2%)
- Gynecomastia
- Hypesthesia (<2%)
- Lipodystrophy
- Lipomatosis
- Myalgia (<2%)
- Paresthesias (<2%)
- Xerostomia (0.5%)

INDOMETHACIN

Trade name: Indocin (Merck)
Other common trade names: Amuno; Durametacin; Imbrilon; Indocid; Indolar SR; Vonum
Category: Nonsteroidal anti-inflammatory (NSAID); antipyretic
Clinically important, potentially serious interactions with: ACE-inhibitors, aminoglycosides, aspirin, beta-blockers, cyclosporine, diuretics, lithium, methotrexate, NSAIDs, triamterene

REACTIONS

SKIN
- Angioedema (<1%)
- Aphthous stomatitis (rare)
- Bullous eruption (<1%)
- Contact dermatitis
- Cutaneous side effects (sic)
- Dermatitis herpetiformis (exacerbation)
- Ecchymoses (<1%)
- Eczematous eruption
- Edema
- Erythema multiforme (<1%)
- Erythema nodosum (<1%)
- Exanthems
- Exfoliative dermatitis (<1%)
- Fixed eruption
- Flushing (>1%)
- Generalized eruption (sic)
- Granulomas (plasma cell)
- Hyperhidrosis (<1%)
- Lichen planus
- Pemphigus (rare)
- Periorbital edema
- Petechiae (>1%)
- Photoallergic reaction
- Pruritus (1–10%)
- Psoriasis
- Purpura (<1%)
- Pustular psoriasis
- Rash (sic) (>10%)
- Reiter's syndrome (exacerbation)
- Stevens-Johnson syndrome (<1%)
- Toxic epidermal necrolysis (<1%)

Urticaria
Urticaria pigmentosa
Vasculitis (<1%)

HAIR
Hair – alopecia (<1%)

NAILS
Nails – onycholysis

OTHER
Ageusia
Anaphylactoid reaction (<1%)
Gynecomastia (<1%)
Hypersensitivity (<1%)
Oral lichenoid eruption
Oral mucosal lesions
Oral ulceration
Paresthesias (<1%)
Serum sickness
Temporal arteritis
Tongue edema
Ulcerative stomatitis (<1%)
Xerostomia (rare)

INSULIN

Trade names: Humulin (Lilly); Iletin Lente (Lilly); Novolin R (Bristol-Myers Squibb); NPH (Lilly); Protamine (Lilly); Velosulin (Novo Nordisk)
Other common trade names: Huminsulin; Humulin; Insuman; Velosuline Humaine; Monotard
Category: Antidiabetic
Clinically important, potentially serious interactions with: beta-blockers, MAO-inhibitors

Note: About 25% of patients with insulin allergy have a concomitant history of penicillin allergy.

REACTIONS

SKIN
Allergic reactions (sic)
Angioedema
Bullous eruption
Contact dermatitis
Edema (1–10%)
Exanthems
Flushing
Granulomas (zinc)
Hyperhidrosis (1–10%)
Hyperkeratotic verrucous papules
Keloid formation
Necrosis
Pigmentation
Pigskin appearance (sic)
Pruritus (1–10%)
Purpura
Urticaria (1–10%)
Vasculitis
Xanthomatosis

OTHER
Anaphylactoid reaction (1–10%)
Dermal atrophy
Dermal reactions (sic) (50%)
Hypersensitivity
Hypertrophic lipodystrophy
Injection-site calcification
Injection-site cancer
Injection-site induration
Injection-site pruritus
Lipoatrophy (1–10%)
Lipodystrophy
Lipohypertrophy (1–10%)
Panniculitis
Tumors (nodules)

INTERFERONS, ALFA

Trade names: Alferon N (Purdue Frederick); Infergen (Amgen); Intron A (Schering); Rebetron (Schering); Roferon-A (Roche)
Other common trade names: Roceron-A; Green-Alpha; Laroferon; Introna; Introne
Category: Biologic response modifiers & antineoplastic
Clinically important, potentially serious interactions with: cimetidine, theophylline, vinblastine

Rebetron is interferon & ribavirin

Nota bene: Many of the adverse reactions depend on the nature of the disease being treated. Either hairy cell leukemia [L] or AIDS-related Kaposi's sarcoma [K].

REACTIONS

SKIN
- Acne (1%)
- Behçet's disease
- Bullous eruption
- Candidiasis (1%)
- Contact dermatitis
- Cutaneous malignancy
- Cutaneous necrosis
- Cutaneous vascular lesions (sic)
- Dermatitis herpetiformis
- Discoloration (sic) (<1%)
- Ecchymoses [L]
- Eczematous eruption (sic)
- Edema (11%) [L]
- Exanthems
- Fungal infection (sic) (<1%)
- Herpes simplex (1%)
- Hot flushes (sic) (1%)
- Hyperhidrosis (22%) [L]; (7%) [K]
- Kaposi's sarcoma
- Keratoses
- Lichen myxedematosus
- Lichen planus
- Linear IgA bullous dermatosis
- Lupus erythematosus
- Melanoma
- Necrosis
- Nodules (painful)
- Pemphigus
- Photosensitivity (<1%)
- Pruritus (13%) [L]; (5%) [K]
- Psoriasis
- Purpura
- Rash (sic) (44%) [L]; (11%) [K]
- Raynaud's phenomenon
- Reiter's syndrome (incomplete)
- Sarcoidosis
- Seborrheic dermatitis
- Sjøgren's syndrome
- Telangiectases
- Ulceration
- Urticaria (<3%) [K]
- Vasculitis
- Vitiligo
- Xerosis (17%) [L]; (22%) [K]

HAIR
- Hair – alopecia (1–10%)
- Hair – discoloration
- Hair – hypertrichosis

OTHER
- Anosmia
- Dysgeusia (25%) (metallic taste) [K]
- Injection-site erythema
- Injection-site induration
- Injection-site necrosis
- Injection-site pruritus
- Injection-site vasculitis
- Lymphoma, malignant
- Myalgia (71%) [L]; (69%) [K]
- Myopathy
- Oral lichen planus
- Paresthesias (12%) [L]; (8%) [K]
- Stomatitis (1–10%)
- Xerostomia (>10%)

INTERLEUKIN-2 (See ALDESLEUKIN)

IPODATE

Trade names: Bilivist (Berlex); Oragrafin (Bristol-Myers Squibb)
Category: Cholecystographic contrast medium
Clinically important, potentially serious interactions with: no data

REACTIONS

SKIN
- Allergic reactions (sic)
- Exanthems
- Pruritus
- Purpura
- Rash (sic)
- Urticaria

OTHER
- Anaphylactoid reaction

IPRATROPIUM

Trade names: Atrovent (Boehringer Ingelheim); Combivent (Boehringer Ingelheim)
Category: Aerosol bronchodilator; anticholinergic
Clinically important, potentially serious interactions with: albuterol, dronabinol

Combivent is albuterol & ipratropium

REACTIONS

SKIN
- Contact dermatitis
- Exanthems
- Flushing (<1%)
- Miliaria profunda
- Pruritus (<1%)
- Rash (sic) (1.2%)
- Urticaria (<1%)

HAIR
- Hair – alopecia (<1%)

OTHER
- Anaphylactoid reaction
- Dysgeusia
- Oral mucosal lesions (1–5%)
- Oral mucosal ulceration (<1%)
- Paresthesias (<1%)
- Stomatitis (<1%)
- Xerostomia (3.2%)

IRBESARTAN

Trade name: Avapro (Bristol-Myers Squibb)
Category: Angiotensin II receptor antagonist
Clinically important, potentially serious interactions with: nifedipine, tolbutamide

REACTIONS

SKIN
- Dermatitis (sic) (<1%)
- Ecchymoses (<1%)
- Erythema (<1%)
- Facial edema (<1%)
- Flushing (<1%)
- Pruritus (<1%)
- Rash (sic) (1%)

OTHER
- Oral lesions (<1%)
- Paresthesias (<1%)

ISOCARBOXAZID

Trade name: Marplan (Roche)
Other common trade name: Enerzer
Category: Monoamine oxidase (MAO) inhibitor; antidepressant & antipanic
Clinically important, potentially serious interactions with: amphetamines, barbiturates, dextroamphetamine, disulfiram, dopamine, ephedrine, fluoxetine, levodopa, meperidine, reserpine, sulfonamides, sympathomimetics, tricyclic antidepressants. Also foods containing tyramine

REACTIONS

SKIN
- Exanthems (7%)
- Hyperhidrosis
- Peripheral edema (1–10%)
- Photosensitivity (4%)
- Pruritus (4%)
- Rash (sic)
- Telangiectases

OTHER
- Black hairy tongue
- Xerostomia (1–10%)

ISONIAZID (INH)

Trade names: Laniazid (Lannett); Nydrazid (Bristol-Myers Squibb)
Other common trade names: Cemidon; Diazid; Isotamine; Isozid; Nicotibine; Nicozid; Tibinide
Category: Tuberculostatic
Clinically important, potentially serious interactions with: anticoagulants, benzodiazepines, carbamazepine, cycloserine, disulfiram, hydantoins, meperidine, phenytoin

REACTIONS

SKIN
- Acne
- Acute generalized exanthematous pustulosis (AGEP)
- Angioedema (<1%)
- Bullous eruption
- Contact dermatitis
- Cutaneous side effects (sic)
- Cutis laxa
- Dermatomyositis
- Erythema multiforme (<1%)
- Exanthems
- Exfoliative dermatitis
- Flushing
- Herpes zoster
- Keratoacanthoma
- Lichenoid eruption
- Lupus erythematosus
- Pellagra
- Photosensitivity
- Pruritus
- Purpura
- Pustular eruption
- Rash (sic) (<1%)
- Stevens-Johnson syndrome
- Striae
- Systemic eczematous contact dermatitis
- Toxic epidermal necrolysis (<1%)
- Urticaria (1–5%)
- Vasculitis

HAIR
- Hair – alopecia

NAILS
- Nails – onycholysis

OTHER
- Acute intermittent porphyria
- Hypersensitivity
- Myopathy
- Oral mucosal lesions
- Oral mucosal ulceration
- Paresthesias
- Serum sickness

ISOPROTERENOL

Trade names: Isuprel (Sanofi Winthrop); Medihaler-ISO (3M); Norisodrine (Abbott)
Other common trade names: Isuprel Mistometer; Isuprel Nebulimetro; Saventrine
Category: Adrenergic bronchodilator; sympathomimetic
Clinically important, potentially serious interactions with: general anesthetics, sympathomimetics

REACTIONS

SKIN
- Edema
- Flushing (1–10%)
- Hyperhidrosis (1–10%)
- Pruritus
- Rash (sic)
- Urticaria

OTHER
- Oral mucosal lesions
- Xerostomia (>10%)

ISOSORBIDE

Trade names: Dilatrate-SR (Schwarz); Imdur (Schering); Ismo (Wyeth); Isordil (Wyeth); Monoket (Schwarz); Sorbitrate (Zeneca)
Other common trade names: Cedocard; Eurecor; ISDN; ISMN; Langoran; Maycor; Monicor
Category: Osmotic diuretic; antianginal
Clinically important, potentially serious interactions with: calcium channel blockers, ergot alkaloids

REACTIONS

SKIN
- Acne
- Ankle edema
- Contact dermatitis
- Cyanosis
- Edema (<1%)
- Exanthems
- Exfoliative dermatitis (1–10%)
- Flushing (>10%)
- Hyperhidrosis
- Nodule (sic)
- Pruritus (<1%)
- Rash (sic) (<1%)
- Urticaria

HAIR
- Hair – abnormal texture

OTHER
- Hypesthesia (<1%)
- Xerostomia

ISOTRETINOIN

Trade name: Accutane (Roche)
Other common trade names: Isotrex; Roaccutane; Roaccutan; Roacutan; Roacuttan
Category: Retinoid; inhibits sebaceous gland function
Clinically important, potentially serious interactions with: acitretin, carbamazepine, dexamethasone, etretinate, fish oil supplements, minocycline, tetracycline, vitamin A

REACTIONS

SKIN
- Acne (fulminans)
- Bruising (sic)
- Cheilitis (>90%)
- Desquamation (palms & soles) (5%)
- Eruptive xanthoma
- Erythema multiforme
- Erythema nodosum
- Exanthems
- Facial cellulitis
- Facial scarring
- Fixed eruption

Flushing
Folliculitis
Fragility
Granulation tissue
Herpes (sic)
Hyperhidrosis
Hyperpigmentation
Keloid formation
Keratolysis exfoliativa
Leucoderma
Melasma
Miliaria
Nummular eczema
Pemphigus
Photosensitivity (>10%)
Pityriasis rosea
Pruritus (1–5%)
Pyoderma gangrenosum
Pyogenic granuloma
Telangiectases
Toxic epidermal necrolysis
Urticaria (rare)
Varicosities
Vasculitis
Xerosis (>10%)

HAIR
Hair – alopecia (16%)
Hair – hirsutism
Hair – pili torti (curly hair)
Hair – trichotillomania

NAILS
Nails – dystrophy
Nails – growth
Nails – onycholysis
Nails – median canaliform dystrophy
Nails – paronychia
Nails – periungual hemorrhage

OTHER
Ageusia
Cellulitis (1–10%)
Dysgeusia
Dysosmia
Galactorrhea
Gynecomastia
Myopathy
Pseudoporphyria
Pseudotumor cerebri
Xerostomia (>10%)

ISRADIPINE

Trade name: Dynacirc (Novartis)
Other common trade names: Dynacirc SRO; Lomir; Lomir SRO; Prescal; Vascal
Category: Calcium channel blocker; antihypertensive
Clinically important, potentially serious interactions with: barbiturates, calcium salts, carbamazepine, cyclosporine, digitalis, propranolol, quinidine, theophylline

REACTIONS

SKIN
Edema (7.2%)
Exanthems
Flushing (2.6%)
Hyperhidrosis (<1%)
Pruritus (<1%)
Rash (sic) (1.5%)
Urticaria (<1%)

OTHER
Oral mucosal lesions
Paresthesias (<1%)
Xerostomia (<1%)

ITRACONAZOLE

Trade name: Sporanox (Janssen)
Other common trade names: Isox; Itranax; Sopronox; Sporacid; Sporal; Sporanox 15 D
Category: Antifungal
Clinically important, potentially serious interactions with: alprazolam, anticoagulants, astemizole, cisapride, cyclosporine, digoxin, felodipine, lovastatin, midazolam, phenytoin, sildenafil, terfenadine, triazolam, warfarin

REACTIONS

SKIN
- Acute generalized exanthematous pustulosis (AGEP)
- Angioedema
- Cutaneous side effects (sic)
- Edema (<1%)
- Erythema multiforme
- Exanthems
- Facial dermatitis (papular, id-like)
- Fixed eruption
- Photoallergic reaction
- Phototoxic reaction
- Pruritus (2.5%)
- Purpura
- Rash (sic) (8.6%)
- Skin eruptions (sic)
- Stevens-Johnson syndrome
- Urticaria
- Vasculitis

HAIR
- Hair – alopecia

NAILS
- Nails – beading

OTHER
- Anaphylactoid reaction
- Gynecomastia
- Myalgia (1%)
- Xerostomia

IVERMECTIN

Trade name: Stromectol (Merck)
Category: Parasiticidal
Clinically important, potentially serious interactions with: no data

REACTIONS

SKIN
- Edema
- Exanthems
- Facial edema
- Pruritus (2.8%)
- Rash (sic) (0.9%)
- Urticaria (0.9%)

OTHER
- Myalgia

KANAMYCIN

Trade name: Kantrex (Mead Johnson)
Other common trade names: Kanamycine; Kanamicina; Kanamytrex; Kanescin; Kannasyn
Category: Aminoglycoside antibiotic
Clinically important, potentially serious interactions with: aminoglycosides, amphotericin B, bumetanide, cephalosporins, diuretics, ethacrynic acid, furosemide, penicillins, torsemide

REACTIONS

SKIN
- Edema (>10%)
- Erythema (<1%)
- Exanthems
- Photosensitivity (<1%)
- Pruritus (1–10%)
- Rash (sic) (1–10%)
- Systemic eczematous contact dermatitis
- Urticaria

OTHER
Injection-site pain (<1%)
Paresthesias
Sialorrhea (<1%)

KETAMINE

Trade name: Ketalar (Parke-David)
Other common trade names: Calypsol; Ketalin; Ketanest; Ketolar; Petar
Category: Anesthetic
Clinically important, potentially serious interactions with: barbiturates, hydroxyzine, narcotics, thyroid

REACTIONS

SKIN
Erythema
Rash (sic) (1–10%)

OTHER
Injection-site erythema
Injection-site pain (1–10%)
Sialorrhea (<1%)

KETOCONAZOLE

Trade name: Nizoral (Janssen)
Other common trade names: Aquarius; Fungarest; Fungoral; Ketoderm; Ketoisidin; Nazoltec
Category: Antifungal
Clinically important, potentially serious interactions with: alcohol, alprazolam, anticoagulants, astemizole, chlordiazepoxide, cimetidine, cisapride, cyclosporine, digoxin, midazolam, omeprazole, phenytoin, ranitidine, rifampin, terfenadine, triazolam, warfarin

REACTIONS

SKIN
Allergic reactions (sic)
Angioedema
Contact dermatitis
Eczema (generalized)
Exanthems
Exfoliative dermatitis
Fixed eruption
Jarisch-Herxheimer reaction
Photosensitivity
Pigmentation
Pruritus (1–5%)
Purpura
Rash (sic)
Urticaria
Vasculitis
Xerosis

HAIR
Hair – alopecia
Hair – trichoptilosis

NAILS
Nails – pigmentation

OTHER
Anaphylactoid reaction
Gingival bleeding
Gingival hyperplasia
Gynecomastia (<1%)
Hypersensitivity
Oral hyperpigmentation
Oral lichenoid eruption
Oral mucosal lesions
Myopathy
Paresthesias
Tongue pigmentation

KETOPROFEN

Trade names: Orudis (Wyeth); Oruvail (Wyeth)
Other common trade names: Alrheumat; Alrheumun; Aneol; Bi-Profenid; Gabrilen Retard
Category: Nonsteroidal anti-inflammatory (NSAID)
Clinically important, potentially serious interactions with: aminoglycosides, cyclosporine, lithium, methotrexate, probenecid

REACTIONS

SKIN
- Allergic reactions (sic) (<1%)
- Angioedema (<1%)
- Aphthous stomatitis
- Bullous eruption (<1%)
- Contact dermatitis
- Cutaneous side effects (sic)
- Eczematous eruption (sic) (<1%)
- Erythema multiforme (<1%)
- Exanthems
- Exfoliative dermatitis (<1%)
- Facial edema (<1%)
- Hyperhidrosis (<1%)
- Photocontact dermatitis
- Photosensitivity (<1%)
- Pigmentation (<1%)
- Pruritus (<1%)
- Psoriasis
- Purpura (<1%)
- Rash (sic) (>10%)
- Stevens-Johnson syndrome (<1%)
- Toxic epidermal necrolysis (<1%)
- Urticaria (<1%)

HAIR
- Hair – alopecia (<1%)

NAILS
- Nails – onycholysis (<1%)

OTHER
- Acute intermittent porphyria
- Anaphylactoid reaction (<1%)
- Dysgeusia (<1%)
- Gynecomastia (<1%)
- Myalgia (<1%)
- Oral mucosal lesions
- Paresthesias (<1%)
- Pseudoporphyria
- Sialorrhea (<1%)
- Stomatitis (<1%)
- Xerostomia (<1%)

KETOROLAC

Trade names: Acular (Allergan); Toradol (Syntex)
Other common trade names: Dolac; Kelac; Ketonic; Nodine; Topadol; Torolac; Torvin
Category: Nonsteroidal anti-inflammatory (NSAID)
Clinically important, potentially serious interactions with: aminoglycosides, cyclosporine, lithium, methotrexate, probenecid, salicylates

REACTIONS

SKIN
- Angioedema
- Aphthous stomatitis (<1%)
- Cutaneous side effects (sic) (0.7%)
- Edema (3–9%)
- Exanthems
- Excoriated papules
- Exfoliative dermatitis (<1%)
- Flushing (<1%)
- Hyperhidrosis (1–10%)
- Pruritus (3–9%)
- Purpura (>1%)
- Rash (sic) (>1%)
- Stevens-Johnson syndrome (<1%)
- Toxic epidermal necrolysis (<1%)
- Urticaria

OTHER
- Anaphylactoid reaction (<1%)
- Dysgeusia
- Hypersensitivity
- Injection-site pain (1–10%)
- Myalgia
- Paresthesias
- Stomatitis (>1%)
- Tongue edema (<1%)
- Xerostomia

LABETALOL

Trade names: Normodyne (Schering); Trandate (Glaxo Wellcome)
Other common trade names: Abetol; Amipress; Hybloc; Ipolab; Labrocol; Presolol; Salmagne
Category: Beta-adrenergic blocking agent; antihypertensive
Clinically important, potentially serious interactions with: beta-blockers, calcium channel blockers, cimetidine, clonidine, flecainide, nifedipine, oral contraceptives, tricyclic antidepressants

REACTIONS

SKIN
- Angioedema
- Contact dermatitis
- Cutaneous side effects (sic) (5.5%)
- Eczematous eruption (sic)
- Exanthems
- Flushing
- Hyperhidrosis (<1%)
- Lichenoid eruption
- Lichen planus (bullous)
- Lupus erythematosus
- Pigmentation (slate-gray)
- Pityriasis rubra pilaris
- Pruritus (1–10%)
- Psoriasis (exacerbation)
- Purpura
- Rash (sic) (<1%)
- Raynaud's phenomenon
- Urticaria

HAIR
- Hair – alopecia (reversible)

OTHER
- Anaphylactoid reaction
- Dysgeusia (1–10%)
- Hypesthesia (1%)
- Myopathy
- Paresthesias (7%)
- Peyronie's disease
- Scalp tingling
- Xerostomia

LAMIVUDINE

Trade names: Combivir (Glaxo Wellcome); Epivir (Glaxo Wellcome)
Category: Reverse transcriptase inhibitor; antiviral
Clinically important, potentially serious interactions with: cotrimoxazole

Combivir is lamivudine & zidovudine

REACTIONS

SKIN
- Angioedema
- Exanthems
- Rash (sic) (9%)
- Urticaria

HAIR
- Hair – alopecia

OTHER
- Myalgia (8%)
- Paresthesias (>10%)

LAMOTRIGINE

Trade name: Lamictal (Glaxo Wellcome)
Category: Anticonvulsant
Clinically important, potentially serious interactions with: acetaminophen, carbamazepine, phenytoin, valproic acid

REACTIONS

SKIN
- Acne (1.3%)
- Angioedema (1–10%)
- Ecchymoses (<1%)

Eczema (sic) (<1%)
Erythema (<1%)
Erythema multiforme
Exanthems (1–10%)
Facial edema (<1%)
Flushing (<1%)
Hyperhidrosis (<1%)
Lupus erythematosus
Petechiae (<1%)
Pruritus (3.1%)
Rash (sic) (10%)
Stevens-Johnson syndrome (1–10%)
Toxic epidermal necrolysis
Urticaria (<1%)
Xerosis (<1%)

HAIR
Hair – alopecia (1.3%)
Hair – hirsutism (<1%)

OTHER
Dysgeusia (<1%)
Foetor ex ore (halitosis) (<1%)
Gingival hyperplasia (<1%)
Gingivitis (<1%)
Hypersensitivity (1–10%)
Hypesthesia (<1%)
Myalgia (>1%)
Oral ulceration (<1%)
Paresthesias (>1%)
Porphyria
Pseudolymphoma
Sialorrhea (<1%)
Stomatitis (<1%)
Vaginal candidiasis (<1%)
Vaginitis (4.1%)
Xerostomia (1%)

LANSOPRAZOLE

Trade name: Prevacid (TAP)
Category: Gastric acid secretion (proton pump) inhibitor
Clinically important, potentially serious interactions with: digoxin, ketoconazole, nifedipine, sucralfate, theophylline

REACTIONS

SKIN
Acne (<1%)
Candidiasis (<1%)
Edema (<1%)
Exanthems
Pruritus (<1%)
Rash (sic) (<1%)
Urticaria (<1%)

HAIR
Hair – alopecia (<1%)

OTHER
Black tongue
Dysgeusia (<1%)
Foetor ex ore (halitosis) (<1%)
Glossitis
Gynecomastia (<1%)
Mastodynia (<1%)
Myalgia (<1%)
Paresthesias (<1%)
Stomatitis (<1%)
Xerostomia (<1%)

LATANOPROST

Trade name: Xalatan (Pharmacia & Upjohn)
Category: Anti-glaucoma agent
Clinically important, potentially serious interactions with: none

REACTIONS

SKIN
Allergic skin reactions (sic) (1.1%)
Blepharitis (0.4%)
Ecchymoses (0.2%
Eczema (sic) (0.7%)
Eyelid burning (1.1%)
Eyelid edema (1–4%)
Eyelid erythema (1–4%)
Eyelid pain (0.4%)
Eyelid pruritus (1.7%)
Eyelid stinging (0.4%)
Facial rash
Pruritus (0.2%)

HAIR
Hair – eyelash hyperpigmentation
Hair – hypertrichosis

OTHER
Gynecomastia (0.2%)

LETROZOLE

Trade name: Femara (Novartis)
Category: Nonsteroidal aromatase inhibitor; advanced breast cancer
Clinically important, potentially serious interactions with: none

REACTIONS

SKIN
Exanthems (5%)
Hot flushes (6%)
Hyperhidrosis (<5%)
Pruritus (2%)
Psoriasis (5%)
Vesicular eruption (5%)

HAIR
Hair – alopecia (<5%)

LEUPROLIDE

Trade name: Lupron (TAP)
Other common trade names: Carcinil; Enantone; Lucrin; Procren Depot; Procrin; Tapros
Category: Gonadotropin-releasing hormone; advanced prostate carcinoma
Clinically important, potentially serious interactions with: none

REACTIONS

SKIN
Dermatitis (sic) (5%)
Ecchymoses (<5%)
Edema (1–10%)
Exanthems
Flushing
Lupus erythematosus
Peripheral edema (12%)
Pigmentation (<5%)
Pruritus (<5%)
Purpura (<1%)
Rash (sic) (1–10%)
Urticaria
Xerosis (<5%)

HAIR
Hair – alopecia (<5%)
Hair – growth (sic) (<1%)

OTHER
Dysgeusia (<5%)
Injection-site inflammation
Injection-site pruritus
Gynecomastia (7%)
Mastodynia (7%)
Myalgia (3%)
Paresthesias (<5%)
Thrombophlebitis (2%)

LEVAMISOLE

Trade name: Ergamisol (Janssen)
Other common trade names: Decaris; Detrax 40; Dewormis 50; Ketrax; Solaskil; Vermisol
Category: Antineoplastic adjunct, immune modulator & anthelmintic
Clinically important, potentially serious interactions with: alcohol, anticoagulants, disulfiram, phenytoin

REACTIONS

SKIN
Angioedema (<1%)
Cutaneous side effects (sic)
Dermatitis (sic) (8%)
Edema (1–10%)
Erythema annulare
Erythema multiforme
Exanthems
Exfoliative dermatitis
Fixed eruption

Hemorrhagic eruption
Lichenoid eruption
Necrosis
Pemphigus
Periorbital edema
Pruritus (1%)
Psoriasis
Purpura
Rash (sic)
Urticaria (<1%)
Vasculitis
Xerosis

HAIR
Hair – alopecia (3%)

OTHER
Anaphylactoid reaction
Dysgeusia (8%) (metallic taste)
Erosive lichen planus
Myalgia (3%)
Oral mucosal lesions
Oral ulceration
Paresthesias (2%)
Parosmia (1%)
Stomatitis (3%)

LEVOBUNOLOL

Trade name: Betagan (Allergan)
Other common trade names: Bunolgan; Gotensin; Vistagan; Vistagen
Category: Ophthalmic beta-adrenergic blocker
Clinically important, potentially serious interactions with: antidiabetics, beta-blockers, quinidine, tacrine, verapamil

REACTIONS

SKIN
Burning
Contact dermatitis
Lichen planus
Pruritus (<1%)
Rash (sic) (<1%)
Stinging
Urticaria

HAIR
Hair – alopecia (1–10%)

OTHER
Hypersensitivity

LEVODOPA

Trade names: Dopar (Roberts); Larodopa (Roche); Sinemet (DuPont)
Other common trade names: Brocadopa; Dopaflex; Doparl; Eldopal; Levodopa-Woelm
Category: Antidyskinetic; anti-parkinsonian
Clinically important, potentially serious interactions with: antacids, MAO inhibitors, phenytoin, vitamin B_6

Sinemet is carbidopa & levodopa

REACTIONS

SKIN
Diaphoresis
Exanthems
Flushing
Hyperhidrosis
Leukoplakia
Lupus erythematosus
Melanoma
Pemphigus
Purpura
Rash (sic)
Urticaria

HAIR
Hair – alopecia
Hair – repigmentation

NAILS
Nails – increased growth

OTHER
Ageusia
Black cartilage
Bruxism
Chromhidrosis (1–10%)

Dysgeusia
Glossopyrosis
Phlebitis
Priapism
Sialorrhea
Xerostomia (1–10%)

LEVOFLOXACIN

Trade name: Levaquin (Ortho-McNeil)
Category: Quinolone antibiotic
Clinically important, potentially serious interactions with: antidiabetics, NSAIDs, theophylline, warfarin

REACTIONS

SKIN
Edema (0.1%)
Erythema
Erythema multiforme
Erythema nodosum (<3%)
Hyperhidrosis (0.1%)
Photosensitivity (<0.1%)
Pruritus (1.6%)
Purpura (<0.5%)
Rash (sic) (1.7%)
Stevens-Johnson syndrome
Urticaria (<0.5%)

OTHER
Anaphylactoid reaction
Candidiasis (0.3%)
Dysgeusia (0.2%)
Myalgia (<0.5%)
Paresthesias
Vaginitis (1.8%)
Xerostomia (<1%)

LEVOTHYROXINE

Trade names: Levothyroid (Forest); Levoxyl (Jones); Synthroid (Knoll)
Other common trade names: Berlthyrox; Droxine; Eferox; Eltroxin; Levothyrox; Thevier
Category: Synthetic thyroid hormone
Clinically important, potentially serious interactions with: anticoagulants, iron, phenytoin, propranolol, tricyclic antidepressants

REACTIONS

SKIN
Acne
Allergic reactions (sic)
Angioedema
Dermatitis herpetiformis
Flushing
Hyperhidrosis (<1%)
Nevi
Pruritus
Rash (sic)
Urticaria

HAIR
Hair – alopecia (<1%)

OTHER
Pseudotumor cerebri (in infants)

LIDOCAINE

Trade names: Anestacon (Alcon); Xylocaine (Astra)
Category: Anesthetic; antiarrhythmic
Clinically important, potentially serious interactions with: beta-blockers, cimetidine, phenytoin, propranolol

REACTIONS

SKIN
Angioedema
Bullous eruption
Contact dermatitis
Eczema (sic)
Edema (<1%)

Erythema multiforme
Exanthems
Exfoliative dermatitis
Fixed eruption
Lupus erythematosus
Pigmentation
Pruritus (<1%)
Purpura
Rash (<1%)
Stevens-Johnson syndrome
Urticaria

OTHER
Acute intermittent porphyria
Anaphylactoid reaction
Embolia cutis medicamentosa (Nicolau syndrome)
Hypersensitivity
Paresthesias (<1%)
Stomatitis

LINCOMYCIN

Trade name: Lincocin (Pharmacia & Upjohn)
Other common trade names: Albiotic; Cillimicina; Cillimycin; Lincocine; Princol; Zumalin
Category: Macrolide antibiotic
Clinically important, potentially serious interactions with: antacids, neuromuscular blocking agents

REACTIONS

SKIN
Allergic reactions (sic)
Angioedema
Contact dermatitis
Erythema multiforme
Exanthems
Exfoliative dermatitis
Photosensitivity
Pruritus
Pruritus ani (<1%)
Purpura
Rash (sic) (<1%)
Stevens-Johnson syndrome (<1%)
Urticaria (<1%)
Vesiculobullous eruptions

OTHER
Anaphylactoid reaction
Glossitis (<1%)
Injection-site erythema
Oral mucosal lesions
Serum sickness
Stomatitis (<1%)
Vaginitis (<1%)

LIOTHYRONINE

Trade name: Cytomel (SmithKline Beecham), Triostat (SmithKline Beecham)
Other common trade names: Cynomel; T3; Tertroxin; Thyronine; Trijodthyronin BCN
Category: Synthetic thyroid hormone
Clinically important, potentially serious interactions with: anticoagulants, iron, metoprolol, phenytoin

REACTIONS

SKIN
Allergic reaction (sic)
Hyperhidrosis (<1%)
Rash (sic)
Urticaria

HAIR
Hair – alopecia (<1%)

OTHER
Phlebitis (1%)

LISINOPRIL

Trade names: Prinivil (Merck); Prinizide (Merck); Zestril (Zeneca)
Other common trade names: Acerbon; Alapril; Carace; Coric; Prinil; Tensopril; Vivatec
Category: Angiotensin-converting enzyme (ACE) inhibitor; antihypertensive
Clinically important, potentially serious interactions with: allopurinol, bumetanide, digitalis, diuretics, furosemide, lithium, salicylates, torsemide

Prinizide is lisinopril & hydrochlorothiazide

REACTIONS

SKIN
- Angioedema (0.1%)
- Bullous eruption
- Diaphoresis (<1%)
- Edema (1%)
- Erythema (1%)
- Exanthems
- Facial edema (<1%)
- Flushing (<1%)
- Lichenoid eruption
- Peripheral edema (<1%)
- Photosensitivity (<1%)
- Pruritus (1.2%)
- Purpura
- Rash (sic) (1.5%)
- Ulceration (ischemic skin ulcer) (sic)
- Urticaria (<1%)
- Vasculitis (<1%)

HAIR
- Hair – alopecia (<1%)

OTHER
- Anaphylactoid reaction (<1%)
- Dysesthesia (<1%)
- Dysgeusia
- Mastodynia (<1%)
- Myalgia (0.5%)
- Paresthesias (0.8%)
- Xerostomia (<1%)

LITHIUM

Trade names: Eskalith (Beecham); Lithobid (Novartis); Lithonate (Solvay); Lithotabs (Solvay)
Other common trade names: Hynorex Retard; Lithicarb; Lithizine; Priadel; Teralithe
Category: Antidepressants, antipsychotic & antimanic
Clinically important, potentially serious interactions with: ACE-inhibitors, CNS depressants, carbamazepine, fluoxetine, haloperidol, indomethacin, iodide salts, NSAIDs, phenothiazines, phenylbutazones, piroxicam, thiazides

REACTIONS

SKIN
- Acanthosis nigricans
- Acne
- Angioedema
- Angular cheilitis
- Atopic dermatitis
- Bullous eruption
- Cutaneous side effects (sic)
- Darier's disease
- Dermatitis (sic)
- Dermatitis herpetiformis
- Discoloration of fingers & toes (sic) (<1%)
- Eczema (sic)
- Edema
- Erythema multiforme
- Exanthems
- Exfoliative dermatitis
- Follicular keratosis (sic)
- Folliculitis
- Hidradenitis suppurativa
- Hyperplasia (verrucous)
- Ichthyosis
- Linear IgA bullous dermatosis
- Keratoderma
- Keratosis pilaris
- Lichen planus
- Lichen simplex chronicus
- Linear IgA bullous dermatosis
- Lupus erythematosus
- Morphea
- Myxedema
- Papular eruption (elbows)
- Port-wine stain
- Prurigo nodularis

Pruritus (<1%)
Psoriasis
Purpura
Pustular eruption
Pustular psoriasis
Rash (sic) (1–10%)
Seborrheic dermatitis
Subcorneal pustular dermatosis (Sneddon-Wilkinson)
Telangiectases
Tinea versicolor
Toxicoderma
Ulceration (lower extremities)
Urticaria
Vasculitis
Verrucous lesions (sic)
Warts
Xerosis

HAIR
Hair – alopecia
Hair – alopecia areata
Hair – brittle
Hair – changes in texture

NAILS
Nails – dystrophy
Nails – onychomadesis
Nails – psoriasis
Nails – transverse bands (Beau's lines)

OTHER
Dysgeusia (>10%)
Geographic tongue
Gingival hyperplasia
Glossodynia
Lichenoid stomatitis
Oral ulceration
Pseudolymphoma
Pseudotumor cerebri (<1%)
Sialorrhea
Stomatitis
Stomatodynia
Vaginal ulceration
Xerostomia (<1%)

LOMEFLOXACIN

Trade name: Maxaquin (Searle)
Other common trade names: Logiflox; Ontop
Category: Broad-spectrum quinolone antibacterial
Clinically important, potentially serious interactions with: azlocillin, betaxolol, caffeine, cimetidine, cyclosporine, metoprolol, probenecid, warfarin

REACTIONS

SKIN
Allergic reactions (sic) (<1%)
Ankle edema
Eczema (sic)
Edema (<1%)
Exanthems
Exfoliation (sic) (<1%)
Facial edema (<1%)
Flushing (<1%)
Genital pruritus (sic)
Hyperhidrosis (<1%)
Photosensitivity (2.4%)
Phototoxic reaction
Pruritus (<1%)
Purpura (<1%)
Pustular eruption
Rash (sic) (<1%)
Stevens-Johnson syndrome
Toxicoderma (sic)
Urticaria (<1%)
Vasculitis

OTHER
Dysgeusia (<1%)
Hypersensitivity
Myalgia (<1%)
Paresthesias (<1%)
Tongue pigmentation (<1%)
Vaginal candidiasis
Vaginitis (<1%)
Xerostomia (<1%)

LOMUSTINE

Trade name: CeeNU (Mead Johnson)
Other common trade names: Belustine; CCNU; Cecenu; Lomeblastin; Lucostine; Lundbeck
Category: Nitrosurea alkylating antineoplastic
Clinically important, potentially serious interactions with: cimetidine, phenobarbital

REACTIONS

SKIN
- Acral erythema
- Flushing
- Neutrophilic eccrine hidradenitis
- Rash (sic) (1–10%)

HAIR
- Hair – alopecia (<1%)

OTHER
- Stomatitis (1–10%)

LOPERAMIDE

Trade name: Imodium (Janssen)
Other common trade names: Brek; Diarstop-L; Imossel; Lop-Dia; Loperhoe; Stopit; Vancotil
Category: Antidiarrheal
Clinically important, potentially serious interactions with: CNS depressants, phenothiazines, tricyclic antidepressants

REACTIONS

SKIN
- Erythema nodosum
- Exanthems
- Rash (sic)
- Urticaria

HAIR
- Hair – alopecia

OTHER
- Gingivitis
- Hypersensitivity
- Oral mucosal lesions (1.1%)
- Xerostomia

LORACARBEF

Trade name: Lorabid (Lilly)
Category: Beta-lactam antibiotic
Clinically important, potentially serious interactions with: aminoglycosides, anticoagulants, cimetidine, cyclosporine, omeprazole, probenecid, ranitidine

REACTIONS

SKIN
- Erythema multiforme (<1%)
- Pruritus (<1%)
- Rash (sic) (1.2%)
- Urticaria (<1%)

OTHER
- Candidal vaginitis (1.3%)

LORATADINE

Trade name: Claritin (Schering)
Other common trade names: Civeran; Claratyne; Claritine; Lisino; Lorastine; Velodan; Zeos
Category: H_1-receptor antihistamine & antiasthmatic
Clinically important, potentially serious interactions with: alcohol, procarbazine

REACTIONS

SKIN
- Angioedema (>2%)
- Dermatitis (sic) (>2%)
- Erythema multiforme (>2%)
- Exanthems
- Flushing (>2%)
- Hyperhidrosis (>2%)
- Peripheral edema (>2%)
- Photosensitivity (>2%)
- Pruritus (>2%)
- Purpura (>2%)
- Rash (sic) (>2%)
- Urticaria (>2%)
- Xerosis (>2%)

HAIR
- Hair – alopecia (>2%)
- Hair – dry (sic) (>2%)

OTHER
- Anaphylactoid reaction (>2%)
- Dysgeusia (>2%)
- Gynecomastia (>2%)
- Hypesthesia (>2%)
- Mastodynia (1–10%)
- Myalgia (>2%)
- Paresthesias (>2%)
- Sialorrhea (>2%)
- Stomatitis (>2%)
- Vaginitis (>2%)
- Xerostomia (>10%)

LORAZEPAM

Trade name: Ativan (Wyeth)
Other common trade names: Durazolam; Laubeel; Merlit; Punktyl; Tavor; Temesta; Titus
Category: Benzodiazepine anxiolytic; anticonvulsant; antiemetic
Clinically important, potentially serious interactions with: alcohol, CNS depressants, clarithromycin, digitalis, fluconazole, itraconazole, ketoconazole, levodopa, loxapine, MAO inhibitors, miconazole, morphine, tricyclic antidepressants, verapamil

REACTIONS

SKIN
- Dermatitis (sic) (1–10%)
- Erythema multiforme
- Exanthems
- Fixed eruption
- Hyperhidrosis (>10%)
- Pruritus
- Purpura
- Rash (sic) (>10%)
- Stevens-Johnson syndrome
- Urticaria

HAIR
- Hair – alopecia
- Hair – hirsutism

OTHER
- Gingival lichenoid reaction
- Injection-site pain (>10%)
- Injection-site phlebitis (>10%)
- Paresthesias
- Pseudolymphoma
- Sialopenia (>10%)
- Sialorrhea
- Xerostomia (>10%)

LOSARTAN

Trade names: Cozaar (Merck); Hyzaar (Merck)
Category: Angiotensin-converting enzyme (ACE) inhibitor; antihypertensive
Clinically important, potentially serious interactions with: cimetidine

Hyzaar is losartan & hydrochlorothiazide

REACTIONS

SKIN
- Angioedema
- Dermatitis (sic) (<1%)
- Ecchymoses (<1%)
- Erythema (<1%)
- Facial edema (<1%)
- Flushing (<1%)
- Hyperhidrosis (<1%)
- Photosensitivity (<1%)
- Pruritus (<1%)
- Purpura
- Rash (<1%)
- Urticaria (<1%)
- Xerosis (<1%)

HAIR
- Hair – alopecia (<1%)

OTHER
- Ageusia
- Dysgeusia (<1%)
- Myalgia (1%)
- Paresthesias (<1%)

LOVASTATIN

Trade name: Mevacor (Merck)
Other common trade names: Lovalip; Mevinacor; Nergadan; Rovacor; Taucor
Category: Antihyperlipidemic; HMG-CoA reductase inhibitor
Clinically important, potentially serious interactions with: anticoagulants, clofibrate, cyclosporine, danazol, erythromycin, gemfibrozil, itraconazole, levothyroxine, niacin

REACTIONS

SKIN
- Erythema multiforme
- Exanthems
- Lupus erythematosus
- Pruritus (5.2%)
- Rash (sic) (5.2%)
- Stevens-Johnson syndrome
- Toxic epidermal necrolysis
- Urticaria
- Vasculitis

HAIR
- Hair – alopecia (>1%)

OTHER
- Dysgeusia (0.8%)
- Gynecomastia (1–10%)
- Hyposmia
- Myalgia (2.4%)
- Myopathy (1–10%)
- Paresthesias (>1%)
- Stomatitis
- Xerostomia (>1%)

LOXAPINE

Trade name: Loxitane (Lederle)
Other common trade names: Desconex; Loxapac
Category: Tricyclic antipsychotic, anxiolytic & antidepressant
Clinically important, potentially serious interactions with: benzodiazepines, bromocriptine, carbamazepine, CNS depressants, guanabenz, MAO inhibitors

REACTIONS

SKIN
- Cutaneous side effects (sic)
- Dermatitis (sic)
- Exanthems
- Facial edema
- Hyperhidrosis
- Photosensitivity (<1%)
- Pigmentation (<1%)
- Pruritus (<1%)
- Purpura
- Rash (sic) (<1%)
- Seborrhea
- Urticaria

HAIR
- Hair – alopecia

OTHER
- Galactorrhea (<1%)
- Gynecomastia (<1%)
- Myopathy
- Paresthesias
- Priapism (<1%)
- Xerostomia (>10%)

MAPROTILINE

Trade name: Ludiomil (Novartis)
Other common trade names: Delgian; Maprostad; Melodil; Mirpan; Psymion; Retinyl
Category: Tetracyclic antidepressant
Clinically important, potentially serious interactions with: anticholinergics, benzodiazepines, CNS antidepressants, guanethidine, MAO inhibitors, phenothiazines, propranolol, sympathomimetics, thyroid

REACTIONS

SKIN
- Acne
- Edema
- Erythema multiforme
- Exanthems (1–5%)
- Flushing
- Hyperhidrosis
- Ichthyosis
- Petechiae
- Photosensitivity
- Pruritus
- Purpura
- Rash (sic) (>10%)
- Stevens-Johnson syndrome
- Urticaria
- Vasculitis

HAIR
- Hair – alopecia

OTHER
- Black tongue
- Dysgeusia
- Galactorrhea
- Gynecomastia (<1%)
- Sialorrhea
- Stomatitis
- Xerostomia (22%)

MARIHUANA (MARIJUANA)

Trade name: Marihuana
Category: Hallucinogen
Clinically important, potentially serious interactions with: no data

REACTIONS

SKIN
- Exanthems
- Pruritus
- Urticaria

OTHER
- Anaphylactoid reaction

MAZINDOL

Trade names: Mazanor (Wyeth); Sanorex (Novartis)
Other common trade names: Diestet; Liofindol; Solucaps; Teronac
Category: Anorexiant (appetite suppressant)
Clinically important, potentially serious interactions with: barbiturates, guanethidine, MAO inhibitors, tricyclic antidepressants

REACTIONS

SKIN
- Edema
- Exanthems
- Hyperhidrosis
- Rash (sic)
- Urticaria

OTHER
- Dysgeusia
- Paresthesias
- Xerostomia

MEBENDAZOLE

Trade name: Vermox (Janssen)
Other common trade names: Amycil; Bantenol; Lomper; Mindol; Nemasol; Pantelmin; Toloxim
Category: Anthelmintic
Clinically important, potentially serious interactions with: carbamazepine, phenytoin

REACTIONS

SKIN
- Allergic reactions (sic)
- Angioedema (rare)
- Exanthems
- Rash (sic) (<1%)
- Urticaria

HAIR
- Hair – alopecia

OTHER
- Xerostomia

MECHLORETHAMINE

Trade name: Mustargen (Merck)
Other common trade names: Mustine; Mustine Hydrochloride Boots
Category: Antineoplastic
Clinically important, potentially serious interactions with: aldesleukin

REACTIONS

SKIN
- Acanthosis nigricans
- Angioedema
- Bullous eruption

Cellulitis
Contact dermatitis
Epidermal cysts
Erythema multiforme (<1%)
Exanthems (<1%)
Fungal infection (sic)
Herpes zoster (<1%)
Hyperpigmentation
Pruritus
Purpura
Rash (sic) (<1%)
Squamous cell carcinoma
Stevens-Johnson syndrome
Urticaria
Xerosis

HAIR
Hair – alopecia (1–10%)

OTHER
Anaphylactoid reaction (1–10%)
Dysgeusia (1–10%)
Hypersensitivity (1–10%)
Injection-site extravasation (1–10%)
Injection-site thrombophlebitis (1–10%)

MECLIZINE

Trade name: Antivert (Roerig-Pfizer)
Other common trade names: Bonamine; Dramine; Peremesin; Postadoxin; Postafen; Suprimal
Category: Antiemetic & antivertigo
Clinically important, potentially serious interactions with: anticholinergics, CNS depressants, neuroleptics

REACTIONS

SKIN
Angioedema (<1%)
Exanthems
Photosensitivity (<1%)
Rash (sic) (<1%)
Urticaria

OTHER
Myalgia (<1%)
Xerostomia (1–10%)

MECLOFENAMATE

Trade name: Meclomen (Parke-Davis)
Other common trade names: Kyroxan; Melvon; Movens
Category: Nonsteroidal anti-inflammatory (NSAID)
Clinically important, potentially serious interactions with: aminoglycosides, anticoagulants, cyclosporine, methotrexate, warfarin

REACTIONS

SKIN
Angioedema (<1%)
Aphthous stomatitis
Edema (>1%)
Erythema multiforme (<1%)
Erythema nodosum (<1%)
Erythroderma
Exanthems (1–5%)
Exfoliative dermatitis (<1%)
Fixed eruption (<1%)
Lupus erythematosus (rare)
Photosensitivity
Pruritus (>1%)
Psoriasis (exacerbation)
Purpura (>1%)
Rash (sic) (3–9%)
Stevens-Johnson syndrome (<1%)
Toxic epidermal necrolysis (<1%)
Urticaria (>1%)
Vasculitis
Vesiculobullous eruption

HAIR
Hair – alopecia (<1%)

OTHER
Dysgeusia (<1%)
Hypersensitivity

- Oral ulceration
- Paresthesias (<1%)
- Serum sickness
- Stomatitis (1–3%)
- Xerostomia

MEDROXYPROGESTERONE

Trade names: Amen (Carnrick); Curretab (Solvay); Cycrin (ESI Lederle); Depo-Provera (Pharmacia & Upjohn); Provera (Pharmacia & Upjohn)
Other common trade names: Aragest 5; Clinofem; Gestapuran; Perlutex; Progevera; Ralovera
Category: Progestin; antineoplastic
Clinically important, potentially serious interactions with: aminoglutethimide, phenytoin, rifampin

REACTIONS

SKIN
- Acne (1–5%)
- Allergic reactions (sic) (<1%)
- Angioedema
- Ankle edema
- Chloasma (<1%)
- Edema (>10%)
- Erythema nodosum
- Exanthems
- Flushing
- Hemorrhagic eruption (sic)
- Hyperhidrosis (<1%)
- Melasma (<1%)
- Mucha-Habermann disease
- Pruritus (1–10%)
- Rash (sic) (1–5%)
- Scleroderma (<1%)
- Urticaria
- Xerosis (<1%)

HAIR
- Hair – alopecia (1–5%)
- Hair – hirsutism (<1%)

OTHER
- Anaphylactoid reaction (<1%)
- Bromhidrosis (<1%)
- Galactorrhea (<1%)
- Gynecomastia (<1%)
- Injection-site pain (<1%)
- Mastodynia (1–5%)
- Paresthesias (<1%)
- Thrombophlebitis (<1%)
- Vaginitis (1–5%)

MEFENAMIC ACID

Trade name: Ponstel (Parke-Davis)
Other common trade names: Dysman; Lysalgo; Mefac; Mefic; Parkemed; Ponstan; Ponstyl
Category: Nonsteroidal anti-inflammatory (NSAID)
Clinically important, potentially serious interactions with: aminoglycosides, anticoagulants, cyclosporine, lithium, methotrexate

REACTIONS

SKIN
- Angioedema (<1%)
- Bullous pemphigoid
- Erythema multiforme (<1%)
- Exanthems
- Exfoliative dermatitis
- Facial edema
- Fixed eruption
- Hyperhidrosis
- Photosensitivity
- Pruritus (1–10%)
- Purpura
- Rash (sic) (>10%)
- Stevens-Johnson syndrome (<1%)
- Toxic epidermal necrolysis (<1%)
- Urticaria (<1%)
- Vasculitis

OTHER
- Anaphylactoid reaction
- Oral ulceration

MEFLOQUINE

Trade name: Lariam (Roche)
Other common trade names: Laricam; Mephaquin; Mephaquine
Category: Antimalarial
Clinically important, potentially serious interactions with: beta-blockers, chloroquine, quinidine, quinine

REACTIONS

SKIN
- Erythema
- Erythema multiforme
- Exanthems
- Exfoliative dermatitis
- Facial dermatitis
- Pruritus
- Rash (sic)
- Stevens-Johnson syndrome
- Toxic epidermal necrolysis
- Urticaria
- Vasculitis

HAIR
- Hair – alopecia (<1%)

OTHER
- Myalgia

MELPHALAN

Trade name: Alkeran (Glaxo Wellcome)
Category: Antineoplastic; nitrogen mustard
Clinically important, potentially serious interactions with: cyclosporine

REACTIONS

SKIN
- Angioedema
- Eccrine squamous syringometaplasia
- Edema
- Exanthems
- Petechiae
- Pruritus (1–10%)
- Purpura
- Rash (sic) (1–10%)
- Urticaria
- Vasculitis (1–10%)

HAIR
- Hair – alopecia (1–10%)

NAILS
- Nails – pigmented bands
- Nails – transverse white bands (Beau's lines)

OTHER
- Anaphylactoid reaction
- Hypersensitivity (1–10%)
- Oral mucosal lesions
- Oral ulceration
- Stomatitis (1–10%)

MEPERIDINE

Trade name: Demerol (Sanofi Winthrop)
Other common trade names: Dolantin; Dolestine; Dolosal; Opistan; Pethidine; Petidin
Category: Narcotic agonist analgesic
Clinically important, potentially serious interactions with: acyclovir, cimetidine, CNS depressants, fluoxetine, furazolidine, isocarboxazid, isoniazid, MAO inhibitors, phenelzine, phenothiazines, phenytoin, ranitidine, ritonavir, selegiline, tranylcypromine, tricyclic antidepressants

REACTIONS

SKIN
- Angioedema
- Diaphoresis
- Flushing

Herpes (sic)
Necrotizing angiitis
Pruritus
Rash (sic)
Toxic epidermal necrolysis
Urticaria

OTHER
Cold microabscesses
Embolia cutis medicamentosa (Nicolau syndrome)
Injection-site erythema
Injection-site pain (1–10%)
Injection-site scarring
Injection-site ulceration
Myopathy
Xerostomia (1–10%)

MEPHENYTOIN

Trade name: Mesantoin (Novartis)
Other common trade names: Epilan-Gerot; Epilanex
Category: Hydantoin anticonvulsant
Clinically important, potentially serious interactions with: chloramphenicol, cyclosporine, disulfiram, dopamine, isoniazid, itraconazole

REACTIONS

SKIN
Acne
Angioedema
Bullous eruption
Cutaneous side effects (sic)
Dermatomyositis
Edema
Erythema multiforme
Exanthems
Exfoliative dermatitis
Lupus erythematosus
Pigmentation
Pruritus
Purpura
Scleroderma
Stevens-Johnson syndrome
Toxic epidermal necrolysis
Urticaria

HAIR
Hair – alopecia

OTHER
Gingival hyperplasia
Oral mucosal eruption
Polyarteritis nodosa
Stomatitis

MEPHOBARBITAL

Trade name: Mebaral (Sanofi Winthrop)
Other common trade name: Prominal
Category: Long-acting barbiturate; anticonvulsant
Clinically important, potentially serious interactions with: benzodiazepines, chloramphenicol, CNS depressants, methylphenidate, propoxyphene, valproic acid

REACTIONS

SKIN
Angioedema (<1%)
Exanthems
Exfoliative dermatitis (<1%)
Purpura
Rash (sic) (<1%)
Stevens-Johnson syndrome (<1%)
Urticaria

OTHER
Serum sickness
Thrombophlebitis (<1%)

MEPROBAMATE

Trade names: Equanil (Wyeth); Miltown (Wallace)
Other common trade names: Harmonin; Meprate; Miltaun; Praol; Probamyl; Urbilat; Visanon
Category: Antianxiety
Clinically important, potentially serious interactions with: CNS depressants

REACTIONS

SKIN
Allergic reactions (sic)
Angioedema (<1%)
Bullous eruption (<1%)
Cutaneous side effects (sic)
Dermatitis (sic) (<1%)
Ecchymoses
Eczematous eruption
Erythema multiforme (<1%)
Erythema nodosum (<1%)
Exanthems
Exfoliative dermatitis
Fixed eruption (<1%)
Lupus erythematosus (aggravated)
Pemphigus
Pemphigus foliaceus
Peripheral edema (<1%)
Petechiae
Photosensitivity
Pityriasis rosea
Pruritus (<1%)
Purpura (<1%)
Rash (sic) (1–10%)
Stevens-Johnson syndrome (<1%)
Toxic epidermal necrolysis (<1%)
Toxic erythema
Urticaria
Vasculitis

OTHER
Acute intermittent porphyria
Anaphylactoid reaction
Gynecomastia
Oral mucosal eruption
Oral ulceration
Paresthesias
Polyarteritis nodosa
Porphyria
Stomatitis
Xerostomia

MERCAPTOPURINE

Trade name: Purinethol (Glaxo Wellcome)
Other common trade names: Classen; Ismipur; Leukerin; Puri-Nethol
Category: Antineoplastic; antimetabolite; immunosuppressant
Clinically important, potentially serious interactions with: allopurinol, anticoagulants, doxorubicin, methotrexate

REACTIONS

SKIN
Acral erythema
Dermatitis
Edema
Exanthems
Lichenoid eruption
Lupus erythematosus
Palmar-plantar erythema
Pellagra
Petechiae
Photosensitivity
Pigmentation (1–10%)
Pruritus
Purpura
Radiation recall
Rash (sic) (1–10%)
Toxic epidermal necrolysis
Urticaria

HAIR
Hair – alopecia

NAILS
Nails – loss (sic)

OTHER
Glossitis (<1%)
Oral mucosal lesions
Stomatitis (1–10%)

MESALAMINE

Trade names: Asacol (Procter Gamble); Pentasa (Hoechst Marion Roussel); Rowasa (Solvay)
Other common trade names: Asacolitin; Claversal; Mesasal; Pentasa SR; Salafalk; Tidocol
Category: Anti-inflammatory; bowel-disease suppressant
Clinically important, potentially serious interactions with: none

REACTIONS

SKIN
- Acne (1.2%)
- Allergic reactions (sic)
- Ecchymoses
- Eczema (sic)
- Edema (1.2%)
- Erythema
- Erythema nodosum
- Exanthems
- Facial edema
- Folliculitis
- Hyperhidrosis (3%)
- Lichen planus
- Lupus erythematosus
- Mucocutaneous lymph node syndrome (Kawasaki syndrome)
- Peripheral edema (0.61%)
- Photosensitivity
- Pruritus (1.2%)
- Psoriasis
- Pyoderma gangrenosum
- Rash (sic) (3%)
- Urticaria
- Vasculitis
- Xerosis

HAIR
- Hair – alopecia (0.86%)

NAILS
- Nails – disorder (sic)

OTHER
- Dysgeusia
- Hypersensitivity
- Myalgia (3%)
- Oral candidiasis
- Oral lichenoid eruption
- Oral ulceration
- Paresthesias

MESNA

Trade name: Mesnex (Mead Johnson)
Other common trade names: Mexan; Uromitexan
Category: Hemorrhagic cystitis prophylactic
Clinically important, potentially serious interactions with: warfarin

REACTIONS

SKIN
- Allergic reactions (sic)
- Angioedema
- Erythema
- Exanthems
- Fixed eruption
- Flushing
- Pruritus (<1%)
- Rash (sic) (<1%)
- Urticaria

OTHER
- Dysgeusia (>10%)
- Oral mucosal lesions
- Oral mucosal ulceration

MESORIDAZINE

Trade name: Serentil (Boehringer)
Other common trade name: Mesorin
Category: Phenothiazine antipsychotic
Clinically important, potentially serious interactions with: barbiturates, CNS depressants, levodopa, piperazine, propranolol

REACTIONS

SKIN
- Angioedema
- Contact dermatitis
- Eczema (sic)
- Edema
- Erythema
- Exfoliative dermatitis
- Flushing
- Hyperhidrosis
- Hypohidrosis (>10%)
- Lupus erythematosus
- Photosensitivity
- Pigmentation (blue-gray) (<1%)
- Pruritus
- Rash (sic) (1–10%)
- Seborrhea
- Urticaria
- Xerosis

HAIR
- Hair – alopecia

OTHER
- Anaphylactoid reaction
- Galactorrhea (<1%)
- Gynecomastia
- Hypertrophic papillae of tongue
- Mastodynia (1–10%)
- Paresthesias
- Priapism (<1%)
- Sialorrhea
- Xerostomia

METAXALONE

Trade name: Skelaxin (Carnrick)
Category: Skeletal muscle relaxant
Clinically important, potentially serious interactions with: no data

REACTIONS

SKIN
- Pruritus
- Rash (sic)
- Urticaria

OTHER
- Anaphylactoid reaction

METFORMIN

Trade name: Glucophage (Bristol-Myers Squibb)
Other common trade names: Diabex; Diaformin; Diformin; Glucomet; Metforal; Metomin
Category: Antidiabetic
Clinically important, potentially serious interactions with: cimetidine, furosemide

REACTIONS

SKIN
- Eczema (sic)
- Erythema (transient)
- Exanthems
- Grinspan's syndrome*
- Lichenoid eruption
- Photosensitivity (1–10%)
- Pruritus
- Purpura
- Rash (sic) (1–10%)
- Urticaria (1–10%)
- Vasculitis

OTHER
- Dysgeusia (3%)

*Grinspan's syndrome: the triad of oral lichen planus, diabetes mellitus, and hypertension.

METHADONE

Trade name: Dolophine (Roxane)
Other common trade names: Eptadone; L-Polamidon; Mephenon; Metadon; Physeptone
Category: Narcotic analgesic; antitussive; suppressant (narcotic abstinence syndrome)
Clinically important, potentially serious interactions with: barbiturates, cimetidine, CNS depressants, MAO inhibitors, phenothiazines, phenytoin, rifampin, tricyclic antidepressants

REACTIONS

SKIN
- Angioedema
- Cellulitis
- Edema (face)
- Exanthems
- Flushing
- Hyperhidrosis
- Pruritus (<1%)
- Purpura
- Rash (sic) (<1%)
- Urticaria (<1%)

OTHER
- Injection-site burning
- Injection-site induration
- Injection-site pain (1–10%)
- Xerostomia (1–10%)

METHAMPHETAMINE

Trade name: Desoxyn (Abbott)
Category: Central nervous system stimulant
Clinically important, potentially serious interactions with: barbiturates, guanethidine, MAO inhibitors

REACTIONS

SKIN
- Acaraphobia
- Hyperhidrosis (1–10%)
- Lichenoid eruption
- Pigmentation
- Rash (sic) (<1%)
- Urticaria (<1%)

OTHER
- Dysgeusia
- Polyarteritis nodosa
- Xerostomia (1–10%)

METHANTHELINE

Trade name: Banthine (SCS)
Other common trade name: Vagantin
Category: Gastrointestinal anticholinergic & antispasmodic
Clinically important, potentially serious interactions with: amantadine, anticholinergics, arbutamine, atenolol, clozapine, digoxin, haloperidol, phenothiazines, tricyclic antidepressants

REACTIONS

SKIN
- Exanthems
- Exfoliative dermatitis
- Flushing
- Hypohidrosis
- Urticaria
- Xerosis

OTHER
- Ageusia
- Anaphylactoid reaction
- Dysgeusia
- Sialopenia
- Xerostomia

METHAZOLAMIDE

Trade name: Neptazane (Storz)
Category: Carbonic anhydrase inhibitor; sulfonamide diuretic
Clinically important, potentially serious interactions with: cyclosporine, digitalis, ephedrine, phenytoin, quinidine, salicylates

REACTIONS

SKIN
- Exanthems (<1%)
- Photosensitivity
- Purpura
- Stevens-Johnson syndrome
- Toxic epidermal necrolysis
- Urticaria
- Vasculitis

OTHER
- Dysgeusia (>10%)
- Paresthesias

METHENAMINE

Trade names: Hiprex; Mandelamine; Urex; Urised (PolyMedica); Uroqid
Other common trade names: Haiprex; Hip-Rex; Hipeksal; Hippramine; Reflux; Urotractan
Category: Urinary tract antibacterial
Clinically important, potentially serious interactions with: carbonic anhydrase inhibitors, sulfonamides

REACTIONS

SKIN
- Erythema multiforme (<1%)
- Exanthems
- Fixed eruption (<1%)
- Photosensitivity
- Pruritus (<1%)
- Rash (sic) (1–10%)
- Systemic eczematous contact dermatitis
- Urticaria

OTHER
- Stomatitis

METHICILLIN

Trade name: Staphcillin (Mead Johnson)
Other common trade names: Estafcilina; Lucoperin; Mechicillin
Category: Penicillinase-resistant penicillin
Clinically important, potentially serious interactions with: anticoagulants, atenolol, cyclosporine, disulfiram, methotrexate, probenecid

REACTIONS

SKIN
- Angioedema
- Bullous eruption
- Ecchymoses
- Erythema multiforme
- Exanthems
- Exfoliative dermatitis
- Hematomas
- Jarisch-Herxheimer reaction
- Pruritus
- Pustular psoriasis
- Rash (sic) (1–10%)
- Stevens-Johnson syndrome
- Urticaria

OTHER
- Anaphylactoid reaction
- Black tongue
- Dysgeusia
- Glossitis
- Glossodynia
- Injection-site pain
- Oral candidiasis
- Phlebitis (<1%)
- Serum sickness (<1%)
- Stomatitis
- Stomatodynia
- Vaginitis
- Xerostomia

METHIMAZOLE

Trade name: Tapazole (Lilly)
Other common trade names: Strumazol; Thacapzol; Thiamazol; Thyrozol; Unimazole
Category: Antithyroid agent
Clinically important, potentially serious interactions with: anticoagulants, digitalis, lithium, metoprolol, potassium iodide, propranolol

REACTIONS

SKIN
- Cutaneous side effects (sic) (28% in high dosages)
- Edema (<1%)
- Exanthems
- Fixed eruption
- Lupus erythematosus (1–10%)
- Pigmentation
- Pruritus
- Purpura
- Rash (sic) (>10%)
- Urticaria
- Vasculitis

HAIR
- Hair – alopecia (<1%)

OTHER
- Ageusia (1–10%)
- Aplasia cutis congenita
- Dysgeusia
- Oral ulceration
- Myalgia
- Paresthesias (<1%)
- Polyarteritis nodosa
- Scalp defects (sic)
- Serum sickness

METHOCARBAMOL

Trade name: Robaxin (Robins)
Other common trade names: Carbametin; Carxin; Lumirelax; Miowas; Ortoton; Robinax; Trolar
Category: Skeletal muscle relaxant
Clinically important, potentially serious interactions with: CNS depressants

REACTIONS

SKIN
- Allergic reactions (sic) (1–10%)
- Exanthems
- Flushing (1–10%)
- Pruritus
- Rash (sic)
- Urticaria

OTHER
- Anaphylactoid reaction
- Dysgeusia
- Injection-site pain (<1%)
- Thrombophlebitis (<1%)

METHOHEXITAL

Trade name: Brevital (Lilly)
Other common trade names: Brietal; Brietal Sodium; Brevimytal
Category: General anesthetic
Clinically important, potentially serious interactions with: CNS depressants, narcotic analgesics, propranolol

REACTIONS

SKIN
- Angioedema
- Erythema
- Exanthems
- Rash (sic)
- Urticaria

OTHER
- Anaphylactoid reaction
- Injection-site edema

Injection-site pain (18%)
Injection-site phlebitis
Sialorrhea
Thrombophlebitis (<1%)

METHOTREXATE

Trade names: Folex (Pharmacia & Upjohn); Mexate (Mead Johnson); Rheumatrex (Lederle)
Other common trade names: Farmitrexat; Lantarel; Ledertrexate; Maxtrex; Metex; Texate
Category: Anti-inflammatory, antiarthritic & antimetabolite
Clinically important, potentially serious interactions with: alcohol, aminoglycosides, amiodarone, cephalothin, chloroquine, cisplatin, colchicine, cyclosporine, diclofenac, ibuprofen, indomethacin, ketoprofen, magnesium trisalicylate, naproxen, NSAIDs, penicillins, phenylbutazone, probenecid, retinoids, salicylates, sulfamethoxazole, sulfapyridine, sulindac, trimethoprim, vincristine

REACTIONS

SKIN
Acne
Acral erythema
Acute inflammation (sic) (reactivation)
Bullous eruption
Burning (palms & soles)
Candidiasis
Capillaritis
Carcinoma (sic)
Cutaneous necrolysis (sic)
Cutaneous side effects (sic)
Dermatitis (sic)
Ecchymoses
Eccrine squamous syringometaplasia
Epidermal necrosis (sic)
Erosion of psoriatic plaques (sic)
Erosions
Erythema (>10%)
Erythema multiforme
Erythroderma
Exanthems (15%)
Folliculitis
Furunculosis
Herpes simplex
Melanoma
Nodules
Photosensitivity (5%)
Pigmentation (1–10%)
Pruritus (1–5%)
Purpura
Radiation recall
Radiodermatitis (reactivation)
Rash (sic) (1–3%)
Scabies (reactivation)
Squamous cell carcinoma
Stevens-Johnson syndrome
Sunburn (reactivation)
Telangiectases
Toxic epidermal necrolysis (<1%)
Ulceration
Urticaria
Vasculitis (>10%)

HAIR
Hair – alopecia (1–3%)
Hair – pigmented bands

NAILS
Nails – discoloration
Nails – onycholysis
Nails – paronychia
Nails – pigmentation

OTHER
Anaphylactoid reaction (1–10%)
Dysgeusia
Gingivitis (>10%)
Glossitis (>10%)
Gynecomastia
Malignant lymphoma
Oral mucositis
Oral ulceration
Peyronie's disease
Porphyria cutanea tarda
Pseudolymphoma
Stomatitis (3–10%)

METHOXSALEN

Trade names: 8-MOP (ICN); Oxsoralen (ICN)
Other common trade names: Geroxalen; Meladinine; Oxsoralon; Puvasoralen; Ultra-MOP
Category: Repigmenting agent & antipsoriatic
Clinically important, potentially serious interactions with: chloroquine, griseofulvin, nalidixic acid, phenothiazines, sulfonamides, tetracyclines, thiazides

REACTIONS

SKIN
- Acne
- Basal cell carcinoma
- Bowen's disease
- Bullous eruption (with UVA)
- Bullous pemphigoid
- Burning (1–10%)
- Burns
- Cancer (sic)
- Cheilitis (1–10%)
- Contact dermatitis
- Eczematous eruption (sic)
- Edema (1–10%)
- Exanthems
- Freckles (1–10%)
- Granuloma annulare
- Herpes simplex
- Herpes zoster
- Hypopigmentation (1–10%)
- Lupus erythematosus
- Miliaria
- Pemphigoid
- Photoallergic reaction
- Photocontact dermatitis
- Photosensitivity
- Phototoxic reaction
- Pigmentation
- Porokeratosis (actinic)
- Prurigo
- Pruritus (>10%)
- Purpura
- Rash (sic) (1–10%)
- Scleroderma
- Seborrheic dermatitis
- Skin pain
- Squamous cell carcinoma
- Tumors (sic)
- Urticaria
- Vasculitis
- Vitiligo
- Warts

HAIR
- Hair – hypertrichosis

NAILS
- Nails – photo-onycholysis
- Nails – pigmentation

OTHER
- Lymphoproliferative disease

METHSUXIMIDE

Trade name: Celontin (Parke-Davis)
Other common trade name: Petinutin
Category: Succinimide anticonvulsant
Clinically important, potentially serious interactions with: phenytoin, valproic acid

REACTIONS

SKIN
- Acanthosis nigricans
- Erythema multiforme
- Exanthems
- Exfoliative dermatitis (<1%)
- Lupus erythematosus (>10%)
- Periorbital edema
- Pruritus
- Purpura
- Rash (sic)
- Stevens-Johnson syndrome (>10%)
- Urticaria (<1%)

HAIR
- Hair – alopecia
- Hair – hirsutism

OTHER
- Gingival hyperplasia
- Oral ulceration

METHYCLOTHIAZIDE

Trade name: Enduron (Abbott)
Other common trade names: Enduron-M; Thiazidil; Urimor
Category: Thiazide diuretic; antihypertensive
Clinically important, potentially serious interactions with: lithium

REACTIONS

SKIN
- Erythema multiforme
- Exanthems
- Photosensitivity (<1%)
- Purpura
- Rash (sic)
- Stevens-Johnson syndrome
- Urticaria

OTHER
- Anaphylactoid reaction
- Dysgeusia
- Paresthesias

METHYLDOPA

Trade names: Aldomet (Merck); Aldoril (Merck)
Other common trade names: Densul; Dopamet; Equibar; Hydopa; Polinal; Presinol; Prodopa
Category: Central alpha-agonist antihypertensive
Clinically important, potentially serious interactions with: beta-blockers, iron, levodopa, lithium, tolbutamide

Aldoril is methyldopa & hydrochlorothiazide

REACTIONS

SKIN
- Ankle edema
- Eczematous eruption
- Erythema multiforme (<1%)
- Erythema nodosum
- Exanthems
- Fixed eruption
- Granulomas
- Lichenoid eruption
- Lichen planus
- Lupus erythematosus (<1%)
- Papulo-vesicular eruption
- Peripheral edema (>10%)
- Petechiae
- Photosensitivity
- Pigmentation
- Pruritus
- Purpura
- Rash (sic) (<1%)
- Seborrheic dermatitis
- Stevens-Johnson syndrome
- Toxic epidermal necrolysis
- Urticaria
- Vasculitis

HAIR
- Hair – alopecia

OTHER
- Acute intermittent porphyria
- Black tongue (<1%)
- Cheilitis
- Galactorrhea
- Gynecomastia (<1%)
- Hypersensitivity
- Myalgia
- Oral lichenoid eruption
- Oral mucosal eruption
- Oral ulceration
- Paresthesias (<1%)
- Xerostomia (1–10%)

METHYLPHENIDATE

Trade name: Ritalin (Novartis)
Other common trade names: Centedrin; Rilatine; Rubifen
Category: Central nervous system stimulant
Clinically important, potentially serious interactions with: guanethidine, MAO inhibitors, phenobarbital, phenytoin, primidone, tricyclic antidepressants, warfarin

REACTIONS

SKIN
- Angioedema
- Edema (eyelids)
- Eosinophilic syndrome
- Erythema multiforme
- Exanthems
- Exfoliative dermatitis
- Fixed eruption
- Hyperhidrosis
- Photosensitivity
- Purpura
- Rash (sic) (<1%)
- Urticaria
- Vasculitis

HAIR
- Hair – alopecia

OTHER
- Hypersensitivity (1–10%)
- Injection-site abscess
- Xerostomia

METHYLTESTOSTERONE

Trade names: Android (ICN); Oreton (ICN); Testred (ICN); Virilon (Star)
Other common trade names: Androral; Enarmon; Teston; Testotonic "B"; Testovis; Viromone
Category: Androgen; antineoplastic
Clinically important, potentially serious interactions with: anticoagulants, cyclosporine

REACTIONS

SKIN
- Acanthosis nigricans
- Acne (>10%)
- Contact dermatitis
- Edema (>10%)
- Exanthems
- Flushing (1–5%)
- Furunculosis
- Lichenoid eruption
- Lupus erythematosus
- Pruritus
- Psoriasis
- Purpura
- Seborrhea
- Seborrheic dermatitis
- Striae
- Urticaria

HAIR
- Hair – alopecia
- Hair – hirsutism (1–10%)

OTHER
- Anaphylactoid reaction
- Gynecomastia (<1%)
- Hypersensitivity (<1%)
- Injection-site pain
- Mastodynia (>10%)
- Paresthesias
- Priapism (>10%)
- Stomatitis

METHYSERGIDE

Trade name: Sansert (Novartis)
Other common trade names: Deseril; Desernil; Deserril; Deseryl
Category: Vascular headache prophylactic; ergot alkaloid
Clinically important, potentially serious interactions with: beta-blockers, clarithromycin, erythromycin, troleandomycin

REACTIONS

SKIN
- Collagenosis (sic)
- Exanthems
- Flushing
- Hypermelanosis
- Lupus erythematosus
- Orange-peel skin (sic)
- Peripheral edema (1–10%)
- Pruritus
- Rash (sic) (1–10%)
- Raynaud's phenomenon
- Scleroderma
- Skin reactions (sic)
- Telangiectases
- Urticaria

HAIR
- Hair – alopecia

OTHER
- Hyperesthesia (<1%)
- Myalgia
- Paresthesias

METOCLOPRAMIDE

Trade names: Octamide (Pharmacia & Upjohn); Reglan (Robins)
Other common trade names: Duraclamid; Emex; Gastronerton; Gastrocil; Mygdalon; Primperan
Category: Dopaminergic blocking agent; peristaltic stimulant; antiemetic
Clinically important, potentially serious interactions with: cyclosporine, digitalis, levodopa, opiate analgesics, procainamide, quinidine, tacrine

REACTIONS

SKIN
- Allergic reactions (sic)
- Angioedema
- Exanthems
- Flushing
- Rash (sic) (1–10%)
- Urticaria

OTHER
- Blue tongue
- Galactorrhea
- Gynecomastia
- Mastodynia (1–10%)
- Paresthesias
- Porphyria
- Xerostomia (1–10%)

METOLAZONE

Trade names: Mykrox (Medeva); Zaroxolyn (Medeva)
Other common trade names: Barolyn; Diondel; Metenix 5; Normelan; Xuret
Category: Thiazide diuretic; antihypertensive
Clinically important, potentially serious interactions with: antidiabetics, bumetanide, digitalis, furosemide, lithium, methotrexate

REACTIONS

SKIN
- Edema (<2%)
- Exanthems
- Photosensitivity (<2%)
- Pruritus (<2%)
- Purpura
- Rash (sic) (<2%)
- Toxic epidermal necrolysis

Urticaria (<2%)
Vasculitis
Xerosis (<2%)
Dysgeusia (<2%)
Paresthesias (<2%)
Xanthopsia (<2%)
Xerostomia (<2%)

OTHER
Anaphylactoid reaction (<2%)

METOPROLOL

Trade names: Lopressor (Novartis); Toprol (Astra)
Other common trade names: Beloc-Zoc; Betaloc; Betazok; Mycol; Seloken-Zok; Selozok
Category: Beta-adrenergic blocking agent; antihypertensive
Clinically important, potentially serious interactions with: calcium channel blockers, clonidine, diltiazem, flecainide, nifedipine, oral contraceptives, salicylates, verapamil

REACTIONS

SKIN
Angioedema
Eczematous eruption
Erythema multiforme
Exanthems
Gangrene (feet)
Hyperhidrosis
Hyperkeratosis (palms & soles)
Lichenoid eruption
Lupus erythematosus
Peripheral edema (1%)
Pityriasis rubra pilaris
Prurigo
Pruritus (1–5%)
Purpura
Psoriasis (induction and aggravation of)
Rash (<5%)
Raynaud's phenomenon (<1%)
Scleroderma
Toxic epidermal necrolysis
Urticaria
Xerosis

HAIR
Hair – alopecia

NAILS
Nails – bluish
Nails – dystrophy
Nails – onycholysis
Nails – transverse depression (sic)

OTHER
Dysgeusia
Oculo-mucocutaneous syndrome
Oral lichenoid eruption
Paresthesias
Peyronie's disease
Polymyalgia
Scalp tingling

METRONIDAZOLE

Trade names: Flagyl (Searle); Metrocream (Galderma); Metrogel (Galderma); Noritate (Dermik)
Other common trade names: Arilin; Ariline; Asuzol; Clont; Fossyol; Rozagel; Rozex; Zadstat
Category: Antiprotozoal, anthelmintic & antibiotic
Clinically important, potentially serious interactions with: alcohol, anticoagulants, astemizole, barbiturates, disulfiram, fluorouracil, phenobarbital, phenytoin, terfenadine, warfarin

REACTIONS

SKIN
Acute generalized exanthematous pustulosis (AGEP)
Angioedema
Candidiasis (exacerbation)
Contact dermatitis
Exanthems
Fixed eruption
Flushing
Pityriasis rosea
Pruritus (1–5%)
Rash (sic)

Toxic epidermal necrolysis
Urticaria

OTHER
Acute intermittent porphyria
Dysgeusia (metallic taste) (<1%)
Glossitis
Gynecomastia
Hypersensitivity (<1%)
Injection-site vasculitis
Oral mucosal eruption
Oral ulceration
Paresthesias
Serum sickness
Stomatitis
Thrombophlebitis (<1%)
Tongue furry (<1%)
Vaginal candidiasis (<1%)
Xerostomia (<1%)

MEXILETINE

Trade name: Mexitil (Boehringer Ingelheim)
Other common trade names: Mexihexal; Mexilen; Mexitec
Category: Antiarrhythmic
Clinically important, potentially serious interactions with: allopurinol, caffeine, phenytoin, rifampin, theophylline

REACTIONS

SKIN
Edema (3.8%)
Exanthems
Exfoliative dermatitis (<1%)
Hyperhidrosis (<1%)
Pruritus
Purpura
Rash (sic) (3.8%)
Stevens-Johnson syndrome (<1%)
Urticaria
Xerosis (<1%)

HAIR
Hair – alopecia (<1%)

OTHER
Dysgeusia (<1%)
Paresthesias (3.8%)
Salivary changes (sic) (<1%)
Xerostomia (2.8%)

MEZLOCILLIN

Trade name: Mezlin (Bayer)
Other common trade name: Baypen
Category: Beta-lactamase-sensitive penicillin
Clinically important, potentially serious interactions with: cyclosporine, heparin, methotrexate, probenecid, tetracycline

REACTIONS

SKIN
Allergic reactions (sic)
Angioedema
Contact dermatitis
Ecchymoses
Erythema multiforme
Exanthems
Exfoliative dermatitis (<1%)
Hematomas
Jarisch-Herxheimer reaction
Pruritus
Rash (sic) (<1%)
Stevens-Johnson syndrome
Urticaria

OTHER
Anaphylactoid reaction
Black tongue
Dysgeusia
Glossitis
Glossodynia
Hypersensitivity
Injection-site pain
Oral candidiasis
Serum sickness (<1%)
Stomatitis
Stomatodynia
Vaginitis
Xerostomia

MIBEFRADIL

Trade name: Posicor (Roche)
Category: Calcium channel ion influx inhibitor
Clinically important, potentially serious interactions with: astemizole, cisapride, cyclosporine, diltiazem, lovastatin, metoprolol, propranolol, quinidine, simvastatin, terfenadine, tricyclic antidepressants, verapamil

REACTIONS

SKIN
- Allergic reaction (sic) (>1%)
- Angioedema (<1%)
- Exfoliative dermatitis (<1%)
- Flushing (>1%)
- Hyperhidrosis (<1%)
- Leg edema (4%)
- Pedal edema (5.1%)
- Rash (sic) (<1%)

OTHER
- Paresthesias (<1%)

MICONAZOLE

Trade name: Monistat (Ortho)
Other common trade names: Aflorix; Aloid; Daktarin; Florid; Funcort; Micotef; Miracol; Zole
Category: Antifungal
Clinically important, potentially serious interactions with: amphotericin B, anticoagulants, astemizole, carbamazepine, cisapride, phenytoin, sulfonylureas, warfarin

REACTIONS

SKIN
- Angioedema
- Bullous eruption
- Contact dermatitis
- Erythema
- Exanthems
- Flushing (<1%)
- Pruritus (21%)
- Purpura
- Rash (sic) (9%)
- Urticaria
- Xanthomas

OTHER
- Injection-site pain (>10%)
- Phlebitis

MIDAZOLAM

Trade name: Versed (Roche)
Other common trade name: Dormicum
Category: Benzodiazepine, sedative-hypnotic; anesthetic
Clinically important, potentially serious interactions with: cimetidine, clarithromycin, CNS depressants, diltiazem, itraconazole, narcotics, verapamil

REACTIONS

SKIN
- Angioedema
- Exanthems
- Peripheral edema (<1%)
- Pruritus (<1%)
- Rash (sic) (<1%)
- Urticaria (<1%)

OTHER
- Anaphylactoid reaction (<1%)
- Dysgeusia (<1%)
- Injection-site pain (>10%)
- Injection-site reactions (>10%)
- Localized flare reaction
- Paresthesias
- Sialorrhea (<1%)

MINOCYCLINE

Trade names: Dynacin (Medicis); Minocin (Lederle); Vectrin
Other common trade names: Mestacine; Minoclir 50; Minogalen; Minomycin; Mynocine
Category: Tetracycline antibiotic
Clinically important, potentially serious interactions with: antacids, anticoagulants, corticosteroids, digitalis, iron salts, isotretinoin, penicillins, retinoids, vitamin A, warfarin

REACTIONS

SKIN
- Acute febrile neutrophilic dermatosis (Sweet's syndrome)
- Angioedema
- Cellulitis
- Eosinophilic pustular folliculitis (Ofuji's disease)
- Erythema multiforme
- Erythema nodosum
- Exanthems
- Exfoliative dermatitis (<1%)
- Fixed eruption (<1%)
- Folliculitis
- Lichenoid eruption
- Lupus erythematosus
- Nodules (facial, blue-gray)
- Photosensitivity (1–10%)
- Pigmentation
- Pigmentation at sites of cutaneous inflammation
- Pruritus (<1%)
- Purpura
- Rash (sic) (<1%)
- Raynaud's phenomenon
- Stevens-Johnson syndrome
- Urticaria
- Vasculitis

NAILS
- Nails – onycholysis
- Nails – photo-onycholysis
- Nails – pigmentation (<1%)

OTHER
- Anaphylactoid reaction (<1%)
- Black hairy tongue
- Black tongue (sic)
- Galactorrhea (black)
- Gingival pigmentation
- Glossitis
- Gynecomastia
- Hypersensitivity
- Oral pigmentation
- Paresthesias (<1%)
- Pseudo-mongolian spot (sic)
- Pseudotumor cerebri
- Serum sickness
- Tongue discoloration
- Tooth discoloration (in children) (>10%)

MINOXIDIL

Trade names: Loniten (Pharmacia & Upjohn); Rogaine (Pharmacia & Upjohn)
Other common trade names: Alopexy; Hairgaine; Lonolox; Lonoten; Minoximen; Regaine
Category: Antihypertensive; vasodilator
Clinically important, potentially serious interactions with: guanethidine

REACTIONS

SKIN
- Acne
- Ankle edema
- Bullous eruption (<1%)
- Contact dermatitis
- Eczematous eruption (sic)
- Edema (>10%)
- Erythema multiforme
- Erythroderma
- Exanthems
- Folliculitis
- Flushing
- Lupus erythematosus
- Pruritus
- Pyogenic granuloma
- Rash (sic) (<1%)
- Stevens-Johnson syndrome (<1%)
- Sunburn (<1%)
- Urticaria

HAIR
- Hair – alopecia

Hair – discoloration
Hair – hirsutism (in women)
Hair – hypertrichosis (>10%)

Dysgeusia
Mastodynia (<1%)
Paresthesias
Polymyalgia

OTHER
Anosmia

MISOPROSTOL

Trade names: Arthrotec (Searle); Cytotec (Searle)
Other common trade name: Symbol
Category: Synthetic prostaglandin E_1 analogue anti-ulcer agent
Clinically important, potentially serious interactions with: no data

Arthrotec is diclofenac & misoprostol

REACTIONS

SKIN
Dermatitis (sic)
Exanthems
Hyperhidrosis
Rash (sic)

HAIR
Hair – alopecia

OTHER
Anaphylactoid reaction
Gingivitis
Gynecomastia

MITOMYCIN

Trade name: Mutamycin (Mead Johnson)
Other common trade names: Ametycine; Mitomycin; Mitomycin-C; Mitomycine
Category: Antineoplastic antibiotic
Clinically important, potentially serious interactions with: doxorubicin

REACTIONS

SKIN
Angioedema
Bullous eruption
Contact dermatitis
Dermatitis (sic)
Edema
Erythema
Erythema multiforme
Exanthems
Exfoliative dermatitis
Photosensitivity
Pigmentation
Pityriasis rosea
Pruritus (<1%)
Purpura
Rash (sic) (<1%)
Ulceration
Urticaria

HAIR
Hair – alopecia (1–10%)

NAILS
Nails – pigmented bands (purple) (1–10%)

OTHER
Injection-site cellulitis (>10%)
Injection-site necrosis (>10%)
Injection-site thrombophlebitis
Oral mucosal lesions
Oral ulceration (1–10%)
Paresthesias (1–10%)
Stomatitis (>10%)
Thrombophlebitis (<1%)

MITOTANE

Trade name: Lysodren (Mead Johnson)
Other common trade name: Opeprim
Category: Antiadrenal; antineoplastic
Clinically important, potentially serious interactions with: phenytoin, spironolactone

REACTIONS

SKIN
- Acral erythema
- Angioedema (<1%)
- Cutaneous side effects (sic)
- Erythema multiforme
- Exanthems
- Flushing (1–10%)
- Hypermelanosis
- Pruritus
- Rash (sic) (15%)
- Urticaria
- Vasculitis (<1%)

HAIR
- Hair – alopecia

OTHER
- Myalgia (1–10%)

MOEXIPRIL

Trade names: Uniretic (Schwarz); Univasc (Schwarz)
Category: Angiotensin converting enzyme inhibitor
Clinically important, potentially serious interactions with: bumetanide, digitalis, lithium, salicylates

Uniretic is moexipril & hydrochlorothiazide

REACTIONS

SKIN
- Angioedema (<1%)
- Exanthems
- Flushing (1.6%)
- Hyperhidrosis (<1%)
- Pemphigus (<1%)
- Peripheral edema (<1%)
- Photosensitivity (<1%)
- Pruritus (1–10%)
- Rash (sic) (1.6%)
- Skin reactions (sic)
- Urticaria (<1%)

HAIR
- Hair – alopecia (1–10%)

OTHER
- Anaphylactoid reaction (<1%)
- Dysgeusia (<1%)
- Myalgia (1.3%)
- Xerostomia (<1%)

MOLINDONE

Trade name: Moban (Gate)
Category: Antipsychotic
Clinically important, potentially serious interactions with: anticonvulsants, antihypertensives, CNS depressants

REACTIONS

SKIN
- Allergic reactions (sic)
- Hypohidrosis (<1%)
- Photosensitivity (<1%)
- Pigmentation (<1%)
- Pruritus (<1%)
- Rash (sic) (<1%)

OTHER
- Galactorrhea (<1%)
- Gynecomastia (1–10%)
- Sialorrhea
- Xerostomia (>10%)

MONTELUKAST

Trade name: Singulair (Merck)
Category: Antiasthmatic (leukotriene receptor antagonist)
Clinically important, potentially serious interactions with: phenobarbital, rifampin

REACTIONS

SKIN
Rash (sic) (1.6%)

MORICIZINE

Trade name: Ethmozine (Roberts)
Category: Antiarrhythmic
Clinically important, potentially serious interactions with: anticoagulants, cimetidine, theophylline

REACTIONS

SKIN
Exanthems (<1%)
Hyperhidrosis (2–5%)
Periorbital edema (1–10%)
Pruritus (<2%)
Rash (sic) (<1%)
Urticaria (<2%)
Xerosis (<2%)

OTHER
Dysgeusia (<2%)
Hypesthesia (2–5%)
Oral mucosal lesions
Paresthesias (2–5%)
Thrombophlebitis (<2%)
Tongue edema (<2%)
Xerostomia (2–5%)

NABUMETONE

Trade name: Relafen (SmithKline Beecham)
Other common trade names: Arthaxan; Consolan; Nabuser; Prodac; Relif; Relifex; Unimetone
Category: Nonsteroidal anti-inflammatory (NSAID)
Clinically important, potentially serious interactions with: aminoglycosides, anticoagulants, cyclosporine, methotrexate, warfarin

REACTIONS

SKIN
Acne (<1%)
Angioedema (<1%)
Bullous eruption (<1%)
Cutaneous side effects (sic)
Edema (3–9%)
Erythema
Erythema multiforme (<1%)
Exanthems (1.2%)
Hyperhidrosis (1–3%)
Photosensitivity (<1%)
Phototoxic reaction
Pruritus (3–9%)
Rash (sic) (3–9%)
Skin reactions (sic)
Stevens-Johnson syndrome (<1%)
Toxic epidermal necrolysis (<1%)
Urticaria (<1%)
Vasculitis (necrotizing)
Xerosis

HAIR
Hair – alopecia (<1%)

OTHER
Anaphylactoid reaction (<1%)
Gingivitis (<1%)
Glossitis (<1%)
Oral ulceration
Paresthesias (<1%)
Porphyria cutanea tarda (<1%)
Pseudoporphyria
Stomatitis (1–3%)
Xerostomia (1–3%)

NADOLOL

Trade names: Corgard (Bristol-Myers Squibb); Corzide (Bristol-Myers Squibb)
Other common trade names: Apo-Nadolol; Farmagard; Nadic; Solgol
Category: Beta-adrenergic blocking agent; antihypertensive; antianginal
Clinically important, potentially serious interactions with: calcium channel blockers, clonidine, epinephrine, flecainide, insulin, nifedipine, oral contraceptives, verapamil

Corzide is nadolol & bendroflumethiazide

REACTIONS

SKIN
- Bullous pemphigoid
- Eczematous eruption (sic)
- Edema (<1%)
- Erythema multiforme
- Exanthems
- Facial edema (<1%)
- Hyperhidrosis (<1%)
- Hyperkeratosis (palms & soles)
- Infiltrative dermatitis of the scalp (sic)
- Lichenoid eruption
- Lupus erythematosus
- Pityriasis rubra pilaris
- Pruritus (1–5%)
- Psoriasis
- Pustular eruption
- Rash (sic) (<1%)
- Raynaud's phenomenon (2%)
- Toxic epidermal necrolysis
- Urticaria
- Xerosis

HAIR
- Hair – alopecia

NAILS
- Nails – bluish
- Nails – dystrophy
- Nails – onycholysis

OTHER
- Dysgeusia
- Oculo-mucocutaneous syndrome
- Oral lichenoid eruption
- Oral mucosal eruption
- Paresthesias (2%)
- Peyronie's disease
- Xerostomia (<1%)

NAFARELIN

Trade name: Synarel (Syntex)
Other common trade name: Synarela
Category: Posterior pituitary hormone
Clinically important, potentially serious interactions with: no data

REACTIONS

SKIN
- Acne (>10%)
- Chloasma (<1%)
- Edema
- Exanthems (<1%)
- Flushing
- Pruritus (1–10%)
- Rash (sic) (1–10%)
- Seborrhea (1–10%)
- Urticaria (1–10%)

HAIR
- Hair – hirsutism

OTHER
- Gynecomastia (<1%)
- Hypersensitivity (0.2%)
- Myalgia (>10%)
- Paresthesias (<1%)

NAFCILLIN

Trade names: Nafcil (Mead Johnson); Nallpen (Beecham); Unipen (Wyeth)
Other common trade name: Vigopen
Category: Penicillinase-resistant penicillin
Clinically important, potentially serious interactions with: anticoagulants, atenolol, cyclosporine, heparin, methotrexate, probenecid, tetracycline

REACTIONS

SKIN
- Allergic reactions (sic)
- Angioedema
- Ecchymoses
- Erythema multiforme
- Exanthems
- Exfoliative dermatitis
- Hematomas
- Jarisch-Herxheimer reaction
- Pruritus
- Rash (sic) (<1%)
- Stevens-Johnson syndrome
- Urticaria

OTHER
- Anaphylactoid reaction
- Black tongue
- Dysgeusia
- Glossitis
- Glossodynia
- Hypersensitivity (<1%)
- Injection-site necrosis
- Injection-site pain
- Oral candidiasis
- Serum sickness
- Stomatitis
- Stomatodynia
- Thrombophlebitis (<1%)
- Vaginitis
- Xerostomia

NALIDIXIC ACID

Trade name: Neggram (Sanofi Winthrop)
Other common trade names: Betaxina; Granexin; Mytacin; Nalidixin; Negram; Nogram; Youdix
Category: Urinary tract anti-infective; quinolone antibiotic
Clinically important, potentially serious interactions with: anticoagulants, warfarin

REACTIONS

SKIN
- Angioedema (<1%)
- Bullous eruption (<1%)
- Erythema multiforme (<1%)
- Exanthems (>5%)
- Exfoliative dermatitis
- Lupus erythematosus
- Photoallergic reaction
- Photosensitivity (<1%)
- Phototoxic bullous eruption
- Pruritus (<1%)
- Purpura
- Rash (sic) (<1%)
- Toxic epidermal necrolysis
- Urticaria (<1%)

HAIR
- Hair – alopecia

OTHER
- Acute intermittent porphyria
- Anaphylactoid reaction
- Paresthesias
- Porphyria cutanea tarda
- Pseudoporphyria

NALOXONE

Trade name: Narcan (DuPont Merck)
Other common trade names: Nalpin; Narcanti; Narcotan; Zynox
Category: Opioid (narcotic) antagonist
Clinically important, potentially serious interactions with: narcotic analgesics

REACTIONS

SKIN
- Angioedema
- Exanthems
- Hyperhidrosis (1–10%)
- Pruritus
- Rash (sic) (1–10%)
- Urticaria

NAPROXEN

Trade names: Aleve (Syntex); Naprosyn (Syntex)
Other common trade names: Apranax; Dymenalgit; Laraflex; Naprogesic; Naprosyne; Synflex
Category: Nonsteroidal anti-inflammatory (NSAID)
Clinically important, potentially serious interactions with: beta-blockers, cyclosporine, furosemide, methotrexate, probenecid

REACTIONS

SKIN
- Angioedema (<1%)
- Aphthous stomatitis
- Bullous eruption
- Cutaneous side effects (sic)
- Ecchymoses (3–9%)
- Edema (3–9%)
- Erythema multiforme (<1%)
- Erythema nodosum
- Exanthems (>5%)
- Exfoliative dermatitis (rare)
- Fixed eruption
- Hyperhidrosis (<3%)
- Lichenoid eruption
- Lichen planus
- Lupus erythematosus
- Photodermatitis (bullous)
- Photosensitivity (<1%)
- Phototoxic reaction
- Pityriasis rosea
- Pruritus (3–9%)
- Pseudo-allergic reaction (sic)
- Purpura (<3%)
- Pustular eruption
- Pyogenic granuloma
- Rash (sic) (3–9%)
- Stevens-Johnson syndrome (<1%)
- Toxic epidermal necrolysis (<1%)
- Urticaria
- Vasculitis
- Vesiculobullous eruption

HAIR
- Hair – alopecia (<1%)

OTHER
- Anaphylactoid reaction (<1%)
- Myalgia (<1%)
- Oral ulceration
- Porphyria cutanea tarda
- Pseudoporphyria
- Salivary gland enlargement
- Stomatitis (<3%)
- Xerostomia

NARATRIPTAN

Trade name: Amerge (Glaxo Wellcome)
Category: Antimigraine
Clinically important, potentially serious interactions with: ergotamines, methysergide, SSRIs (fluoxetine, fluvoxamine, paroxetine, sertraline)

REACTIONS

SKIN
Acne (<1%)
Allergic reactions (sic) (<1%)
Atypical sensations (sic) (<1)%
Dermatitis (sic) (<1%)
Edema (<1%)
Erythema (<1%)
Exanthems (<1%)
Folliculitis (<1%)
Hyperhidrosis (<1%)
Photosensitivity (<1%)
Purpura (<1%)
Rash (sic) (<1%)
Urticaria (<1%)
Xerosis (<1%)

HAIR
Hair – alopecia (<1%)

OTHER
Dysgeusia (<1%)
Hyperesthesia (<1%)
Hypesthesia (<1%)
Paresthesias (2%)
Photophobia (<1%)
Sialopenia (<1%)

NEFAZODONE

Trade name: Serzone (Bristol-Myers Squibb)
Category: Phenylpiperazine antidepressant
Clinically important, potentially serious interactions with: alprazolam, astemizole, cisapride, CNS depressants, digoxin, fluoxetine, haloperidol, MAO inhibitors, phenytoin, terfenadine, trazodone, triazolam

REACTIONS

SKIN
Acne (<1%)
Allergic reactions (sic) (<1%)
Cellulitis (<1%)
Ecchymoses (<1%)
Eczema (sic) (<1%)
Exanthems (<1%)
Facial edema (<1%)
Flushing
Peripheral edema (3%)
Photosensitivity (<1%)
Pruritus (2%)
Rash (sic) (2%)
Urticaria (<1%)
Vesiculobullous eruption (<1%)
Xerosis (<1%)

HAIR
Hair – alopecia (<1%)

OTHER
Ageusia (<1%)
Dysgeusia (2%)
Foetor ex ore (halitosis) (<1%)
Gingivitis (<1%)
Glossitis (<1%)
Gynecomastia (<1%)
Hyperesthesia (<1%)
Mastodynia (1%)
Myalgia
Oral candidiasis (<1%)
Oral ulceration (<1%)
Paresthesias (4%)
Priapism (<1%)
Sialorrhea (<1%)
Stomatitis (<1%)
Vaginitis (2%)
Xerostomia (25%)

NELFINAVIR

Trade name: Viracept (Agouron)
Category: Protease inhibitor
Clinically important, potentially serious interactions with: astemizole, barbiturates, benzodiazepines, carbamazepine, cisapride, delavirdine, indinavir, nevirapine, rifabutin, rifampin, ritonavir, terfenadine

REACTIONS

SKIN
- Allergy (sic) (<1%)
- Dermatitis (sic) (<1%)
- Diaphoresis (<1%)
- Pruritus (<1%)
- Rash (sic) (1–10%)
- Urticaria (<1%)

OTHER
- Paresthesias (<1%)
- Myalgia (<1%)
- Oral ulceration (<1%)

NEOMYCIN

Trade name: Mycifradin (Pharmacia & Upjohn)
Other common trade names: Gemicina; Neomicina; Neomycine Diamant; Neosulf; Nivemycin
Category: Aminoglycoside antibiotic
Clinically important, potentially serious interactions with: aldesleukin, aminoglycosides, bumetanide, digitalis, ethacrynic acid, fenoprofen, furosemide, indomethacin, ketoprofen, naproxen, NSAIDs, piroxicam, succinylcholine, torsemide, vancomycin

REACTIONS

SKIN
- Allergic reaction (sic)
- Angioedema
- Bullous eruption
- Contact dermatitis
- Dermatitis (sic)
- Eczematous eruption (sic)
- Erythema multiforme
- Exanthems
- Fixed eruption
- Pruritus
- Toxic epidermal necrolysis
- Ulceration
- Urticaria

HAIR
- Hair – alopecia

OTHER
- Anaphylactoid reaction

NEVIRAPINE

Trade name: Viramune (Roxane)
Category: Non-nucleoside reverse transcriptase inhibitor; antiviral
Clinically important, potentially serious interactions with: estrogens, indinavir, nelfinavir, ritonavir, saquinavir

REACTIONS

SKIN
- Exanthems
- Rash (sic) (39.6%)
- Stevens-Johnson syndrome

OTHER
- Myalgia (1%)
- Paresthesias (1%)

NIACIN; NIACINAMIDE (VITAMIN B_3)

Trade names: Niaspan (Kos); Nicolar (Rhône-Poulenc Rorer); Nicotinamide
Other common trade names: Apo-Nicotinamide; Nicobion; Nicovital; Pepeom Amide
Category: Water-soluble nutritional supplement; antihyperlipidemic
Clinically important, potentially serious interactions with: adrenergic blocking agents, carbamazepine, lovastatin

REACTIONS

SKIN
- Acanthosis nigricans
- Contact dermatitis
- Erythema
- Exanthems
- Fixed eruption (<1%)
- Flushing (1–10%)
- Hyperpigmentation
- Ichthyosis
- Keratoses, pigmented
- Pruritus (1–5%)
- Rash (sic)
- Scaling (sic)
- Urticaria
- Xerosis

OTHER
- Anaphylactoid reaction
- Burning mouth syndrome
- Myopathy
- Paresthesias (1–10%)

NICARDIPINE

Trade name: Cardene (Roche; Syntex))
Other common trade names: Antagonil; Dagan; Loxen; Nicardal; Nicodel; Ranvil; Rydene
Category: Calcium channel blocker; antianginal & antihypertensive
Clinically important, potentially serious interactions with: beta-blockers, carbamazepine, cimetidine, cyclosporine, digitalis, fentanyl, quinidine, theophylline

REACTIONS

SKIN
- Allergic reactions (sic)
- Cutaneous side effects (sic)
- Edema (1%)
- Exanthems
- Flushing (5.6%)
- Peripheral edema (7.1%)
- Rash (sic) (1.2%)
- Urticaria (rare)

OTHER
- Erythromelalgia
- Myalgia (1%)
- Paresthesias (1%)
- Xerostomia (1.4%)

NIFEDIPINE

Trade names: Adalat (Bayer); Procardia (Pfizer)
Other common trade names: Adalate; Apo-Nifed; Aprical; Calcilat; Coracten; Nifecor; Pidilat
Category: Calcium channel blocker; antianginal & antihypertensive
Clinically important, potentially serious interactions with: beta-blockers, carbamazepine, cyclosporine, digitalis, fentanyl, prazosin, quinidine, theophylline

REACTIONS

SKIN
- Acute generalized exanthematous pustulosis (AGEP)
- Angioedema
- Ankle edema
- Bullous eruption
- Cutaneous side effects (sic)
- Dermatitis (sic) (<2%)
- Edema
- Erysipelas
- Erythema
- Erythema multiforme

Erythema nodosum
Exanthems
Exfoliative dermatitis
Facial edema (1%)
Fixed eruption
Flushing (dose related) (25%)
Hyperhidrosis (<2%)
Lichenoid eruption
Lupus erythematosus
Painful edema of extremities
Pemphigus foliaceus
Periorbital edema (1%)
Peripheral edema (7%)
Photosensitivity
Prurigo nodularis
Pruritus (<2%)
Purpura (<2%)
Rash (sic) (<3%)
Stevens-Johnson syndrome
Telangiectases
Toxic epidermal necrolysis
Urticaria (<1%)
Vasculitis

HAIR
Hair – alopecia (1%)
Hair – discoloration

NAILS
Nails – dystrophy

OTHER
Dysgeusia (<1%)
Erythromelalgia (<0.5%)
Erythromyalgia
Gingival hyperplasia (<0.5%)
Gynecomastia
Paresthesias (<3%)
Xerostomia (<3%)

NIMODIPINE

Trade name: Nimotop (Bayer)
Other common trade names: Admon; Periplum; Vasotop
Category: Calcium channel blocker
Clinically important, potentially serious interactions with: barbiturates, beta-blockers, carbamazepine, cimetidine, cyclosporine, digitalis, fentanyl, omeprazole, prazosin, quinidine, theophylline

REACTIONS

SKIN
Acne (<1%)
Edema (2%)
Exanthems (2.4%)
Flushing (2.1%)
Hyperhidrosis (<1%)
Peripheral edema
Pruritus (<1%)
Purpura
Rash (sic) (3%)

HAIR
Hair – alopecia

NISOLDIPINE

Trade name: Sular (Zeneca)
Other common trade names: Baymycard; Syscor
Category: Calcium channel blocker
Clinically important, potentially serious interactions with: beta-blockers, carbamazepine, cimetidine, cyclosporine, digitalis, fentanyl, quinidine, theophylline. Also with grapefruit

REACTIONS

SKIN
Acne (<1%)
Angioedema
Cellulitis (<1%)
Cutaneous side effects (sic)
Ecchymoses (<1%)
Exanthems (<1%)
Exfoliative dermatitis (<1%)
Facial edema (<1%)
Flushing
Herpes simplex (<1%)
Herpes zoster (<1%)

Hyperhidrosis (<1%)
Peripheral edema (22%)
Petechiae (<1%)
Photosensitivity
Pigmentation (<1%)
Pruritus (<1%)
Pustular eruption (<1%)
Rash (sic) (2%)
Ulceration (<1%)
Urticaria (<1%)
Xerosis (<1%)

HAIR
Hair – alopecia (<1%)

OTHER
Dysgeusia (<1%)
Gingival hyperplasia (<1%)
Glossitis (<1%)
Hypesthesia (<1%)
Oral ulceration (<1%)
Paresthesias (<1%)
Vaginitis (<1%)
Xerostomia (<1%)

NITROFURANTOIN

Trade names: Furadantin (Procter Gamble); Macrobid (Procter Gamble); Macrodantin (Procter Gamble)
Other common trade names: Furadantina; Furadoine; Furobactina; Infurin; Urofuran
Category: Urinary tract anti-infective
Clinically important, potentially serious interactions with: probenecid

REACTIONS

SKIN
Angioedema
Bullous eruption
Contact dermatitis
Eczematous eruption (sic)
Erythema multiforme
Erythema nodosum
Exanthems (1–5%)
Exfoliative dermatitis
Fixed eruption
Flushing
Lupus erythematosus
Panniculitis, nodular nonsuppurative
Photosensitivity
Pruritus (<1%)
Purpura
Rash (sic) (<1%)
Reticular hyperplasia
Stevens-Johnson syndrome
Toxic epidermal necrolysis
Urticaria

HAIR
Hair – alopecia

NAILS
Nails – onycholysis

OTHER
Anaphylactoid reaction
Galactorrhea
Hypersensitivity
Mastodynia
Myalgia
Paresthesias (1–10%)
Tooth discoloration
Xerostomia

NITROGLYCERIN

Trade names:
Buccal tablets: Nitrogard
Lingual aerosol: Nitrolingual
Oral capsules: Nitro-Bid; Nitrocap; Nitrocine; Nitroglyn; Nitrospan
Oral tablets: Klavikordal; Niong; Nitronet; Nitrong
Parenteral: Nitro-Bid; Nitroject; Nitrol; Nitrostat; Tridil
Sublingual tablets: Nitrostat
Topical ointment: Nitro-Bid; Nitrol; Nitrong; Nitrostat
Topical transdermal systems: Deponit; Minitran; Nitrocine; Nitrodisc; Nitro-Dur; Transderm-Nitro.

(Various pharmaceutical companies.)

Other common trade names: Corditrine; Lenitral; Nitradisc; Nitroglin; Suscard; Sustac
Category: Anti-anginal vasodilator; antihypertensive
Clinically important, potentially serious interactions with: alcohol, alteplase, beta-blockers, calcium channel blockers, ergot, heparin

REACTIONS

SKIN
- Angioedema
- Contact dermatitis (to topical systems) (<1%)
- Cyanosis
- Eczematous eruption (sic)
- Erythema (to transdermal delivery system)
- Erythroderma
- Exanthems
- Exfoliative dermatitis (1–10%)
- Flushing (>10%)
- Hyperhidrosis (<1%)
- Purpura
- Rash (sic) (1–10%)
- Rosacea (exacerbation)
- Urticaria

OTHER
- Xerostomia

NIZATIDINE

Trade name: Axid (Lilly)
Other common trade names: Calmaxid; Gastrax; Nizax; Nizaxid; Panaxid; Tazac; Zanizal
Category: Histamine H_2-receptor antagonist & anti-ulcer
Clinically important, potentially serious interactions with: cephalosporins, ketoconazole, nifedipine, nisoldipine, quinolones

REACTIONS

SKIN
- Acne (<1%)
- Contact dermatitis
- Edema
- Exanthems
- Exfoliative dermatitis
- Hyperhidrosis (1%)
- Pruritus (1.7%)
- Rash (sic) (1.9%)
- Urticaria (<1%)
- Vasculitis
- Xerosis (<1%)

OTHER
- Gynecomastia
- Myalgia (1.7%)
- Paresthesias (<1%)
- Pseudolymphoma
- Serum sickness
- Xerostomia (1.4%)

NORFLOXACIN

Trade names: Chibroxin (Merck); Noroxin (Roberts)
Other common trade names: Barazan; Chibroxine; Chibroxol; Lexinor; Noroxine; Utinor; Zoroxin
Category: Broad-spectrum fluoroquinolone antibiotic
Clinically important, potentially serious interactions with: azlocillin, betaxolol, caffeine, cimetidine, cyclosporine, metoprolol, omeprazole, probenecid, propranolol, theophylline, warfarin

REACTIONS

SKIN
- Angioedema
- Bullous eruption
- Edema
- Erythema (sic) (<1%)
- Erythema multiforme
- Exanthems
- Exfoliative dermatitis
- Fixed eruption
- Hyperhidrosis (<1%)

Photosensitivity
Phototoxic reaction
Pruritus (<1%)
Pustular eruption
Rash (sic) (<1%)
Stevens-Johnson syndrome
Subcorneal pustular dermatosis (Sneddon-Wilkinson)
Toxic epidermal necrolysis
Toxic pustuloderma
Urticaria
Vasculitis

NAILS
Nails – photo-onycholysis

OTHER
Anaphylactoid reaction
Dysgeusia (<1%) (bitter taste)
Myalgia
Paresthesias
Stomatitis
Vaginal candidiasis
Xerostomia (<1%)

NORTRIPTYLINE

Trade names: Aventyl (Lilly); Pamelor (Novartis)
Other common trade names: Allegron; Aventyl; Noritren; Norpress; Nortrilen; Paxtibi; Vividyl
Category: Tricyclic antidepressant & antipanic
Clinically important, potentially serious interactions with: cimetidine, clonidine, CNS depressants, diltiazem, epinephrine, guanethidine, isoproterenol, MAO inhibitors, warfarin

REACTIONS

SKIN
Allergic reactions (sic) (<1%)
Edema
Exanthems
Flushing
Hyperhidrosis (1–10%)
Petechiae
Photosensitivity (<1%)
Phototoxic reaction
Pruritus
Purpura
Rash (sic)
Urticaria

HAIR
Hair – alopecia (<1%)

OTHER
Acute intermittent porphyria
Black hairy tongue
Dysgeusia (>10%)
Galactorrhea (<1%)
Gynecomastia (<1%)
Paresthesias
Stomatitis
Tongue edema
Xerostomia (>10%)

NYSTATIN

Trade names: Mycostatin (Bristol-Myers Squibb); Nilstat (Lederle); Nystex (Savage)
Other common trade names: Biofanal; Candio-Hermal; Moronal; Nystacid; Nystan; Oranyst
Category: Antifungal (anti-candidal) antibiotic
Clinically important, potentially serious interactions with: methotrexate

REACTIONS

SKIN
Acrodermatitis perstans (exacerbation)
Acute generalized exanthematous pustulosis (AGEP)
Contact dermatitis (<1%)
Eczematous eruption (sic)
Erythema multiforme
Erythroderma
Exanthems
Fixed eruption
Pruritus
Rash (sic)
Stevens-Johnson syndrome (<1%)
Urticaria

OTHER
Hypersensitivity (<1%)
Tongue edema

OCTREOTIDE

Trade name: Sandostatin (Novartis)
Other common trade names: Sandostatina; Sandostatine
Category: Antidiarrheal; antihypotensive; growth hormone suppressant; antihypoglycemic
Clinically important, potentially serious interactions with: cyclosporine

REACTIONS

SKIN
- Allergic reactions (sic)
- Cellulitis (1–4%)
- Edema (1–10%)
- Exanthems
- Flushing (1–4%)
- Hyperhidrosis
- Petechiae (1–4%)
- Pruritus (1–4%)
- Purpura (1–4%)
- Rash (sic) (<1%)
- Raynaud's phenomenon (1–4%)
- Urticaria (1–4%)

HAIR
- Hair – alopecia (<1%)

OTHER
- Anaphylactoid reaction
- Galactorrhea (1–4%)
- Gynecomastia (1–4%)
- Hyperesthesia
- Injection-site erythema (1%)
- Injection-site local reaction
- Injection-site pain (7.5%)
- Thrombophlebitis (1–4%)
- Vaginitis (1–4%)
- Xerostomia

OFLOXACIN

Trade names: Floxin (Ortho); Ocuflox (Allergan)
Other common trade names: Exocine; Flobasin; Floxan; Oflocet; Oflocin; Tabrin; Taravid
Category: Broad-spectrum fluoroquinoline antibiotic
Clinically important, potentially serious interactions with: anticoagulants, azlocillin, betaxolol, caffeine, cimetidine, cyclosporine, metoprolol, NSAIDs, omeprazole, probenecid, propranolol, theophylline, warfarin

REACTIONS

SKIN
- Angioedema
- Bullous eruption
- Candidiasis (sic)
- Cutaneous side effects (sic) (0.4%)
- Dermatitis (sic)
- Ecchymoses
- Edema (<1%)
- Erythema multiforme
- Erythema nodosum
- Exanthems
- Exfoliative dermatitis
- Fixed eruption
- Genital pruritus in women (1–3%)
- Hyperhidrosis
- Petechiae
- Photosensitivity
- Phototoxic reaction
- Pigmentation
- Pruritus (1–3%)
- Purpura
- Rash (sic) (1–10%)
- Stevens-Johnson syndrome
- Toxic epidermal necrolysis
- Toxic pustuloderma
- Urticaria (<1%)
- Vasculitis (<1%)

NAILS
- Nails – photo-onycholysis

OTHER
- Anaphylactoid reaction
- Dysgeusia (1–3%)
- Injection-site pain
- Myalgia (<1%)
- Oral mucosal eruption
- Paresthesias (<1%)
- Parosmia
- Serum sickness
- Vaginitis (1–10%)
- Xerostomia (1–3%)

OLANZAPINE

Trade name: Zyprexa (Lilly)
Category: Benzodiazepine antipsychotic
Clinically important, potentially serious interactions with: carbamazepine

REACTIONS

SKIN
- Aphthous stomatitis (<1%)
- Candidiasis (<1%)
- Contact dermatitis (<1%)
- Ecchymoses (>1%)
- Eczema (sic) (<1%)
- Exanthems (<1%)
- Facial edema (<1%)
- Hyperhidrosis (>1%)
- Peripheral edema (2%)
- Photosensitivity (<1%)
- Pigmentation (<1%)
- Pruritus (>1%)
- Rash (>1%)
- Seborrhea (<1%)
- Ulceration (<1%)
- Urticaria (<1%)
- Vesiculobullous eruption (2%)
- Xerosis (<1%)

HAIR
- Hair – alopecia (<1%)
- Hair – hirsutism (<1%)

OTHER
- Dysgeusia (<1%)
- Gingivitis (<1%)
- Glossitis (<1%)
- Hypesthesia (<1%)
- Myalgia (>1%)
- Oral candidiasis (<1%)
- Oral ulceration (<1%)
- Sialorrhea (<1%)
- Stomatitis (<1%)
- Tongue discoloration (<1%)
- Tongue edema (<1%)
- Twitching (2%)
- Vaginitis (>1%)
- Xerostomia (13%)

OLSALAZINE

Trade name: Dipentum (Pharmacia & Upjohn)
Category: Inflammatory bowel disease suppressant
Clinically important, potentially serious interactions with: none

REACTIONS

SKIN
- Acne
- Exanthems (0.4%)
- Lupus erythematosus
- Pruritus (1.1%)
- Rash (sic) (2.3%)
- Urticaria (4.3%)

OTHER
- Stomatitis (1%)

OMEPRAZOLE

Trade name: Prilosec (Astra)
Other common trade names: Antra; Audazol; Gastroloc; Logastric; Mopral; Omed; Parizac
Category: Anti-ulcer; gastric acid secretion inhibitor
Clinically important, potentially serious interactions with: cyclosporine, diazepam, digoxin, itraconazole, ketoconazole, methotrexate, phenytoin, quinolones, warfarin

REACTIONS

SKIN
- Allergic edema (sic)
- Angioedema (<1%)
- Bullous eruption
- Bullous pemphigoid
- Burning (sic)
- Eczema (sic)
- Edema (1–10%)
- Erythema (sic)
- Erythema multiforme (<1%)

Erythema nodosum
Exanthems
Exfoliative dermatitis
Hyperhidrosis (<1%)
Lichen planus
Lichen spinulosus
Lupus erythematosus
Pemphigoid (exacerbation)
Pityriasis rosea
Pruritus (1–10%)
Psoriasis
Purpura
Rash (sic) (1.5%)
Stevens-Johnson syndrome (<1%)
Toxic epidermal necrolysis (<1%)
Urticaria (1–10%)
Xerosis (<1%)

HAIR
Hair – alopecia (<1%)
Hair – discoloration

OTHER
Dysgeusia (<1%)
Gynecomastia (<1%)
Myalgia (1–10%)
Oral candidiasis
Paresthesias
Xerostomia (1–10%)

ONDANSETRON

Trade name: Zofran (Glaxo Wellcome)
Other common trade names: Emeset; Oncoden; Zofron
Category: Antiemetic
Clinically important, potentially serious interactions with: allopurinol, barbiturates, carbamazepine, cimetidine, disulfiram, phenylbutazone, phenytoin, rifampin

REACTIONS

SKIN
Angioedema
Exanthems
Fixed eruption
Flushing
Pruritus (5%)
Rash (sic) (<1%)
Urticaria

HAIR
Hair – alopecia

OTHER
Anaphylactoid reaction (rare)
Hypersensitivity
Injection-site burning
Injection-site erythema
Injection-site pain
Injection-site reaction (4%)
Paresthesias (2%)
Porphyria
Xerostomia (1–10%)

ORAL CONTRACEPTIVES

Trade names: Brevicon; Demulen; Desogen; Enovid; Estrostep; Jenest; Levlen; Loestrin; Lo/Ovral; Modicon; Nordette; Norinyl; Norlestrin; Ortho-Cept; Ortho-Novum; Ortho-Cyclen; Ortho Tri-Cyclen; Ovcon; Ovral; Tri-Levlen; Tri-Norinyl; Triphasil. (Various pharmaceutical companies.)
Clinically important, potentially serious interactions with: anticonvulsants, danazol, theophylline, troleandomycin, tuberculostatics

REACTIONS

SKIN
Acanthosis nigricans
Acne
Angioedema
Autoimmune progesterone dermatitis
Bullous eruption
Candidiasis
Chloasma
Cold urticaria
Dermatitis herpetiformis
Eczema (sic)
Edema
Erythema
Erythema multiforme

Erythema nodosum
Exanthems
Fixed eruption
Fox-Fordyce disease
Herpes genitalis (sic)
Herpes gestationis
Lichenoid eruption
Livedo racemosa (Sneddon's syndrome)
Lupus erythematosus
Melanoma
Melasma
Mucha-Habermann disease
Perioral dermatitis
Photosensitivity
Pigmentation
Polymorphous light eruption
Pruritus (<1%)
Psoriasis
Purpura (rare)
Seborrhea
Spider angiomas
Stevens-Johnson syndrome
Telangiectases
Urticaria
Varicosities

HAIR
Hair – alopecia
Hair – alopecia areata
Hair – hirsutism

NAILS
Nails – onycholysis

OTHER
Acute intermittent porphyria
Galactorrhea
Gingival hyperplasia
Oral mucosal pigmentation
Porphyria cutanea prematura
Porphyria cutanea tarda
Porphyria variegata
Thrombophlebitis

ORPHENADRINE

Trade names: Banflex (Forest); Norflex (3M)
Other common trade names: Biorfen; Biorphen; Distalene; Disipal; Opheryl; Prolongatum
Category: Skeletal muscle relaxant
Clinically important, potentially serious interactions with: propoxyphene

REACTIONS

SKIN
Exanthems
Flushing (1–10%)
Pigment disorder (sic)
Pruritus
Rash (sic) (1–10%)
Urticaria

OTHER
Anaphylactoid reaction
Embolia cutis medicamentosa (Nicolau syndrome)
Hypersensitivity
Paresthesias
Xerostomia

OXACILLIN

Trade names: Bactocill (Beecham); Prostaphlin (Mead Johnson)
Other common trade names: Bristopen; Stapenor
Category: Penicillinase-resistant penicillin
Clinically important, potentially serious interactions with: anticoagulants, cyclosporine, disulfiram, methotrexate, tetracycline

REACTIONS

SKIN
Angioedema
Bullous eruption
Ecchymoses
Erythema multiforme
Exanthems
Exfoliative dermatitis
Hematomas
Jarisch-Herxheimer reaction
Necrosis
Pruritus
Rash (sic) (<1%)

Stevens-Johnson syndrome
Urticaria

OTHER
Anaphylactoid reaction (0.04%)
Black tongue
Dysgeusia
Glossitis
Glossodynia
Injection-site pain
Oral candidiasis
Serum sickness (<1%)
Stomatitis
Stomatodynia
Vaginitis
Xerostomia

OXAPROZIN

Trade name: Daypro (Searle)
Other common trade names: Deflam; Duraprox
Category: Non-steroidal anti-inflammatory (NSAID)
Clinically important, potentially serious interactions with: anticoagulants, aspirin, cyclosporine, diuretics, methotrexate

REACTIONS

SKIN
Angioedema (<1%)
Ecchymoses
Edema
Erythema multiforme (<1%)
Exanthems
Exfoliative dermatitis (<1%)
Hyperhidrosis (<1%)
Phototoxic reaction
Pruritus (1–10%)
Purpura
Rash (sic) (1–10%)
Stevens-Johnson syndrome (<1%)
Urticaria (<1%)

HAIR
Hair – alopecia

OTHER
Anaphylactoid reaction (<1%)
Dysgeusia
Pseudoporphyria
Stomatitis (<1%)

OXAZEPAM

Trade name: Serax (Wyeth)
Other common trade names: Adumbran; Azutranquil; Durazepam; Murelax; Praxiten; Serepax
Category: Benzodiazepine antianxiety & sedative-hypnotic; anticonvulsant
Clinically important, potentially serious interactions with: alcohol, barbiturates, clarithromycin, CNS depressants, diltiazem, levodopa, MAO inhibitors, narcotics, phenothiazines, verapamil

REACTIONS

SKIN
Dermatitis (sic) (1–10%)
Edema
Erythema multiforme
Exanthems
Fixed eruption
Hyperhidrosis (>10%)
Pruritus
Purpura
Rash (sic) (>10%)
Urticaria

OTHER
Paresthesias
Sialopenia (>10%)
Sialorrhea (1–10%)
Xerostomia (>10%)

OXYTETRACYCLINE

Trade name: Terramycin (Pfizer)
Other common trade names: Aknin; Cotet; Macocyn; Oxacycle; Oxy; Rorap; Terramycine
Category: Tetracycline antibiotic; antiprotozoal
Clinically important, potentially serious interactions with: antacids, anticoagulants, digitalis, penicillin, warfarin

REACTIONS

SKIN
Angioedema
Contact dermatitis
Exanthems
Exfoliative dermatitis (<1%)
Fixed eruption
Lupus erythematosus
Photosensitivity
Pigmentation
Pruritus (<1%)
Purpura
Pustular eruption
Sensitivity (sic)
Urticaria
Vasculitis

NAILS
Nails – pigmentation (<1%)

OTHER
Anaphylactoid reaction (<1%)
Black hairy tongue
Hypersensitivity (<1%)
Oral mucosal lesions
Paresthesias (<1%)
Porphyria cutanea tarda
Pseudotumor cerebri (<1%)
Thrombophlebitis (<1%)
Tooth discoloration (>10%) (in infants)

PACLITAXEL

Trade name: Taxol (Mead Johnson)
Category: Antineoplastic
Clinically important, potentially serious interactions with: cisplatin, ketoconazole

REACTIONS

SKIN
Acral erythema
Angioedema
Cutaneous manifestations (sic)
Edema (21%)
Erythema
Erythrodysesthesia
Exanthems
Fixed eruption
Flushing (28%)
Pruritus
Purpura
Radiation-recall
Rash (sic) (12%)
Urticaria

HAIR
Hair – alopecia (87%)

NAILS
Nails – pigmentation (2%)

OTHER
Hypersensitivity (41%)
Injection-site cellulitis (>10%)
Injection-site extravasation (>10%)
Injection-site pain (>10%)
Injection-site reaction (13%)
Mucocutaneous toxicity (sic)
Myalgia (60%)
Oral mucosal lesions
Paresthesias (>10%)
Recall at site of prior extravasation

PAMIDRONATE

Trade name: Aredia (Novartis)
Category: Antidote (hypercalcemia)
Clinically important, potentially serious interactions with: none

REACTIONS

SKIN
- Angioedema (<1%)
- Edema (1%)
- Exanthems
- Rash (sic) (<1%)

OTHER
- Dysgeusia (<1%)
- Hypersensitivity (<1%)
- Infusion-site reaction (4%)
- Myalgia (1%)
- Stomatitis (1%)

PAPAVERINE

Trade name: Pavabid (Hoechst Marion Roussel)
Other common trade names: Angioverin; Optenyl; Pameion; Papaverine 60; Papaverini
Category: Peripheral vasodilator
Clinically important, potentially serious interactions with: CNS depressants, levodopa, morphine

REACTIONS

SKIN
- Exanthems
- Fixed eruption
- Flushing (<1%)
- Hyperhidrosis (<1%)
- Pyogenic granuloma
- Pruritus (<1%)
- Rash (sic)
- Toxic epidermal necrolysis
- Urticaria

OTHER
- Injection-site thrombophlebitis (<1%)
- Priapism
- Xerostomia (<1%)

PARA-AMINOSALICYLIC ACID (PAS) (See AMINOSALICYLATE SODIUM)

PARAMETHADIONE

Trade name: Paradione (Abbott)
Category: Anticonvulsant
Clinically important, potentially serious interactions with: phenytoin, valproic acid

REACTIONS

SKIN
- Acne
- Erythema multiforme
- Exanthems
- Exfoliative dermatitis
- Lupus erythematosus
- Pruritus

HAIR
- Hair – alopecia

OTHER
- Bleeding gums
- Oral mucosal eruption
- Paresthesias

PAROXETINE

Trade name: Paxil (SmithKline Beecham)
Other common trade name: Aropax 20
Category: Selective serotonin reuptake inhibitor (SSRI); antidepressant
Clinically important, potentially serious interactions with: alcohol, anticoagulants, cimetidine, fluoxetine, MAO inhibitors, phenothiazines, phenytoin, sertraline, trazodone, tricyclic antidepressants, warfarin

REACTIONS

SKIN
- Acne (<1%)
- Allergic reactions (sic) (<1%)
- Angioedema (<1%)
- Aphthous stomatitis (<1%)
- Candidiasis
- Contact dermatitis (<1%)
- Cutaneous reaction (sic)
- Ecchymoses (<1%)
- Eczema (sic)
- Edema (<1%)
- Erythema nodosum (<1%)
- Exanthems (<1%)
- Facial edema (<1%)
- Furunculosis (<1%)
- Hyperhidrosis (11.2%)
- Lymphedema
- Melanoma (<1%)
- Peripheral edema (<1%)
- Photosensitivity (<1%)
- Pigmentation (<1%)
- Pruritus (<1%)
- Purpura (<1%)
- Rash (sic) (1.7%)
- Toxic epidermal necrolysis
- Urticaria (<1%)
- Xerosis (<1%)

HAIR
- Hair – alopecia (<1%)

OTHER
- Ageusia (<1%)
- Anosmia
- Bruxism (<1%)
- Dysgeusia (2.4%)
- Galactorrhea
- Gingivitis (<1%)
- Glossitis (<1%)
- Myalgia (1.7%)
- Oral ulceration
- Paresthesias (3.8%)
- Priapism
- Sialorrhea (<1%)
- Stomatitis (<1%)
- Tongue edema (<1%)
- Vaginal candidiasis (<1%)
- Vaginitis
- Xerostomia (18.1%)

PEMOLINE

Trade name: Cylert (Abbott)
Other common trade names: Betanamin; Tradon
Category: Central nervous system stimulant; anorexient
Clinically important, potentially serious interactions with: CNS depressants, CNS stimulants, sympathomimetics

REACTIONS

SKIN
- Exanthems (<1%)
- Rash (sic) (>10%)

PENBUTOLOL

Trade name: Levatol (Schwarz)
Other common trade names: Betapresin; Betapressin
Category: Beta-adrenergic blocking agent
Clinically important, potentially serious interactions with: clonidine, epinephrine, insulin, naproxen, salicylates, verapamil

REACTIONS

SKIN
- Allergic reactions (sic)
- Ankle edema
- Exanthems
- Flushing
- Hyperhidrosis (1.6%)
- Pruritus
- Psoriasis
- Purpura
- Rash (sic)

HAIR
- Hair – alopecia

NAILS
- Nails – bluish

OTHER
- Dysgeusia
- Peyronie's disease

PENICILLAMINE

Trade names: Cuprimine (Merck); Depen (Wallace)
Other common trade names: Artamin; Distamine; D-Penamine; Kelatin; Pendramine
Category: Chelating agent & antirheumatic
Clinically important, potentially serious interactions with: antacids, antimalarials, chloroquine, digoxin, gold, immunosuppressants, iron, oxyphenbutazone, phenylbutazone, probenecid

REACTIONS

SKIN
- Anetoderma
- Aphthous stomatitis
- Atrophy
- Bullous eruption
- Bullous pemphigoid
- Contact dermatitis
- Cutis laxa
- Dermatomyositis
- Dermopathy
- Discoid lupus erythematosus
- Edema (1–10%)
- Ehlers-Danlos syndrome
- Elastosis perforans serpiginosa
- Epidermal inclusion cysts
- Epidermolysis bullosa
- Erythema multiforme (1–5%)
- Erythema nodosum (<1%)
- Exanthems
- Exfoliative dermatitis
- Facial edema
- Flushing
- Guillain-Barré syndrome
- Lathyrism
- Lichenoid eruption
- Lichen planus
- Lupus erythematosus (<1%)
- Morphea
- Papular lesions at site of trauma
- Pemphigoid
- Pemphigus (<1%)
- Pemphigus erythematodes (Senear-Usher)
- Pemphigus foliaceus
- Pemphigus herpetiformis
- Pruritus (<1%)
- Pseudoxanthoma elasticum
- Psoriasis
- Purpura
- Rash (sic) (>10%)
- Scleroderma
- Sjøgren's syndrome
- Stevens-Johnson syndrome
- Toxic epidermal necrolysis (<1%)
- Urticaria (<1%)
- Vasculitis
- Vesicular eruption
- Wrinkling (sic)
- Xerosis

HAIR
Hair – alopecia
Hair – hirsutism

NAILS
Nails – dystrophy
Nails – elkonyxis (punched-out appearance of the nail at lunulae)
Nails – leukonychia
Nails – longitudinal ridges
Nails – onychoschizia
Nails – yellow nail syndrome

OTHER
Ageusia (12%)
Benign mucous membrane pemphigoid
Bromhidrosis
Dysgeusia (metallic taste)
Glossitis
Gynecomastia
Hypersensitivity
Hypogeusia (>10%)
Mucosal lesions (pemphigus-like)
Mucosal ulceration
Oral lichenoid eruption
Oral ulceration
Polymyositis
Serum sickness
Stomatitis

PENICILLINS

Generic names:

Amoxicillin
Trade names: Amoxil; Augmentin; Larotid; Polymox; Trimox; Wymox
Ampicillin
Trade names: Omnipen; Olycillin; Principen; Unasyn
Azlocillin
Trade name: Azlin
Bacampicillin
Trade name: Spectrobid
Carbenicillin
Trade name: Geopen
Cloxacillin
Trade names: Cloxapen; Tegopen
Cyclacillin
Trade name: None
Dicloxacillin
Trade names: Dycil; Dynapen; Pathocil
Methicillin
Trade name: Staphcillin
Mexlocillin
Trade name: Mezlin
Nafcillin
Trade name: Unipen
Oxacillin
Trade names: Bactocill; Prostaphlin
Penicillin G
Trade names: Bicillin; Crysticillin; Wycillin
Penicillin V
Trade names: Beepen; Betapen; Ledercillin; Pen Vee K; V-Cillin; etc.
Piperacillin
Trade name: Pipracil
Ticarcillin
Trade name: Ticar

(Various pharmaceutical companies.)

Category: Antibiotic

Clinically important, potentially serious interactions with: aminoglycosides, atenolol, cyclosporine, doxycycline, methotrexate, minocycline, probenecid, tetracyclines

Note: "Patients with a history of penicillin allergy are about ten times more likely than the general population to experience a potentially fatal reaction to subsequent therapy with most other haptenating drugs." The degradation products of penicillin can bind with tissue or serum proteins to form an immunogenic complex that can elicit an immune response.

REACTIONS

SKIN
Acute generalized exanthematous pustulosis (AGEP)
Angioedema
Bullous pemphigoid
Contact dermatitis
Contact urticaria
Cutis laxa
Eczematous eruption
Erythema annulare centrifugum
Erythema multiforme
Erythema nodosum

Exanthems
Exfoliative dermatitis
Fixed eruption
Hyperhidrosis
Jarisch-Herxheimer reaction (<1%)
Linear IgA bullous dermatosis
Lupus erythematosus
Pemphigoid
Pemphigus
Pityriasis rosea
Pruritus
Purpura
Pustular psoriasis
Rash (sic) (<1%)
Stevens-Johnson syndrome
Toxic epidermal necrolysis
Toxic erythema
Urticaria
Vasculitis

HAIR
Hair – alopecia

OTHER
Anaphylactoid reaction (<1%)
Black hairy tongue
Embolia cutis medicamentosa (Nicolau syndrome)
Hypersensitivity (<1%)
Injection-site aseptic necrosis
Injection-site reactions (1–10%)
Injection-site urticaria
Oral candidiasis (>10%)
Oral ulceration
Serum sickness
Thrombophlebitis (<1%)

PENTAGASTRIN

Trade name: Peptavlon (Ayerst)
Other common trade name: Gastrodiagnost
Category: Diagnostic aid (gastric function)
Clinically important, potentially serious interactions with: no data

REACTIONS

SKIN
Angioedema
Exanthems
Flushing
Hyperhidrosis
Pruritus
Purpura
Rash (sic)
Urticaria

OTHER
Hypersensitivity
Injection-site pain
Paresthesias

PENTAMIDINE

Trade names: Nebupent (Fujisawa); Pentam 300 (Fujisawa)
Other common trade name: Pentacarinat
Category: Antiprotozoal; also indicated in the treatment of *Pneumocystis carinii* pneumonia
Clinically important, potentially serious interactions with: no data

Note: The rate of adverse side effects is increased in patients with AIDS.

REACTIONS

SKIN
Bullous eruption
Cutaneous side effects (sic)
Exanthems
Jarisch-Herxheimer reaction
Pruritus
Purpura
Rash (sic) (3.3%)
Stevens-Johnson syndrome (0.2%)
Toxic epidermal necrolysis
Ulceration
Urticaria
Vasculitis
Xerosis

OTHER
Ageusia
Anosmia

Dysgeusia (metallic taste) (1.7%)
Gingivitis
Injection-site calcification
Injection-site cutaneous reaction (sic) (>10%)
Injection-site irritation
Injection-site ulceration
Myalgia (<5%)
Xerostomia

PENTAZOCINE

Trade name: Talwin (Sanofi Winthrop)
Other common trade names: Fortral; Fortwin; Liticon; Ospronim; Pentafen; Sosegon; Susevin
Category: Narcotic analgesic; sedative
Clinically important, potentially serious interactions with: alcohol, anxiolytics, cimetidine, CNS depressants, hypnotics, tranquilizers, tripelennamine

REACTIONS

SKIN
Cellulitis
Dermatitis (sic)
Exanthems
Facial edema
Flushing
Generalized eruption (sic)
Hyperhidrosis
Hyperpigmentation (surrounding ulcers)
Pruritus (<1%)
Rash (sic) (1–10%)
Scleroderma
Sclerosis (sic)
Toxic epidermal necrolysis (<1%)
Tricotropism (sic)
Ulceration
Urticaria

OTHER
Acute intermittent porphyria
Dysgeusia
Embolia cutis medicamentosa (Nicolau syndrome)
Fibrous myopathy
Injection-site calcification
Injection-site fibrosis
Injection-site granulomas & induration
Injection-site induration & ulcers
Injection-site pain
Injection-site pigmentation
Lipogranulomas
Panniculitis (chronic)
Paresthesias
Phlebitis
Sclerosis (sic)
Soft tissue calcification
Xerostomia (1–10%)

PENTOBARBITAL

Trade name: Nembutal (Abbott)
Other common trade names: Medinox Mono; Mintal; Pentobarbitone; Prodromol; Sombutol
Category: Hypnotic & sedative barbiturate; anticonvulsant
Clinically important, potentially serious interactions with: acetaminophen, anticoagulants, CNS depressants, cimetidine, diltiazem, MAO-inhibitors, metoprolol, nifedipine

REACTIONS

SKIN
Angioedema (<1%)
Bullous eruption
Erythema multiforme
Exanthems
Exfoliative dermatitis (<1%)
Fixed eruption
Herpes simplex (activation)
Lupus erythematosus
Necrosis
Photoallergic reaction
Pruritus
Purpura
Rash (sic) (<1%)
Stevens-Johnson syndrome (<1%)
Toxic epidermal necrolysis
Urticaria
Vasculitis

OTHER
Injection-site reactions (<1%)
Oral ulceration
Porphyria
Porphyria variegata
Thrombophlebitis (<1%)

PENTOSTATIN

Trade name: Nipent (Parke-Davis)
Category: Antineoplastic
Clinically important, potentially serious interactions with: allopurinol, fludarabine, vidarabine

REACTIONS

SKIN
Acne (<3%)
Allergic reactions (sic) (>10%)
Bullous eruption (3–10%)
Candidiasis (<3%)
Contact dermatitis (<3%)
Dermatitis (sic) (<1%)
Ecchymoses (3–10%)
Eczema (sic) (3–10%)
Exanthems (3–10%)
Exfoliative dermatitis (<3%)
Facial edema (<3%)
Flushing (<3%)
Herpes simplex (3–10%)
Herpes zoster (3–10%)
Hyperhidrosis (3–10%)
Peripheral edema (3–10%)
Petechiae (3–10%)
Photosensitivity (<3%)
Pigmentation (3–10%)
Pruritus (3–10%)
Psoriasis (<3%)
Purpura (<3%)
Rash (sic) (26%)
Reactivation of pruritus & erythema of preexisting keratoses (sic)
Seborrhea (3–10%)
Skin disorder (sic) (17%)
Urticaria (<1%)
Xerosis (3–10%)

HAIR
Hair – alopecia (<3%)

OTHER
Anaphylactoid reaction (<3%)
Dysgeusia (<3%)
Gingivitis (<3%)
Gynecomastia (<3%)
Injection-site hemorrhage (<3%)
Injection-site inflammation (<3%)
Leukoplakia (<3%)
Myalgia (>10%)
Paresthesias (3–10%)
Stomatitis (1–10%)
Thrombophlebitis (3–10%)
Vaginitis (<3%)

PENTOXIFYLLINE

Trade name: Trental (Hoechst Marion Roussel)
Other common trade names: Artal; Azupentat; Elorgan; Hemovas; Pentoxi; Pexal; Torental
Category: Blood viscosity-reducing agent
Clinically important, potentially serious interactions with: antihypertensives, cimetidine, warfarin

REACTIONS

SKIN
Allergic reactions (sic)
Angioedema (<1%)
Edema (<1%)
Exanthems
Flushing
Hyperhidrosis
Pruritus (<1%)
Purpura
Rash (sic) (<1%)
Urticaria

NAILS
Nails – brittle (<1%)

OTHER
- Dysgeusia (<1%)
- Dysphagia
- Paresthesias
- Serum sickness
- Sialorrhea (<1%)
- Xerostomia (<1%)

PERGOLIDE

Trade name: Permax (Athena)
Other common trade names: Celance; Parkotil; Pergolide
Category: Anti-parkinsonian; dopamine receptor agonist
Clinically important, potentially serious interactions with: none

REACTIONS

SKIN
- Acne
- Discoloration (sic)
- Edema (1.6%)
- Exanthems
- Facial edema (1.1%)
- Hyperhidrosis (2.1%)
- Peripheral edema (1–10%)
- Pruritus
- Rash (sic) (3.2%)
- Seborrhea
- Ulceration
- Urticaria
- Vasculitis
- Xerosis

HAIR
- Hair – alopecia
- Hair – hirsutism

OTHER
- Dysgeusia (1.6%)
- Erythromelalgia
- Gingivitis (<1%)
- Mastodynia
- Myalgia (<1%)
- Paresthesias (1.6%)
- Priapism
- Xerostomia (1–10%)

PERPHENAZINE

Trade name: Trilafon (Schering)
Other common trade names: Decentan; Fentazin; Peratsin; Perphenan; Trilifan Retard; Triomin
Category: Phenothiazine antipsychotic & antiemetic
Clinically important, potentially serious interactions with: anticonvulsants, bromocriptine, CNS depressants, levodopa, piperazine

REACTIONS

SKIN
- Angioedema
- Contact dermatitis
- Eczema (sic)
- Erythema
- Exanthems
- Exfoliative dermatitis
- Hypohidrosis (>10%)
- Lupus erythematosus
- Peripheral edema
- Photosensitivity
- Pigmentation (blue-gray) (<1%)
- Pruritus
- Purpura
- Rash (sic) (1–10%)
- Urticaria

OTHER
- Anaphylactoid reaction
- Galactorrhea (black) (<1%)
- Gynecomastia
- Mastodynia (1–10%)
- Priapism (<1%)
- Pseudolymphoma
- Sialorrhea
- Xerostomia

PHENAZOPYRIDINE

Trade name: Pyridium (Parke-Davis)
Other common trade names: Azodine; Phenazo; Pyronium; Sedural; Urohman; Uropyridin
Category: Analgesic (urinary)
Clinically important, potentially serious interactions with: none

REACTIONS

SKIN
- Allergic reactions (sic)
- Edema
- Exanthems
- Pigmentation (<1%)
- Pruritus
- Rash (sic) (<1%)

NAILS
- Nails – lemon-yellow

OTHER
- Anaphylactoid reaction

PHENDIMETRAZINE

Trade names: Bontril (Carnrick); Plegine (Ayerst)
Other common trade name: Obesan-X
Category: Appetite suppressant
Clinically important, potentially serious interactions with: diltiazem, doxycycline, MAO-inhibitors, nifedipine, quinidine, tetracycline, tricyclic antidepressants

REACTIONS

SKIN
- Flushing
- Hyperhidrosis
- Urticaria

OTHER
- Dysgeusia
- Xerostomia

PHENELZINE

Trade name: Nardil (Parke-Davis)
Other common trade name: Nardelzine
Category: Monoamine oxidase (MAO) inhibitor; antidepressant & antipanic
Clinically important, potentially serious interactions with: barbiturates, CNS depressants, dextroamphetamine, disulfiram, fluoxetine, levodopa, meperidine, phenothiazines, psychotropics, sumatriptan, sympathomimetics, venlafaxine. Also tyramine-containing foods

REACTIONS

SKIN
- Angioedema
- Ankle edema
- Diaphoresis
- Edema
- Exanthems
- Hyperhidrosis
- Lupus erythematosus
- Peripheral edema (1–10%)
- Photosensitivity
- Pruritus (13%)
- Rash (sic)
- Telangiectases
- Urticaria

OTHER
- Black tongue
- Glossitis
- Xerostomia (1–10%)

PHENINDAMINE

Trade name: Nolahist (Carnrick)
Category: H_1-receptor antihistamine & appetite stimulant
Clinically important, potentially serious interactions with: no data

REACTIONS

SKIN
- Angioedema
- Dermatitis (sic)
- Erythema
- Flushing
- Hyperhidrosis
- Lupus erythematosus
- Photosensitivity
- Purpura
- Rash (sic)
- Urticaria

OTHER
- Xerostomia

PHENOBARBITAL

Trade names: Luminal (Sanofi Winthrop); Solfoton (ECR)
Other common trade names: Gardenal; Luminal; Luminaletten; Phenaemal; Phenobarbitone
Category: Sedative-hypnotic & anticonvulsant barbiturate
Clinically important, potentially serious interactions with: acetaminophen, anticoagulants, benzodiazepines, CNS depressants, chloramphenicol, diltiazem, methylphenidate, metoprolol, propoxyphene, tricyclic antidepressants, valproic acid

REACTIONS

SKIN
- Acne
- Allergic reactions (sic)
- Angioedema (<1%)
- Bullous eruption
- Depigmentation
- Erythema multiforme
- Erythroderma
- Exanthems
- Exfoliative dermatitis (<1%)
- Fixed eruption
- Herpes simplex (activation)
- Lupus erythematosus
- Necrosis
- Pellagra
- Pemphigus
- Photoallergic reaction
- Pruritus
- Purpura
- Pustules (generalized)
- Rash (sic) (<1%)
- Stevens-Johnson syndrome (<1%)
- Toxic epidermal necrolysis
- Urticaria
- Vasculitis

HAIR
- Hair – depigmentation

NAILS
- Nails – hypoplasia

OTHER
- Hypersensitivity (<1%)
- Hypoplasia of phalanges
- Injection-site bullous eruption
- Injection-site pain (>10%)
- Oral ulceration
- Porphyria cutanea tarda
- Porphyria variegata
- Xerostomia

PHENOLPHTHALEIN

Trade names: Alophen; Espotabs; Ex-Lax; Feen-A-Mint; Modane; Phenolax; etc. (Various pharmaceutical companies.)
Other common trade names: Bom-Bon; Bonomint; Darmol; Easylax; Purganol; Ruguletts
Category: Laxative
Clinically important, potentially serious interactions with: no data

REACTIONS

SKIN
- Angioedema
- Bullous eruption
- Erythema annulare (sic)
- Erythema multiforme
- Exanthems
- Exfoliative dermatitis
- Fixed eruption
- Lupus erythematosus
- Pigmentation
- Pruritus
- Stevens-Johnson syndrome
- Toxic epidermal necrolysis
- Urticaria

NAILS
- Nails – discoloration of lunulae

OTHER
- Oral mucosal fixed eruption
- Oral mucosal pigmentation
- Oral mucosal ulceration

PHENSUXIMIDE

Trade name: Milontin (Parke-Davis)
Category: Anticonvulsant
Clinically important, potentially serious interactions with: phenytoin, valproic acid

REACTIONS

SKIN
- Erythema multiforme (<1%)
- Lupus erythematosus
- Periorbital edema
- Pruritus
- Purpura
- Rash (sic)
- Stevens-Johnson syndrome

HAIR
- Hair – alopecia
- Hair – hirsutism

OTHER
- Acute intermittent porphyria
- Gingival hyperplasia
- Oral ulceration

PHENTERMINE

Trade names: Adipex-P (Gate); Fastin (Beecham); Ionamin (Medeva)
Other common trade names: Behapront; Minobese-Forte; Panbesy; Panbesyl; Redusa; Umine
Category: Appetite suppressant
Clinically important, potentially serious interactions with: barbiturates, CNS stimulants, MAO inhibitors, sympathomimetics, tricyclic antidepressants

REACTIONS

SKIN
- Hyperhidrosis (<1%)
- Purpura
- Rash (sic)
- Raynaud's phenomenon
- Urticaria

HAIR
- Hair – alopecia (<1%)

OTHER
- Dysgeusia
- Myalgia (<1%)
- Xerostomia

PHENTOLAMINE

Trade name: Regitine (Novartis)
Other common trade names: Regitin; Rogitene; Rogitine
Category: Alpha-adrenergic blocking agent; antihypertensive; diagnostic aid for pheochromocytoma
Clinically important, potentially serious interactions with: ethanol

REACTIONS

SKIN
Flushing (1–10%)

PHENYTOIN (DIPHENYLHYDANTOIN)

Trade name: Dilantin (Parke-Davis)
Other common trade names: Di-Hydran; Epanutin; Fenytoin; Phenhydan; Pyoredol; Zentropil
Category: Hydantoin anticonvulsant; antiarrhythmic
Clinically important, potentially serious interactions with: amiodarone, chloramphenicol, cimetidine, corticosteroids, cyclosporine, diazoxide, dicumarol, disopyramide, disulfiram, doxycycline, ethosuximide, fluconazole, isoniazid, itraconazole, meperidine, mexiletine, oral contraceptives, phenylbutazone, primidone, quinidine, rifampin, saquinavir, theophylline, valproic acid, warfarin

Note: About 19% of patients receiving phenytoin develop skin reactions. They typically develop 10 to 14 days after the start of treatment.

REACTIONS

SKIN
Acne
Acute generalized exanthematous pustulosis (AGEP)
Angioedema
Bullous eruption
Eosinophilic fasciitis
Epidermolysis bullosa
Erythema multiforme
Erythroderma
Exanthems
Exfoliative dermatitis
Fixed eruption
Heel pad thickening
Lichenoid eruption
Lichen planus
Linear IgA bullous dermatosis
Lupus erythematosus (<1%)
Mycosis fungoides
Pellagra
Pemphigus
Pigmentation
Pruritus
Pseudoacanthosis nigricans
Purple glove syndrome (sic)
Purpura
Pustular eruption
Rash (sic) (1–10%)
Reticular hyperplasia
Scleroderma
Sezary syndrome
Sjøgren's syndrome
Stevens-Johnson syndrome (<1%)
Toxic dermatitis (sic)
Toxic epidermal necrolysis
Urticaria
Vasculitis
Warts

HAIR
Hair – alopecia
Hair – hirsutism
Hair – hypertrichosis

NAILS
Nails – disorder
Nails – hypoplasia
Nails – malformation
Nails – onychopathy
Nails – pigmentation

OTHER
- Acromegaloid-like
- Acute intermittent porphyria
- Coarse facies (sic)
- Digital malformations
- Fetal hydantoin syndrome*
- Gingival hyperplasia (>10%)
- Gynecomastia
- Hypersensitivity syndrome**
- Injection-site necrosis
- Injection-site pain
- Lymphadenopathy
- Lymphoma (<1%)
- Lymphoproliferative disease
- Mucocutaneous eruptions
- Mucocutaneous lymph node syndrome
- Myopathy
- Oral ulceration
- Paresthesias (<1%)
- Periarteritis nodosa
- Peyronie's disease
- Polyfibromatosis
- Polymyositis
- Porphyria
- Porphyria cutanea tarda
- Pseudolymphoma (<1%)
- Serum sickness
- Thrombophlebitis (<1%)

*Note: The fetal hydantoin syndrome (FHS) – Children whose mothers receive phenytoin during pregnancy are born with FHS. The main features of this syndrome are mental and growth retardation, unusual facies, digital and nail hypoplasia, and coarse scalp hair. Occasionally neonatal acne will be present.

**Note: The phenytoin hypersensitivity reaction (also known as the anticonvulsant hypersensitivity syndrome) is described in detail in (1978): Stanley J+, *Arch Dermatol* 114, 1350. The salient features of this reaction, which characteristically occur within the first 2 to 4 weeks of phenytoin therapy, are fever, generalized tender lymphadenopathy, hepatitis, leukocytosis, and a widespread, pruritic, irregular eruption consisting of ill-defined patches of macular erythema. Periorbital edema is common. The mucous membranes are frequently involved with erythema of the oral mucosa and pharynx. Papules, vesicles and pustules occasionally develop.

PHYTONADIONE (VITAMIN K)

Trade names: Aquamephyton (Merck); Mephyton (Merck); Phytomenadione; Vitamin K_1 (Abbott)
Other common trade names: Kaywan; Vitak
Category: Fat-soluble nutritional supplement & antihemorrhagic
Clinically important, potentially serious interactions with: anticoagulants

REACTIONS

SKIN
- Allergic reactions (sic)
- Contact dermatitis
- Eczematous plaques
- Erythema (annular)
- Exanthems
- Flushing
- Hyperhidrosis (<1%)
- Rash (sic)
- Scleroderma
- Urticaria
- Vasculitis

OTHER
- Anaphylactoid reaction (<1%)
- Dysgeusia (<1%)
- Hypersensitivity (<1%)
- Injection-site eczematous eruption
- Injection-site erythema
- Injection-site indurated plaques (Texier's syndrome) (<1%)

PIMOZIDE

Trade name: Orap (Gate)
Other common trade names: Frenal; Neurap; Orap; Pimodac
Category: Antipsychotic & antidyskinetic (Tourette's syndrome)
Clinically important, potentially serious interactions with: alfentanil, amphetamines, azithromycin, clarithromycin, CNS depressants, dirithromycin, erythromycin, fluoxetine, guanabenz, MAO inhibitors, methylphenidate

REACTIONS

SKIN
- Exanthems
- Facial edema (1–10%)
- Hyperhidrosis (rare)
- Hyperpigmentation
- Periorbital edema
- Photosensitivity
- Pruritus
- Rash (sic) (8.3%)
- Urticaria

OTHER
- Dysgeusia
- Galactorrhea
- Gynecomastia (>10%)
- Myalgia (2.7%)
- Sialorrhea (13.8%)
- Xerostomia (>10%)

PINDOLOL

Trade name: Visken (Novartis)
Other common trade names: Barbloc; Durapindol; Nonspi; Pinbetol; Pinden; Vypen
Category: Beta-adrenergic blocking agent; antihypertensive
Clinically important, potentially serious interactions with: calcium channel blockers, clonidine, flecainide, insulin, nifedipine, oral contraceptives, verapamil

REACTIONS

SKIN
- Eczematous eruption (sic)
- Edema (6%)
- Erythema multiforme
- Exanthems
- Hyperhidrosis (2%)
- Hyperkeratosis (palms & soles)
- Lichenoid eruption
- Lupus erythematosus
- Pityriasis rubra pilaris
- Pruritus (1–5%)
- Psoriasis
- Purpura
- Rash (sic) (1–10%)
- Raynaud's phenomenon
- Toxic epidermal necrolysis
- Urticaria
- Xerosis

HAIR
- Hair – alopecia

NAILS
- Nails – dystrophy
- Nails – onycholysis

OTHER
- Dysgeusia
- Myopathy
- Oculo-mucocutaneous syndrome
- Oral lichenoid eruption
- Paresthesias
- Peyronie's disease

PIPERACILLIN

Trade names: Pipracil (Lederle); Zosyn (Lederle)
Other common trade names: Avocin; Ivacin; Picillin; Pipcil; Piperilline; Pipril; Piprilin; Pitamycin
Category: Beta-lactamase-sensitive penicillin antibiotic
Clinically important, potentially serious interactions with: aminoglycosides, anticoagulants, methotrexate, neuromuscular blockers, probenecid, tetracycline

Zosyn is piperacillin & tazobactam

REACTIONS

SKIN
- Allergic reactions (sic) (2–4%)
- Exanthems
- Jarisch-Herxheimer reaction (<1%)
- Pruritus
- Rash (sic) (1%)
- Stevens-Johnson syndrome
- Urticaria
- Vesicular eruptions

OTHER
- Anaphylactoid reaction (<1%)
- Glossodynia
- Hypersensitivity (<1%)
- Injection-site pain (2%)
- Injection-site phlebitis (2%)
- Oral candidiasis
- Serum sickness
- Stomatodynia
- Thrombophlebitis (<1%)

PIROXICAM

Trade name: Feldene (Pfizer)
Other common trade names: Antiflog; Baxo; Doblexan; Felden; Larapam; Sotilen; Zunden
Category: Nonsteroidal anti-inflammatory (NSAID)
Clinically important, potentially serious interactions with: anticoagulants, aspirin, beta-blockers, diuretics, lithium, methotrexate, warfarin

REACTIONS

SKIN
- Angioedema (<1%)
- Aphthous stomatitis
- Contact dermatitis
- Cutaneous side effects (46.9%)
- Dyshidrosis
- Ecchymoses (<1%)
- Edema (>1%)
- Erythema (<1%)
- Erythema annulare centrifugum
- Erythema multiforme (<1%)
- Erythroderma
- Exanthems (>5%)
- Exfoliative dermatitis (<1%)
- Fixed eruption
- Hyperhidrosis (<1%)
- Lichenoid eruption
- Linear IgA bullous dermatosis
- Lupus erythematosus
- Pemphigus
- Pemphigus foliaceus
- Petechiae (<1%)
- Photoallergic reaction (<1%)
- Photocontact dermatitis
- Photosensitivity
- Pruritus (1–10%)
- Purpura (<1%)
- Rash (sic) (>10%)
- Stevens-Johnson syndrome (<1%)
- Toxic dermatitis (sic)
- Toxic epidermal necrolysis (<1%)
- Urticaria (<1%)
- Vasculitis (<1%)
- Vesicular eruption (<1%)

HAIR
- Hair – alopecia

NAILS
- Nails – onycholysis

OTHER
- Anaphylactoid reaction (<1%)
- Buccal ulceration

Paresthesias
Serum sickness (<1%)
Stomatitis (>1%)
Xerostomia (<1%)

PLICAMYCIN (MITHRAMYCIN)

Trade name: Mithracin (Bayer)
Other common trade name: Mithraline
Category: Antineoplastic; antihypercalcemic; antihypercalciuric; bone resorption inhibitor
Clinically important, potentially serious interactions with: calcitonin, etidronate, glucagon

REACTIONS

SKIN
Bleeding tendency (5–12%)
Ecchymoses
Exanthems
Flushing (1–10%)
Petechiae
Purpura
Seborrheic keratoses (inflammation of)
Toxic epidermal necrolysis

OTHER
Injection-site cellulitis (1–10%)
Injection-site erythema (1–10%)
Injection-site pain
Oral mucosal lesions
Stomatitis (>10%)

POLYTHIAZIDE

Trade names: Minizide (Pfizer); Renese (Pfizer)
Other common trade names: Drenusil; Nephril
Category: Thiazide diuretic; antihypertensive
Clinically important, potentially serious interactions with: antidiabetics, digitalis, lithium, methotrexate

Minizide is prazosin & polythiazide

REACTIONS

SKIN
Exanthems
Photosensitivity (<1%)
Purpura
Rash (sic) (<1%)
Urticaria
Vasculitis

OTHER
Paresthesias

POTASSIUM IODIDE

Trade names: Pima (Fleming); SSKI (Upsher Smith)
Other common trade names: Jodatum; Jodid; Kalium
Category: Antihyperthyroid; thyroid inhibitor; antifungal; expectorant
Clinically important, potentially serious interactions with: lithium

REACTIONS

SKIN
Acne (1–10%)
Angioedema (1–10%)
Bullous pemphigoid
Dermatitis herpetiformis
Exanthems
Hyperhidrosis
Iododerma
Lupus erythematosus
Pustular psoriasis
Rash (sic)
Systemic eczematous contact dermatitis
Urticaria (1–10%)
Vasculitis

OTHER
Dysgeusia (metallic taste) (1–10%)
Paresthesias
Sialorrhea
Stomatodynia

PRAMIPEXOLE

Trade name: Mirapex (Pharmacia & Upjohn)
Category: Anti-parkinsonian
Clinically important, potentially serious interactions with: cimetidine, diltiazem, haloperidol, levodopa, metoclopramide, phenothiazines, quinidine, quinine, ranitidine, thiothixene, triamterene, verapamil

REACTIONS

SKIN
- Allergic reactions (sic) (>1%)
- Edema (5%)
- Hyperhidrosis (>1%)
- Peripheral edema (5%)
- Pruritus (>1%)
- Rash (sic) (>1%)
- Skin disorders (sic) (2%)

OTHER
- Dysgeusia (>1%)
- Hypesthesia (3%)
- Myalgia (>1%)
- Paresthesias (>1%)
- Sialorrhea (>1%)
- Tooth disease (sic) (>1%)
- Twitching (sic) (2%)
- Xerostomia (7%)

PRAVASTATIN

Trade name: Pravachol (Bristol-Myers Squibb)
Other common trade names: Elisor; Lipostat; Pravasin; Pravasine; Selectin; Selektine; Selipran
Category: Antihyperlipidemic; HMG-CoA reductase inhibitor
Clinically important, potentially serious interactions with: anticoagulants, cholestyramine, clofibrate, gemfibrozil

REACTIONS

SKIN
- Allergic reactions (sic)
- Angioedema
- Dermatomyositis
- Eczematous eruption (generalized)
- Erythema multiforme
- Exanthems
- Flushing
- Lichenoid eruption
- Lupus erythematosus
- Photosensitivity
- Pruritus
- Purpura
- Rash (sic) (1–10%)
- Stevens-Johnson syndrome
- Toxic epidermal necrolysis
- Urticaria
- Vasculitis

HAIR
- Hair – alopecia

OTHER
- Anaphylactoid reaction
- Dysgeusia (<1%)
- Gynecomastia
- Myalgia (2.7%)
- Myopathy
- Paresthesias
- Porphyria cutanea tarda
- Stomatitis

PRAZEPAM

Trade name: Centrax (Parke-Davis)
Other common trade names: Centrac; Demetrin; Lysanxia; Prazene; Sedapran; Trepidan
Category: Benzodiazepine sedative-hypnotic, anxiolytic & antidepressant; anticonvulsant
Clinically important, potentially serious interactions with: anticonvulsants, CNS depressants, cimetidine, clarithromycin, digoxin, disulfiram, verapamil

Reactions

SKIN
- Ankle edema
- Dermatitis (sic) (1–10%)
- Exanthems
- Facial edema
- Hyperhidrosis (>10%)
- Pruritus
- Purpura
- Rash (sic) (>10%)
- Urticaria

HAIR
- Hair – alopecia
- Hair – hirsutism

OTHER
- Gingivitis
- Paresthesias
- Sialopenia (>10%)
- Sialorrhea (1–10%)
- Xerostomia (>10%)

PRAZIQUANTEL

Trade name: Biltricide (Bayer)
Other common trade names: Cisticid; Distocide; Flukacide; Kalcide; Prazite; Tecprazin; Teniken
Category: Anthelmintic
Clinically important, potentially serious interactions with: aminoquinolines, carbamazepine, phenytoin

Reactions

SKIN
- Edema
- Urticaria

PRAZOSIN

Trade names: Minipress (Pfizer); Minizide (Pfizer)
Other common trade names: Duramipress; Eurex; Hypovase; Peripress; Pratisol; Pressin
Category: Alpha-adrenergic blocker, peripheral vasodilator & antihypertensive
Clinically important, potentially serious interactions with: beta-blockers, diltiazem, diuretics, nifedipine, verapamil

Minizide is prazosin & polythiazide

Reactions

SKIN
- Angioedema
- Edema (1–4%)
- Exanthems (1–5%)
- Hyperhidrosis (<1%)
- Lichenoid eruption
- Lichen planus (<1%)
- Lupus erythematosus
- Pruritus (<1%)
- Rash (sic) (1–4%)
- Urticaria

HAIR
- Hair – alopecia (<1%)

OTHER
- Anaphylactoid reaction
- Myopathy
- Paresthesias (<1%)
- Priapism (<1%)
- Xerostomia (1–4%)

PRIMAQUINE

Trade name: Primaquine (Sanofi Winthrop)
Other common trade names: Neo-Quipenyl; Palum
Category: Antiprotozoal; antimalarial
Clinically important, potentially serious interactions with: quinacrine

REACTIONS

SKIN
Angioedema
Exanthems
Pruritus (<1%)
Psoriasis
Urticaria

PRIMIDONE

Trade name: Mysoline (Ayerst)
Other common trade names: Midone; Mylepsin; PMS Primidone; Prysoline
Category: Anticonvulsant; barbiturate
Clinically important, potentially serious interactions with: acetaminophen, anticoagulants, MAO inhibitors, methylphenidate, valproic acid

REACTIONS

SKIN
Acne
Allergic reactions (sic)
Erythema multiforme (<1%)
Exanthems (1–5%)
Exfoliative dermatitis
Lupus erythematosus (<1%)
Rash (sic) (<1%)
Toxic epidermal necrolysis
Urticaria

OTHER
Acute intermittent porphyria
Gingival hyperplasia
Mucocutaneous syndrome

PROBENECID

Trade names: Benemid (Merck); Colbenemid (Merck)
Other common trade names: Bencid; Benecid; Benuryl; Panuric; Procid; Solpurin; Urocid
Category: Antigout; antihyperuricemic
Clinically important, potentially serious interactions with: acyclovir, benzodiazepines, beta-lactams, dapsone, ketorolac, methotrexate, penicillamine, sulfonylureas, thiopental, zidovudine

REACTIONS

SKIN
Allergic reactions (sic)
Dermatitis (sic)
Erythema multiforme
Exanthems
Flushing (1–10%)
Pruritus (1–10%)
Rash (sic) (1–10%)
Urticaria

HAIR
Hair – alopecia

OTHER
Anaphylactoid reaction (<1%)
Gingivitis (1–10%)
Hypersensitivity

PROCAINAMIDE

Trade names: Procan (Parke-Davis); Pronestyl (Bristol-Myers Squibb)
Other common trade names: Amisalen; Biocoryl; Ritmocamid
Category: Antiarrhythmic
Clinically important, potentially serious interactions with: amiodarone, astemizole, beta-blockers, cimetidine, lidocaine, quinidine, ranitidine, terfenadine, trimethoprim

REACTIONS

SKIN
- Angioedema (<1%)
- Dermatitis (sic)
- Eczematous eruption (sic)
- Exanthems (1–5%)
- Flushing
- Lichen planus
- Lupus erythematosus (>10%)
- Pruritus
- Purpura
- Rash (sic) (<1%)
- Sjøgren's syndrome
- Urticaria (1–5%)
- Vasculitis

OTHER
- Dysgeusia
- Myopathy (<1%)
- Oral mucosal eruption

PROCARBAZINE

Trade name: Matulane (Roche)
Other common trade name: Natulan
Category: Antineoplastic
Clinically important, potentially serious interactions with: amphetamines, digitalis, epinephrine, MAO inhibitors, methotrexate, tricyclic antidepressants. Also tyramine-containing foods

REACTIONS

SKIN
- Allergic reactions (sic) (<1%)
- Angioedema
- Dermatitis (sic) (<1%)
- Edema
- Exanthems
- Exfoliative dermatitis
- Fixed eruption
- Flushing
- Herpes zoster
- Hyperhidrosis
- Petechiae
- Photosensitivity
- Pigmentation (1–10%)
- Pruritus (<1%)
- Purpura
- Rash (sic)
- Toxic epidermal necrolysis
- Urticaria

HAIR
- Hair – alopecia (1–10%)

OTHER
- Gynecomastia
- Hypersensitivity (2%)
- Oral mucosal lesions
- Myalgia (<1%)
- Paresthesias (>10%)
- Stomatitis (>10%)
- Xerostomia

PROCHLORPERAZINE

Trade name: Compazine (SmithKline Beecham)
Other common trade names: Novamin; Novomit; Pasotomin; Stella; Stemetil; Tementil; Vertigon
Category: Phenothiazine antipsychotic & antiemetic
Clinically important, potentially serious interactions with: anticonvulsants, CNS depressants, epinephrine, levodopa, piperazine, trazodone

REACTIONS

SKIN
- Erythema
- Exanthems
- Exfoliative dermatitis
- Fixed eruption (<1%)
- Hypohidrosis (>10%)
- Lupus erythematosus
- Peripheral edema
- Photosensitivity (1–10%)
- Phototoxic reaction
- Pigmentation (<1%) (blue-gray)
- Pruritus (1–10%)
- Purpura
- Rash (sic) (1–10%)
- Toxic epidermal necrolysis
- Urticaria

OTHER
- Anaphylactoid reaction (1–10%)
- Blue tongue (sic)
- Galactorrhea (<1%)
- Gynecomastia (1–10%)
- Lip ulceration
- Priapism (<1%)
- Xerostomia (>10%)

PROCYCLIDINE

Trade name: Kemadrin (Glaxo Wellcome)
Other common trade names: Apricolin; Kemadren; Onservan
Category: Anticholinergic, antidyskinetic, anti-parkinsonian
Clinically important, potentially serious interactions with: anticholinergics, atenolol, digitalis, meperidine, phenothiazines, tricyclic antidepressants

REACTIONS

SKIN
- Hypohidrosis (>10%)
- Rash (sic) (<1%)

OTHER
- Xerostomia (>10%)

PROGESTINS

Generic names:
- Hydroxyprogesterone
  - Trade names: Delta-Lutin; Duralutin; Hylutin; Pro-Depo; Prodrox
- Medroxyprogesterone
  - Trade names: Amen; Curretab; Cycrin; Provera
- Megestrol
  - Trade name: Megace
- Norethindrone
  - Trade names: Aygestin; Micronor; Norlutin; Norlutate; Nor-QD
- Norgestrol
  - Trade name: Ovrette
- Progesterone
  - Trade names: Gesterol 50; Progestaject

(Various pharmaceutical companies.)

Categories: Progestin; antineoplastic; contraceptive (systemic)

REACTIONS

SKIN
- Acne
- Angioedema
- Ankle edema
- Autoimmune dermatitis
- Dermatitis

Edema
Erythema multiforme
Erythema nodosum
Exanthems
Flushing
Hemorrhagic eruption (sic)
Hyperhidrosis
Melasma
Pruritus
Rash (sic)
Telangiectases
Urticaria

HAIR
Hair – alopecia
Hair – hirsutism

OTHER
Anaphylactoid reaction
Galactorrhea
Gynecomastia (painful)

PROMAZINE

Trade name: Sparine (Wyeth)
Other common trade names: Liranol; Prazine; Protactyl; Savamine; Talofen
Category: Phenothiazine antipsychotic; antiemetic
Clinically important, potentially serious interactions with: levodopa, piperazine, sympathomimetics, trazodone, tricyclic antidepressants

REACTIONS

SKIN
Dermatitis (sic)
Edema
Exanthems
Hypohidrosis (>10%)
Photoallergic reaction
Photosensitivity (1–10%)
Phototoxic reaction
Pigmentation (<1%) (blue-gray)
Purpura
Rash (sic)
Urticaria
Xerosis

OTHER
Galactorrhea (<1%)
Gynecomastia
Mastodynia (1–10%)
Priapism (<1%)
Xerostomia

PROMETHAZINE

Trade names: Anergan (Forest); Phenergan (Wyeth)
Other common trade names: Atosil; Bonnox; Closin; Goodnight; Histantil; Prothiazine; Pyrethia
Category: Phenothiazine H_1-receptor antihistamine & antiemetic, antivertigo & sedative-hypnotic
Clinically important, potentially serious interactions with: anticholinergics, bromocriptine, CNS depressants, epinephrine, MAO inhibitors

REACTIONS

SKIN
Angioedema (<1%)
Bullous eruption (<1%)
Contact dermatitis
Eczematous eruption (sic)
Erythema multiforme
Exanthems
Fixed eruption
Hyperhidrosis
Lupus erythematosus
Photoallergic reaction
Photosensitivity (<1%)
Purpura
Rash (sic) (<1%)
Stevens-Johnson syndrome
Systemic eczematous contact dermatitis
Toxic epidermal necrolysis (<1%)
Urticaria

OTHER
Anaphylactoid reaction (with temazepam)
Embolia cutis medicamentosa (Nicolau syndrome)
Hypersensitivity

Myalgia (<1%)
Oral ulceration
Paresthesias (<1%)
Xerostomia (1–10%)

PROPAFENONE

Trade name: Rythmol (Knoll)
Other common trade names: Arythmol; Norfenon; Normorytmin; Rythmex; Rytmonorm
Category: Antiarrhythmic
Clinically important, potentially serious interactions with: anticoagulants, beta-blockers, cyclosporine, digoxin, quinidine, ritonavir, tricyclic antidepressants, warfarin

REACTIONS

SKIN
Acne (1%)
Diaphoresis
Edema
Exanthems
Lupus erythematosus (<1%)
Pruritus (<1%)
Purpura (<1%)
Rash (sic) (>10%)
Urticaria

HAIR
Hair – alopecia (<1%)

OTHER
Dysgeusia (1–10%)
Oral mucosal lesions
Paresthesias (<1%)
Parosmia (<1%)
Xerostomia (>10%)

PROPANTHELINE

Trade name: Pro-Banthine (Roberts)
Other common trade names: Bropantil; Corrigast; Ercoril; Ercotina; Norproban; Propantel
Category: Gastrointestinal anticholinergic antispasmodic
Clinically important, potentially serious interactions with: adenosine, amiodarone, amoxapine, analgesics, anticholinergics, beta-blockers, bretylium, CNS depressants, corticosteroids, disopyramide, phenothiazines, tricyclic antidepressants

REACTIONS

SKIN
Contact dermatitis
Exanthems
Hyperhidrosis (>10%)
Hypohidrosis
Rash (sic) (<1%)
Urticaria
Xerosis (>10%)

OTHER
Ageusia
Anaphylactoid reaction
Dysgeusia
Sialopenia
Xerostomia (>10%)

PROPOFOL

Trade name: Diprivan (Zeneca)
Category: Anesthetic; sedative
Clinically important, potentially serious interactions with: atracurium, benzodiazepines, theophylline

REACTIONS

SKIN
Allergic reactions (sic)
Edema (<1%)
Exanthems
Fixed eruption (1%)
Flushing (>1%)
Pruritus (>1%)
Rash (sic) (5%)

Urticaria

HAIR
Hair – color change

OTHER
Anaphylactoid reaction (1–10%)
Dysgeusia (<1%)
Injection-site erythema (<1%)
Injection-site pain (>10%)
Injection-site pruritus (<1%)
Myalgia (>1%)
Sialorrhea (>1%)
Xerostomia (<1%)

PROPOXYPHENE

Trade names: Darvocet-N (Lilly); Darvon (Lilly); Darvon Compound (Lilly)
Other common trade names: Algafan; Antalvic; Develin; Dolotard; Doloxene; Liberan; Parvon
Category: Narcotic analgesic
Clinically important, potentially serious interactions with: alprazolam, carbamazepine, CNS depressants, MAO inhibitors, phenobarbital, ritonavir, tricyclic antidepressants, warfarin

Darvocet is propoxyphene & acetaminophen; Darvon Compound is propoxyphene & aspirin

REACTIONS

SKIN
Exanthems
Facial edema
Flushing
Hyperhidrosis
Pruritus
Rash (sic) (<1%)
Urticaria (<1%)

OTHER
Ano-recto-vaginal ulcerations
Injection-site nodules
Injection-site pain (1–10%)
Xerostomia (1–10%)

PROPRANOLOL

Trade name: Inderal (Ayerst)
Other common trade names: Acifol; Apsolol; Betabloc; Cinlol; Inderex; Prosin; Sinal; Tesnol
Category: Beta-adrenergic blocking agent; antianginal; antihypertensive
Clinically important, potentially serious interactions with: antidiabetics, calcium channel blockers, clonidine, flecainide, haloperidol, insulin, nifedipine, oral contraceptives, verapamil

REACTIONS

SKIN
Acne
Angioedema
Bullous eruption
Contact dermatitis
Eczematous eruption (sic)
Erythema multiforme
Exanthems
Exfoliative dermatitis
Flushing
Hyperhidrosis
Hyperkeratosis (palms & soles)
Lichenoid eruption
Lupus erythematosus
Pemphigus
Peripheral skin necrosis (sic)
Photosensitivity
Phototoxic reaction
Pruritus
Psoriasis
Purpura
Pustular psoriasis
Rash (sic) (1–10%)
Raynaud's phenomenon
Sclerosis
Stevens-Johnson syndrome
Systemic erythematous eruption (sic)
Toxic epidermal necrolysis
Toxicoderma
Urticaria

HAIR
Hair – alopecia

NAILS
Nails – discoloration
Nails – onycholysis
Nails – pitting (psoriasiform)
Nails – thickening

OTHER
Anaphylactoid reaction
Cheilostomatitis (sic)
Dupuytren's contracture
Dysgeusia
Myopathy
Oral ulceration
Paresthesias
Peyronie's disease
Serum sickness
Tongue pigmentation
Xerostomia

PROPYLTHIOURACIL

Trade name: Propylthiouracil
Other common trade names: Propacil; Propycil; Propyl-Thyracil; Tiotil
Category: Antihyperthyroid
Clinically important, potentially serious interactions with: anticoagulants, digitalis, metoprolol

Reactions

SKIN
Angioedema
Dermatitis (sic)
Edema (<1%)
Erythema nodosum
Exanthems
Exfoliative dermatitis (<1%)
Lichenoid eruption
Lupus erythematosus (1–10%)
Pigmentation
Pruritus (<1%)
Purpura
Rash (sic) (>10%)
Ulceration
Urticaria (<1%)
Vasculitis (<1%)
Vesicular eruption (in newborn)

HAIR
Hair – alopecia (<1%)

OTHER
Ageusia (1–10%)
Dysgeusia (metallic taste)
Myalgia
Oral mucosal lesions
Oral ulceration
Paresthesias (<1%)

PROTAMINE

Trade name: Protamine Sulfate (Lilly, others)
Category: Antidote (to heparin)
Clinically important, potentially serious interactions with: none

Reactions

SKIN
Angioedema
Exanthems
Flushing (<1%)
Urticaria

OTHER
Anaphylactoid reaction
Hypersensitivity (<1%)

PROTRIPTYLINE

Trade name: Vivactil (Merck)
Other common trade names: Concordin; Triptil
Category: Tricyclic antidepressant & antinarcolepsy adjunct
Clinically important, potentially serious interactions with: alcohol, anticholinergics, CNS depressants, cimetidine, clonidine, epinephrine, guanethidine, MAO inhibitors, sympathomimetics

REACTIONS

SKIN
- Allergic reactions (sic) (<1%)
- Angioedema
- Dermatitis (sic) (3%)
- Edema
- Exanthems
- Flushing
- Hyperhidrosis (1–10%)
- Petechiae
- Photosensitivity (<1%)
- Phototoxic reaction
- Pruritus (1–5%)
- Purpura
- Rash (sic)
- Urticaria

HAIR
- Hair – alopecia (<1%)

OTHER
- Black hairy tongue
- Dysgeusia (>10%)
- Galactorrhea (<1%)
- Glossitis
- Gynecomastia (<1%)
- Oral mucosal eruption
- Paresthesias
- Stomatitis
- Xerostomia (>10%)

PSEUDOEPHEDRINE

Trade names: Actifed; Afrinol; Allerid; Cenafed; Decofed; Drixoral; Entex; Novafed; Seldane-D, Sudafed; Trinalin; etc. (Various pharmaceutical companies.)
Other common trade name: Maxiphed
Category: Nasal decongestant; sympathomimetic
Clinically important, potentially serious interactions with: bromocriptine, furazolidone, MAO inhibitors, propranolol, sympathomimetics, tricyclic antidepressants

REACTIONS

SKIN
- Angioedema
- Dermatitis (sic)
- Eczematous eruption
- Exanthems
- Exfoliative dermatitis
- Fixed eruption:
- Hyperhidrosis (1–10%)
- Pseudo-scarlatina (sic)
- Systemic contact dermatitis
- Toxic shock syndrome
- Urticaria

PSORALENS

Trade names: 8-MOP (ICN); Oxsoralen (ICN); Trisoralen (ICN)
Category: Repigmenting agents
Clinically important, potentially serious interactions with: other photosensitizing agents

REACTIONS

SKIN
- Acne
- Blistering (sic)
- Bowen's disease
- Bullous pemphigoid (with UVA)
- Burning (1–10%)
- Cheilitis (1–10%)
- Contact dermatitis
- Eczematous eruption (sic)
- Edema (1–10%)

Folliculitis
Freckles (1–10%)
Granuloma annulare
Herpes simplex
Herpes zoster
Hypopigmentation (1–10%)
Keratoacanthoma
Lichen planus
Lupus erythematosus
Melanoma
Miliaria
Pemphigoid
Pemphigus vulgaris
Photoallergic reaction
Photocontact dermatitis
Photosensitivity
Phototoxic reaction
Phytophotodermatitis
Pigmentation
Porokeratosis (actinic)
Prurigo
Pruritus (>10%)
Psoriasis
Rash (sic) (1–10%)
Rosacea
Scleroderma
Seborrheic dermatitis
Skin pain
Squamous cell carcinoma
Tumors (malignant for the most part)
Urticaria
Vasculitis
Vitiligo
Warts

HAIR
Hair – hypertrichosis

NAILS
Nails – photo-onycholysis
Nails – pigmentation

OTHER
Lymphoproliferative disease

PYRAZINAMIDE

Trade name: Pyrazinamide (Lederle)
Other common trade names: Dipimide; Isopas; Lynamide; Pirilene; Pyrazide; Rozide; Zinastat
Category: Antibacterial; antitubercular
Clinically important, potentially serious interactions with: cyclosporine, rifampin

REACTIONS

SKIN
Acne (<1%)
Erythema multiforme
Exanthems
Fixed eruption
Flushing
Pellagra
Photosensitivity (<1%)
Pruritus (<1%)
Purpura
Rash (sic) (<1%)
Urticaria

OTHER
Acute intermittent porphyria
Myalgia (1–10%)
Oral mucosal lesions
Porphyria cutanea tarda (<1%)

PYRIDOXINE

Trade names: Hexabetalin (Lilly); Vitamin B_6
Other common trade names: B(6)-Vicotrat; Godabion B6
Category: Water-soluble nutritional supplement & antidote
Clinically important, potentially serious interactions with: levodopa

REACTIONS

SKIN
Acne
Allergic reactions (sic) (<1%)
Bullous eruption
Contact dermatitis
Fixed eruption
Photosensitivity
Purpura

Toxic epidermal necrolysis
Vasculitis
Vesicular eruption

HAIR
Hair – pigmentation

OTHER
Hypersensitivity
Paresthesias (<1%)
Porphyria cutanea tarda
Pseudoporphyria

PYRILAMINE

Trade name: Triaminic (Novartis)
Category: H_1-receptor antihistamine
Clinically important, potentially serious interactions with: no data

REACTIONS

SKIN
Angioedema
Dermatitis (sic)
Flushing
Hyperhidrosis
Lupus erythematosus
Photosensitivity
Purpura
Rash (sic)
Urticaria

OTHER
Anaphylactoid reaction
Gynecomastia
Paresthesias
Stomatitis
Xerostomia

PYRIMETHAMINE

Trade names: Daraprim (Glaxo Wellcome); Fansidar (Roche)
Other common trade names: Erbaprelina; Malocide; Pirimecidan
Category: Antimalarial
Clinically important, potentially serious interactions with: cotrimoxazole, folic acid, methotrexate, sulfonamides

Fansidar is pyrimethamine & sulfadoxine

REACTIONS

SKIN
Acute generalized exanthematous pustulosis (AGEP)
Angioedema
Bullous eruption
Dermatitis (sic) (<1%)
Erythema multiforme (<1%)
Exanthems
Exfoliative dermatitis
Fixed eruption
Lichenoid eruption
Photosensitivity (>10%)
Pigmentation (<1%)
Pruritus
Purpura
Pustular eruption
Rash (sic) (<1%)
Stevens-Johnson syndrome (1–10%)
Toxic dermatitis (sic)
Toxic epidermal necrolysis (<1%)
Urticaria

HAIR
Hair – alopecia

OTHER
Dysgeusia
Glossitis (atrophic) (<1%)
Hypersensitivity (>10%)
Lymphoproliferative disease
Xerostomia (<1%)

QUAZEPAM

Trade name: Doral (Wallace)
Other common trade names: Oniria; Pamerex; Quazium; Quiedorm; Selepam; Temodal
Category: Benzodiazepine sedative-hypnotic; antidepressant
Clinically important, potentially serious interactions with: alcohol, anesthetics, barbiturates, CNS depressants, cimetidine, clarithromycin, diltiazem, levodopa, MAO inhibitors, narcotics, phenothiazines, tricyclic antidepressants, verapamil

REACTIONS

SKIN
- Dermatitis (sic) (1–10%)
- Hyperhidrosis (>10%)
- Pruritus
- Purpura
- Rash (sic) (>10%)
- Urticaria

HAIR
- Hair – alopecia
- Hair – hirsutism

OTHER
- Dysgeusia
- Oral ulceration
- Paresthesias
- Sialopenia (>10%)
- Sialorrhea (1–10%)
- Xerostomia (1–5%)

QUETIAPINE

Trade name: Seroquel (Zeneca)
Category: Antipsychotic
Clinically important, potentially serious interactions with: cimetidine, levodopa, phenothiazines, phenytoin

REACTIONS

SKIN
- Candidiasis (<1%)
- Facial edema (<1%)
- Photosensitivity (<1%)
- Rash (sic) (4%)
- Xerosis (<1%)

OTHER
- Bruxism (<1%)
- Gingivitis (<1%)
- Glossitis (<1%)
- Myalgia (<1%)
- Oral ulceration (<1%)
- Paresthesias (1%)
- Sialorrhea (<1%)
- Stomatitis (<1%)
- Tongue edema (<1%)
- Thrombophlebitis (<1%)
- Xerostomia (7%)

QUINACRINE

Trade name: Atabrine (Sanofi-Winthrop)
Other common trade names: Atabil
Category: Anthelmintic; antimalarial
Clinically important, potentially serious interactions with: none

REACTIONS

SKIN
- Erythema dyschromicum perstans
- Erythematous plaques
- Exanthems
- Exfoliative dermatitis
- Fixed eruption
- Hypomelanosis
- Keratoderma
- Lichenoid eruption
- Ochronosis
- Photosensitivity
- Pigmentation

Pruritus (<1%)
Squamous cell carcinoma
Urticaria

HAIR
Hair – alopecia

NAILS
Nails – changes (sic)
Nails – pigmentation

OTHER
Oral pigmentation

QUINAPRIL

Trade name: Accupril (Parke-Davis)
Other common trade names: Accuprin; Accupro; Acuitel; Acupril; Asig; Korec; Quinazil
Category: Angiotensin-converting enzyme (ACE) inhibitor; antihypertensive & vasodilator
Clinically important, potentially serious interactions with: allopurinol, bumetanide, digitalis, lithium, potassium-sparing diuretics, salicylates, tetracycline

REACTIONS

SKIN
Angioedema (0.1%)
Ankle edema
Bullous eruption
Edema
Exanthems
Exfoliative dermatitis (<1%)
Facial edema (sic)
Flushing (<1%)
Hyperhidrosis (<1%)
Peripheral edema (<1%)
Photosensitivity (<1%)
Pruritus (<1%)
Rash (sic)
Urticaria (<1%)
Vasculitis (<1%)

OTHER
Dysgeusia
Myalgia (1.5%)
Paresthesias
Xerostomia (<1%)

QUINESTROL

Trade name: Estrovis (Parke-Davis)
Category: Estrogen
Clinically important, potentially serious interactions with: corticosteroids

REACTIONS

SKIN
Angioedema
Chloasma (<1%)
Edema (<1%)
Melasma (<1%)
Peripheral edema (>10%)
Rash (sic) (<1%)
Urticaria

OTHER
Gynecomastia (>10%)
Mastodynia (>10%)
Thrombophlebitis

QUINETHAZONE

Trade name: Hydromox (Lederle)
Other common trade name: Aquamox
Category: Thiazide diuretic & antihypertensive
Clinically important, potentially serious interactions with: antidiabetics, digitalis, furosemide, lithium, loop diuretics

REACTIONS

SKIN
Bullous eruption (<1%)
Exanthems
Photoallergic reaction

Photosensitivity (<1%)
Pruritus
Purpura
Rash (sic) (<1%)
Urticaria
Vasculitis

OTHER
Hypersensitivity
Paresthesias
Xanthopsia
Xerostomia

QUINIDINE

Trade names: Cardioquin (Purdue Frederick); Quinaglute (Berlex); Quinidex (Robins)
Other common trade names: Cardine; Cardioquin; Gluquine; Kinidin; Quinate; Quinidex
Category: Antiarrhythmic
Clinically important, potentially serious interactions with: amiodarone, anticoagulants, astemizole, beta-blockers, cimetidine, coumarin, digoxin, ritonavir, terfenadine, verapamil

REACTIONS

SKIN
Acne
Acute generalized exanthematous pustulosis (AGEP)
Allergic reactions (sic)
Angioedema (<1%)
Bullous eruption
Contact dermatitis
Cutaneous side effects (sic)
Eczematous eruption (sic)
Erythema multiforme
Exanthems
Exfoliative dermatitis
Exudative dermatitis (sic)
Fixed eruption
Flushing
Granuloma annulare
Lichenoid eruption
Lichen planus
Livedo reticularis
Lupus erythematosus
Palmoplantar keratosis
Photoallergic reaction
Photosensitivity
Pigmentation
Pruritus
Psoriasis
Purpura
Pustular eruption
Rash (sic) (1–10%)
Subcorneal pustular dermatosis (Sneddon-Wilkinson)
Toxic epidermal necrolysis
Urticaria
Vasculitis

HAIR
Hair – alopecia

OTHER
Dysgeusia (bitter taste) (>10%)
Lymphoproliferative disease
Oral mucosal eruption
Oral mucosal pigmentation
Oral ulceration
Polymyalgia
Porphyria
Pseudoporphyria
Sicca syndrome

QUININE

Trade names: Legatrin (Columbia), Quinamm (Marion Merrill Dow); Quiphile (Geneva)
Other common trade names: Adaquin; Chinine; Genin; Quinate; Quinoctal; Quinsan; Quinsul
Category: Antiprotozoal & antimyotonic
Clinically important, potentially serious interactions with: amiodarone, anticoagulants, astemizole, beta-blockers, cimetidine, coumarin, digoxin, quinidine, terfenadine, verapamil

REACTIONS

SKIN
Acne
Angioedema (<1%)
Bullous eruption
Contact dermatitis
Eczematous eruption (sic)

Erythema multiforme (<1%)
Exanthems (1–5%)
Exfoliative dermatitis
Facial edema
Fixed eruption
Flushing (<1%)
Hyperhidrosis
Hyperpigmentation
Lichenoid eruption
Lichen planus
Livedo racemosa (photosensitive)
Lupus erythematosus
Ochronosis
Photoallergic reaction
Photosensitivity
Pigmentation
Pruritus (<1%)
Psoriasis
Purpura
Rash (sic) (<1%)
Stevens-Johnson syndrome
Toxic epidermal necrolysis (<1%)
Urticaria
Vasculitis
Vitiligo

NAILS
Nails – photo-onycholysis

OTHER
Hypersensitivity (<1%)
Oral mucosal eruption
Oral ulceration
Porphyria

RALOXIFENE

Trade name: Evista (Lilly)
Category: Selective estrogen receptor modulator (prevents osteoporosis in postmenopausal women)
Clinically important, potentially serious interactions with: anticoagulants, cholestyramine

REACTIONS

SKIN
Hot flashes (24.6%)
Hyperhidrosis (3.1%)
Peripheral edema (3.3%)
Rash (sic) (5.5%)

OTHER
Mastodynia (4.4%)
Myalgia (7.7%)
Vaginitis (4.3%)

RAMIPRIL

Trade name: Altace (Hoechst Marion Roussel)
Other common trade names: Delix; Hytren; Pramace; Quark; Ramace; Triatec; Tritace; Unipril
Category: Angiotensin-converting enzyme (ACE) inhibitor; antihypertensive & vasodilator
Clinically important, potentially serious interactions with: allopurinol, digitalis, furosemide, lithium, potassium-sparing diuretics, salicylates

REACTIONS

SKIN
Acne
Angioedema (0.3%)
Dermatitis (sic) (<1%)
Dry feeling on face (sic)
Edema (<1%)
Erythema (circumscribed) (sic)
Erythema multiforme (<1%)
Exanthems
Flushing
Hyperhidrosis (<1%)
Lichen planus pemphigoides
Pemphigus
Photosensitivity (<1%)
Pruritus (<1%)
Purpura (<1%)
Rash (sic) (<1%)
Urticaria (<1%)
Vasculitis (<1%)

HAIR
Hair – alopecia (1–10%)

OTHER
Ageusia (<1%)
Anaphylactoid reaction (<1%)

Dysgeusia (<1%)
Hypersensitivity (<1%)
Paresthesias (<1%)
Sialorrhea (<1%)
Xerostomia (<1%)

RANITIDINE

Trade name: Zantac (Glaxo Wellcome)
Other common trade names: Axoban; Azantac; Raniben; Raniplex; Sostril; Zantab; Zantic
Category: Histamine H_2-antagonist; antiulcer drug
Clinically important, potentially serious interactions with: cyclosporine, fentanyl, gentamicin, glipizide, glyburide, metoprolol, midazolam, nifedipine, pentoxifylline, phenytoin, quinidine, quinolones

REACTIONS

SKIN
Acute generalized exanthematous pustulosis (AGEP)
Angioedema (<1%)
Contact dermatitis
Eczematous eruption (sic)
Erythema multiforme
Exanthems
Fixed eruption
Lichenoid eruption
Photosensitivity
Pruritus (<1%)
Psoriasis
Purpura
Pustular eruption
Rash (sic) (<2%)
Toxic epidermal necrolysis
Urticaria
Vasculitis
Xerosis

HAIR
Hair – alopecia

OTHER
Anaphylactoid reaction
Dysgeusia
Gynecomastia (>10%)
Hypersensitivity
Injection-site burning
Injection-site pain
Myalgia
Porphyria
Pseudolymphoma

REPAGLINIDE

Trade name: Prandin (Novo Nordisk)
Category: Antidiabetic
Clinically important, potentially serious interactions with: barbiturates, carbamazepine, erythromycin, ketoconazole, miconazole, rifampin, troglitazone

REACTIONS

SKIN
Allergy (sic) (2%)

OTHER
Anaphylactoid reaction (<1%)
Paresthesias (3%)

RESERPINE

Trade names: Ser-Ap-Es (Novartis); Serpasil (Ciba)
Other common trade names: Anserpin; Inerpin; Reserfia; Sedaraupin; Serpasol; Tionsera
Category: Nondiuretic antihypertensive rauwolfia alkaloid
Clinically important, potentially serious interactions with: MAO inhibitors, sympathomimetics, tricyclic antidepressants

Ser-Ap-Es is reserpine, hydralazine & hydrochlorothiazide

REACTIONS

SKIN
- Ankle edema
- Bullous eruption
- Exanthems
- Flushing
- Lupus erythematosus (exacerbation)
- Peripheral edema (1–10%)
- Pruritus
- Purpura
- Rash (sic) (<1%)
- Toxic epidermal necrolysis
- Urticaria

OTHER
- Gynecomastia
- Xerostomia (>10%)

RIBAVIRIN

Trade names: Rebetron (Schering); Virazole (Viratek)
Other common trade names: Viramid; Virazid
Category: Antiviral (against respiratory syncytial virus (RSV)
Clinically important, potentially serious interactions with: none

Rebetron is interferon & ribavirin

REACTIONS

SKIN
- Erythema multiforme
- Exanthems
- Fixed eruption
- Herpes simplex (activation)
- Rash (sic) (<1%)

RIBOFLAVIN

Trade names: Riboflavin; Riobin; Vitamin B_2
Category: Water-soluble nutritional supplement
Clinically important, potentially serious interactions with: probenecid

REACTIONS

SKIN
- Acne
- Allergic reactions (sic)
- Angioedema
- Ichthyosis
- Urticaria

RIFABUTIN

Trade name: Mycobutin (Pharmacia & Upjohn)
Category: Antitubercular antibiotic
Clinically important, potentially serious interactions with: anticoagulants, bisoprolol, corticosteroids, cyclosporine, tacrolimus

REACTIONS

SKIN
- Lupus erythematosus
- Pigmentation
- Rash (sic) (11%)

OTHER
Ageusia
Dysgeusia (3%)
Myalgia (2%)
Paresthesias (<1%)

RIFAMPIN

Trade names: Rifadin (Hoechst Marion Roussel); Rifampicin; Rimactane (Novartis)
Other common trade names: Abrifam; Corifam; Ramicin; Rifaldin; Rifamed; Rimpin; Rimycin
Category: Tuberculostatic & antileprotic
Clinically important, potentially serious interactions with: anticoagulants, barbiturates, chloramphenicol, corticosteroids, cyclosporine, digoxin, diltiazem, ketoconazole, methadone, oral contraceptives, phenytoin, quinidine, tacrolimus, theophylline, verapamil

REACTIONS

SKIN
Acne
Angioedema
Bullous eruption (<1%)
Contact dermatitis
Cutaneous side effects (sic)
Erythema multiforme (<1%)
Exanthems (1–5%)
Exfoliative dermatitis
Facial edema
Fixed eruption
Flushing
Hyperhidrosis (1–10%)
Linear IgA bullous dermatosis
Pemphigus
Pruritus (<1%)
Purpura
Rash (sic) (<1%)
Red man syndrome
Stevens-Johnson syndrome
Toxic epidermal necrolysis
Urticaria
Vasculitis

OTHER
Anaphylactoid reaction
Glossodynia
Injection-site erythema
Mucosal bleeding (sic)
Oral mucosal eruption
Porphyria
Porphyria cutanea tarda
Serum sickness
Stomatitis (<1%)

RIMANTADINE

Trade name: Flumadine (Forest)
Other common trade name: Ruflual
Category: Antiviral
Clinically important, potentially serious interactions with: acetaminophen, aspirin, cimetidine

REACTIONS

SKIN
Edema (pedal) (1–10%)
Rash (sic) (<1%)

OTHER
Ageusia (<0.3%)
Dysgeusia
Hypesthesia
Parosmia (<0.3%)
Stomatitis
Xerostomia (1.6%)

RISPERIDONE

Trade name: Risperdal (Janssen)
Category: Antipsychotic
Clinically important, potentially serious interactions with: carbamazepine, clozapine, levodopa, quinidine, warfarin

REACTIONS

SKIN
- Acne (<1%)
- Allergic reactions (<1%)
- Angioedema
- Bullous eruption (<1%)
- Bullous pemphigoid
- Dermatitis (sic)
- Edema
- Exfoliative dermatitis (0.1–1%)
- Flushing (<1%)
- Furunculosis (<1%)
- Galactorrhea (1–10%)
- Gynecomastia (1–10%)
- Hyperhidrosis (<1%)
- Hyperkeratosis (sic) (<1%)
- Hypohidrosis (<1%)
- Lichenoid eruption (<1%)
- Photosensitivity (1–10%)
- Pigmentation (1%)
- Priapism (1–10%)
- Pruritus (<1%)
- Psoriasis (<1%)
- Purpura (<1%)
- Rash (sic) (5%)
- Seborrhea
- Ulceration (<1%)
- Urticaria (<0.1%)
- Warts (<1%)
- Xerosis (2%)

HAIR
- Hair – alopecia (<1%)
- Hair – hypertrichosis (<1%)

OTHER
- Anaphylactoid reaction
- Dysgeusia (<1%)
- Gingivitis (<1%)
- Gynecomastia (<1%)
- Hypesthesia (<1%)
- Mastodynia (<1%)
- Myalgia (<1%)
- Paresthesias (<1%)
- Sialopenia (5%)
- Sialorrhea (2%)
- Stomatitis (<1%)
- Thrombophlebitis (<1%)
- Tongue edema (<1%)
- Tongue pigmentation (<1%)
- Xerostomia (1–10%)

RITONAVIR

Trade name: Norvir (Abbott)
Category: Antiviral; protease inhibitor
Clinically important, potentially serious interactions with: amiodarone, astemizole, benzodiazepines, bepridil, cisapride, clozapine, desipramine, flecainide, ketoconazole, propoxyphene, quinidine, terfenadine, theophylline

REACTIONS

SKIN
- Acne (<2%)
- Allergic reactions (sic) (<2%)
- Angioedema
- Bullous eruption (<2%)
- Cheilitis (<2%)
- Contact dermatitis (<2%)
- Ecchymoses (<2%)
- Eczema (sic) (<2%)
- Exanthems (<2%)
- Facial edema (<2%)
- Folliculitis (<2%)
- Hyperhidrosis
- Peripheral edema (<2%)
- Photosensitivity (<2%)
- Pruritus (<2%)
- Psoriasis (<2%)
- Rash (sic) (<1%)
- Seborrhea (<2%)
- Stevens-Johnson syndrome
- Urticaria (<2%)
- Xerosis (<2%)

OTHER
- Ageusia (<2%)
- Anaphylactoid reaction
- Dysgeusia (10.3%)
- Gingivitis (<2%)
- Hyperesthesia (<2%)
- Oral candidiasis (<2%)
- Oral ulceration (<2%)
- Paresthesias (2.6%)
- Parosmia (<2%)
- Xerostomia (<2%)

RITORDINE

Trade name: Yutopar (Astra)
Category: Tocolytic (uterine relaxant)
Clinically important, potentially serious interactions with: none

REACTIONS

SKIN
- Erythema (10–15%)
- Erythema multiforme
- Exanthems
- Hyperhidrosis (1–3%)
- Rash (sic) (1–3%)
- Urticaria
- Vasculitis

OTHER
- Anaphylactoid reaction (1–3%)

ROPINIROLE

Trade name: Requip (SmithKline Beecham)
Category: Anti-parkinsonian
Clinically important, potentially serious interactions with: ciprofloxacin

REACTIONS

SKIN
- Basal cell carcinoma (>1%)
- Cellulitis (<1%)
- Dermatitis (sic) (<1%)
- Eczema (sic) (<1%)
- Edema (<1%)
- Exanthems (<1%)
- Flushing (3%)
- Fungal dermatitis (sic) (<1%)
- Furunculosis (<1%)
- Herpes simplex (<1%)
- Herpes zoster (<1%)
- Hyperhidrosis (6%)
- Hyperkeratosis (<1%)
- Hypertrophy (sic) (<1%)
- Peripheral edema (<1%)
- Photosensitivity (<1%)
- Pigmentation (<1%)
- Pruritus (<1%)
- Psoriasis (<1%)
- Purpura (<1%)
- Rash (sic) (>1%)
- Ulceration (<1%)
- Urticaria (<1%)

HAIR
- Alopecia (<1%)

OTHER
- Balanoposthitis (<1%)
- Gingivitis (>1%)
- Glossitis (<1%)
- Gynecomastia (<1%)
- Hypesthesia (4%)
- Mastitis (<1%)
- Paresthesias (>1%)
- Peyronie's disease (<1%)
- Sialorrhea (>1%)
- Stomatitis (<1%)
- Thrombophlebitis (<1%)
- Tongue edema (<1%)
- Ulcerative stomatitis (<1%)
- Vaginal candidiasis (<1%)
- Xerostomia (5%)

SACCHARIN

Trade names: Saccharin; Sweet 'n Low
Category: Sulfonamide sweetening agent
Clinically important, potentially serious interactions with: none

REACTIONS

SKIN
- Dermatitis (sic)
- Exanthems
- Fixed eruption
- Notalgia paresthetica
- Photosensitivity
- Pruritus
- Sensitivity (sic)
- Urticaria

OTHER
- Dysgeusia

SALMETEROL

Trade name: Serevent (Glaxo Wellcome)
Other common trade names: Salmeter; Serobid
Category: Sympathomimetic bronchodilator; adrenergic agonist
Clinically important, potentially serious interactions with: beta-blockers, MAO inhibitors, tricyclic antidepressants

REACTIONS

SKIN
- Angioedema
- Eczematoid eruption (sic)
- Exanthems
- Pruritus
- Rash (sic) (1–3%)
- Urticaria (1–3%)

OTHER
- Hypersensitivity (<1%)
- Myalgia (1–3%)
- Paresthesias

SALSALATE

Trade names: Disalcid (3M); Mono-Gesic (Schwarz); Salflex (Carnrick); Salsitab (Upsher Smith)
Other common trade names: Atisuril; Disalgesic; Nobegyl; Salina; Umbradol
Category: Nonsteroidal anti-inflammatory (NSAID)
Clinically important, potentially serious interactions with: ACE-inhibitors, anticoagulants, beta-blockers, heparin, hypoglycemics, methotrexate

REACTIONS

SKIN
- Angioedema
- Dermatitis (sic)
- Exanthems
- Pruritus
- Purpura
- Rash (sic) (1–10%)
- Urticaria

OTHER
- Anaphylactoid reaction (1–10%)

SAQUINAVIR

Trade name: Invirase (Roche); Fortovase (Roche)
Category: Antiviral; HIV protease inhibitor
Clinically important, potentially serious interactions with: calcium channel blockers, clindamycin, dapsone, ketoconazole, quinidine, rifampin, ritonavir, triazolam

REACTIONS

SKIN
- Acne (<2%)
- Candidiasis (<2%)
- Cheilitis (<2%)
- Dermatitis (<2%)
- Eczema (sic) (<2%)
- Erythema (<2%)
- Exanthems (<2%)
- Folliculitis (<2%)
- Furunculosis
- Herpes simplex (<2%)
- Herpes zoster (<2%)
- Hyperhidrosis (<2%)
- Photosensitivity (<2%)
- Pigmentary changes (<2%)
- Rash (sic) (1.3%)
- Seborrheic dermatitis (<2%)
- Ulceration (<2%)
- Urticaria (<2%)
- Warts (<2%)
- Xerosis (<2%)

HAIR
- Hair – changes (<2%)

OTHER
- Dysesthesia (<2%)
- Dysgeusia (<2%)
- Gingivitis (<2%)
- Glossitis (<2%)
- Hyperesthesia (<2%)
- Oral ulceration (2.5%)
- Paresthesias (2.6%)
- Stomatitis (<2%)
- Xerostomia (<2%)

SCOPOLAMINE

Trade name: Transderm-Scop (Novartis)
Other common trade name: Scopoderm-TTS
Category: Anticholinergic, antispasmodic
Clinically important, potentially serious interactions with: acetaminophen, amantadine, anticholinergics, digoxin, ketoconazole, levodopa, riboflavin, tacrine, tricyclic antidepressants

REACTIONS

SKIN
- Contact dermatitis
- Dermatitis (from transdermal patch)
- Edema (<1%)
- Erythema
- Erythema multiforme
- Exanthems
- Fixed eruption
- Flushing
- Hypohidrosis (>10%)
- Rash (sic) (<1%)
- Xerosis

OTHER
- Anaphylactoid reaction
- Injection-site irritation (>10%)
- Oral mucosal lesions
- Xerostomia (>60%)

SECOBARBITAL

Trade name: Seconal (Lilly)
Other common trade names: Immenoctal; Novosecobarb; Secanal
Category: Short-acting barbiturate; hypnotic-sedative
Clinically important, potentially serious interactions with: acetaminophen, anticoagulants, CNS depressants, chloramphenicol, chlorpropamide, MAO inhibitors

REACTIONS

SKIN
- Angioedema (<1%)
- Exanthems
- Exfoliative dermatitis (<1%)
- Purpura
- Rash (sic) (<1%)
- Stevens-Johnson syndrome (<1%)
- Urticaria

OTHER
- Injection-site pain (>10%)
- Serum sickness
- Thrombophlebitis (<1%)

SECRETIN

Trade name: Secretin-Ferring (Ferring)
Category: Gastrointestinal peptide hormone
Clinically important, potentially serious interactions with: no data

REACTIONS

SKIN
- Allergic reactions (sic)
- Urticaria

OTHER
- Injection-site allergic reaction (sic)

SELEGILINE

Trade name: Eldepryl (Somerset)
Other common trade names: Eldeprine; Jumex; Movergan; Plurimen
Category: Monoamine oxidase inhibitor; anti-parkinsonian
Clinically important, potentially serious interactions with: dopamine, ephedrine, fluoxetine, levodopa, meperidine, opioids, paroxetine, sertraline, sympathomimetics, tricyclic antidepressants, venlafaxine

REACTIONS

SKIN
- Hyperhidrosis
- Peripheral edema
- Photosensitivity
- Rash (sic)

HAIR
- Hair – alopecia
- Hair – hypertrichosis (facial)

OTHER
- Bruxism (1–10%)
- Dysgeusia
- Paresthesias
- Xerostomia (>10%)

SERTRALINE

Trade name: Zoloft (Roerig)
Other common trade name: Atruline
Category: Selective serotonin reuptake inhibitor (SSRI); antidepressant
Clinically important, potentially serious interactions with: beta-blockers, lithium, MAO inhibitors, trazodone, tricyclic antidepressants, warfarin

REACTIONS

SKIN
- Acne (<1%)
- Allergic reactions (sic)
- Angioedema
- Aphthous stomatitis (<1%)
- Balanoposthitis (<1%)
- Bullous eruption (<1%)
- Cutaneous reaction (sic)
- Dermatitis (sic) (<1%)
- Discoloration (sic) (<1%)
- Edema (<1%)
- Erythema multiforme (<1%)
- Exanthems (<1%)
- Fixed eruption
- Flushing (2.2%)
- Hyperhidrosis (8.4%)
- Periorbital edema (<1%)
- Peripheral edema (<1%)
- Photosensitivity (<1%)
- Pruritus (<1%)
- Purpura (<1%)
- Rash (sic) (2.1%)
- Urticaria (<1%)
- Xerosis (<1%)

HAIR
- Hair – abnormal texture (sic) (<1%)
- Hair – alopecia (<1%)
- Hair – hirsutism (<1%)

OTHER
- Bromhidrosis (<1%)
- Bruxism (<1%)
- Dysgeusia
- Galactorrhea
- Gingival hyperplasia (<1%)
- Glossitis (<1%)
- Gynecomastia (<1%)
- Halitosis (<1%)
- Hyperesthesia (<1%)
- Hypesthesia (2%)
- Paresthesias (2%)
- Sialorrhea (<1%)
- Stomatitis (<1%)
- Tongue edema (<1%)
- Tongue ulceration (<1%)
- Vaginitis (atrophic)
- Xerostomia (16.3%)

SIBUTRAMINE

Trade name: Meridia (Knoll)
Category: Obesity management; anorexiant
Clinically important, potentially serious interactions with: erythromycin, fentanyl, ketoconazole, lithium, MAO inhibitors, meperidine, SSRIs, sumatriptan, venlafaxine

REACTIONS

SKIN
- Acne (1.0%)
- Allergic reactions (sic) (1.5%)
- Ecchymoses (0.7%)
- Edema (2%)
- Herpes simplex (1.3%)
- Hyperhidrosis (2.5%)
- Peripheral edema (>1%)
- Pruritus (>1%)
- Rash (sic) (3.8%)

OTHER
- Dysgeusia (2.2%)
- Myalgia (1.9%)
- Paresthesias (2.0%)
- Vaginal candidiasis (1.2%)
- Xerostomia (17.2%)

SILDENAFIL

Trade name: Viagra (Pfizer)
Category: Erectile dysfunction agent
Clinically important, potentially serious interactions with: cimetidine, erythromycin

REACTIONS

SKIN
- Allergic reactions (sic) (<2%)
- Contact dermatitis (<2%)
- Edema (<2%)
- Exfoliative dermatitis (<2%)
- Flushing (10%)
- Facial edema (<2%)
- Fixed eruption (urticarial)
- Genital edema (<2%)
- Herpes simplex (<2%)
- Hyperhidrosis (<2%)
- Peripheral edema (<2%)
- Photosensitivity (<2%)
- Pruritus (<2%)
- Rash (sic) (2%)
- Ulceration (<2%)
- Urticaria (<2%)

OTHER
- Dyschromatopsia (blue-green vision) (3%)
- Gingivitis (<2%)
- Glossitis (<2%)
- Gynecomastia (<2%)
- Hypesthesia (<2%)
- Myalgia (<2%)
- Paresthesias (<2%)
- Photophobia (<2%)
- Stomatitis (<2%)
- Xerostomia (<2%)

SIMVASTATIN

Trade name: Zocor (Merck)
Other common trade names: Denan; Lipex; Liponorm; Lodales; Simovil; Sivastin; Zocord
Category: Antihyperlipidemic (cholesterol-lowering)
Clinically important, potentially serious interactions with: anticoagulants, cyclosporine, erythromycin, gemfibrozil, niacin, warfarin

REACTIONS

SKIN
- Angioedema
- Ankle edema
- Dermatomyositis
- Eczema (sic)
- Eczematous eruption (generalized)
- Erythema multiforme
- Erythematous scaly plaques
- Exanthems
- Flushing
- Hyperhidrosis
- Lichenoid eruption
- Lichen planus
- Lupus erythematosus
- Petechiae
- Photosensitivity
- Pruritus
- Purpura
- Pustular eruption
- Radiation recall
- Rash (sic) (1–10%)
- Rosacea
- Stevens-Johnson syndrome
- Toxic epidermal necrolysis
- Urticaria
- Vasculitis

HAIR
- Hair – alopecia

OTHER
- Anaphylactoid reaction
- Dysgeusia (<1%)
- Gynecomastia
- Myopathy (1–10%)
- Paresthesias
- Porphyria cutanea tarda

SOTALOL

Trade name: Betapace (Berlex)
Other common trade names: Beta-Cardone; Betades; Cardol; Sotahexal; Sotalex; Sotapor
Category: Beta-adrenergic blocking agent; antiarrhythmic
Clinically important, potentially serious interactions with: antidiabetics, calcium channel blockers, clonidine, flecainide, naproxen, nifedipine, oral contraceptives, sertraline

REACTIONS

SKIN
- Cold extremities (sic)
- Cutaneous thickening (sic)
- Edema (5%)
- Exanthems
- Hyperhidrosis (<1%)
- Lichenoid eruption
- Photosensitivity
- Pruritus (1–10%)
- Psoriasis
- Rash (sic) (3%)
- Raynaud's phenomenon (<1%)
- Scleroderma
- Skin irritation (sic)
- Urticaria

HAIR
- Hair – alopecia

OTHER
- Myalgia
- Myopathy
- Paresthesias (3%)
- Phlebitis (<1%)

SPARFLOXACIN

Trade name: Zagam (Rhône-Poulenc Rorer)
Other common trade names: Spara; Sparlox; Torospar
Category: Quinolone antibiotic
Clinically important, potentially serious interactions with: bumetanide, digitalis, lithium, salicylates, zinc/iron salts

REACTIONS

SKIN
- Acne (<1%)
- Allergic reactions (sic) (<1%)
- Angioedema (<1%)
- Bullous eruption (<1%)
- Cellulitis (<1%)
- Contact dermatitis (<1%)
- Ecchymoses (<1%)
- Edema (<1%)
- Erythema nodosum
- Exanthems (<1%)
- Exfoliative dermatitis (<1%)
- Facial edema (<1%)
- Furunculosis (<1%)
- Herpes simplex (<1%)
- Hyperhidrosis (<1%)
- Lichenoid eruption
- Peripheral edema (<1%)
- Petechiae (<1%)
- Photosensitivity (3.6%)
- Phototoxic reaction (7.9%)
- Pigmentation (<1%)
- Pruritus (3.3%)
- Purpura
- Pustular eruption (<1%)
- Rash (sic) (1.1%)
- Stevens-Johnson syndrome
- Toxic epidermal necrolysis
- Urticaria (<1%)
- Vasculitis
- Xerosis (<1%)

HAIR
- Hair – alopecia (<1%)

OTHER
- Anaphylactoid reaction (<1%)
- Anosmia
- Dysgeusia (1.4%)
- Gingivitis (<1%)
- Hyperesthesia (<1%)
- Hypersensitivity
- Hypesthesia (<1%)
- Mastodynia (<1%)
- Myalgia (<1%)
- Oral candidiasis (<1%)

Oral ulceration (<1%)
Paresthesias (<1%)
Serum sickness
Stomatitis (<1%)
Tongue disorder (<1%)
Vaginal candidiasis (2.8%)
Vaginitis (<1%)
Xerostomia (1.4%)

SPECTINOMYCIN

Trade name: Trobicin (Pharmacia & Upjohn)
Category: Antibiotic
Clinically important, potentially serious interactions with: none

REACTIONS

SKIN
Contact dermatitis
Exanthems
Pruritus (<1%)
Rash (sic) (<1%)
Urticaria (<1%)

OTHER
Anaphylactoid reaction
Hypersensitivity
Injection-site induration
Injection-site pain (<1%)
Oral mucosal lesions

SPIRONOLACTONE

Trade name: Aldactone (Searle)
Other common trade names: Aldopur; Almatol; Diram; Merabis; Osiren; Spiroctan; Tensin
Category: Potassium-sparing antihypertensive diuretic
Clinically important, potentially serious interactions with: ACE inhibitors, benazepril, digitalis, diuretics, enalapril, fosinopril, indomethacin, lisinopril, NSAIDs, potassium chloride, triamterene

REACTIONS

SKIN
Chloasma
Contact dermatitis
Cutaneous side effects (sic)
Eczematous eruption
Erythema annulare centrifugum
Erythema multiforme
Exanthems
Flushing (<1%)
Lichenoid eruption
Lichen planus
Lupus erythematosus
Necrotizing angiitis
Photosensitivity
Pigmentation
Pruritus
Purpura
Rash (sic) (1–10%)
Raynaud's phenomenon (rare)
Urticaria
Vasculitis
Xerosis

HAIR
Hair – alopecia
Hair – hirsutism

OTHER
Acute intermittent porphyria
Ageusia
Anaphylactoid reaction
Gynecomastia (<1%)
Oral lichen planus
Paresthesias
Xerostomia

STANOZOLOL

Trade name: Winstrol (Sanofi Winthrop)
Other common trade names: Menabol; Stromba
Category: Anabolic steroid; androgen
Clinically important, potentially serious interactions with: ACTH, adrenal steroids, anticoagulants, antidiabetics, insulin, sulfonylureas

REACTIONS

SKIN
- Acne (>10%)
- Edema
- Exanthems
- Folliculitis
- Hyperpigmentation (1–10%)
- Rosacea
- Seborrheic dermatitis
- Urticaria

HAIR
- Hair – alopecia (in women)
- Hair – hirsutism (in women)

OTHER
- Gynecomastia (>10%)
- Priapism (>10%)

STREPTOKINASE

Trade names: Kabikinase (Pharmacia & Upjohn); Streptase (Astra)
Category: Thrombolytic
Clinically important, potentially serious interactions with: anticoagulants

REACTIONS

SKIN
- Allergic reactions (sic) (4.4%)
- Angiitis
- Angioedema (>10%)
- Cutaneous bleeding
- Exanthems (1–5%)
- Flushing (<1%)
- Hyperhidrosis (<1%)
- Periorbital edema (>10%)
- Pruritus (<1%)
- Purpura
- Rash (sic) (<1%)
- Urticaria (1–5%)
- Vasculitis

OTHER
- Anaphylactoid reaction
- Injection-site bleeding
- Injection-site phlebitis
- Serum sickness
- Stomatitis (after local application)
- Tongue edema (with hemorrhagic swelling)

STREPTOMYCIN

Trade name: Streptomycin (Lilly)
Category: Aminoglycoside antibiotic; tuberculostatic
Clinically important, potentially serious interactions with: aminoglycosides, amphotericin B, bumetanide, ethacrynic acid, furosemide, loop diuretics, polypeptide antibiotics, torsemide

REACTIONS

SKIN
- Acute generalized exanthematous pustulosis (AGEP)
- Allergic reactions (sic)
- Angioedema (<1%)
- Bullous eruption (<1%)
- Contact dermatitis
- Eczematous eruption (sic)
- Edema
- Erythema multiforme (<1%)
- Erythema nodosum (<1%)
- Exanthems (>5%)
- Exfoliative dermatitis
- Fixed eruption (<1%)
- Follicular pustular eruption (sic)
- Lichenoid eruption

Lupus erythematosus
Photosensitivity
Pruritus (<1%)
Purpura
Pustular eruption
Rash (sic) (<1%)
Stevens-Johnson syndrome
Systemic eczematous contact dermatitis
Toxic epidermal necrolysis
Toxic erythema (sic)
Urticaria
Vasculitis

HAIR
Hair – hypertrichosis

OTHER
Anaphylactoid reaction
Black hairy tongue
Cheilitis (2%)
Glossitis (2%)
Injection-site granuloma
Oral mucosal eruption
Oral ulceration
Paresthesias (<1%)
Stomatitis

STREPTOZOCIN

Trade name: Zanosar (Pharmacia & Upjohn)
Category: Antineoplastic
Clinically important, potentially serious interactions with: doxorubicin

REACTIONS

SKIN
Edema
Exanthems
Pruritus
Purpura
Toxic epidermal necrolysis

OTHER
Injection-site erythema
Injection-site necrosis
Injection-site pain (1–10%)

SUCCINYLCHOLINE

Trade names: Anectine (Glaxo Wellcome); Quelicin (Abbott)
Category: Skeletal muscle relaxant
Clinically important, potentially serious interactions with: aminoglycosides, anticholinesterase drugs, cimetidine, cyclophosphamide, digitalis, ketamine, lidocaine, MAO inhibitors, oral contraceptives, quinidine, quinine, tacrine, vancomycin

REACTIONS

SKIN
Contact dermatitis
Erythema (<1%)
Exanthems
Pruritus (<1%)
Rash (sic) (<1%)
Urticaria

OTHER
Anaphylactoid reaction
Hypersensitivity
Myalgia (<1%)
Myopathy
Sialorrhea (1–10%)

SUCRALFATE

Trade name: Carafate (Hoechst Marion Roussel)
Other common trade names: Antepsin; Sucrabest; Sulcrate; Ulcar; Ulcogant; Ulcyte; Urbal
Category: Antiulcer; gastric mucosa protectant
Clinically important, potentially serious interactions with: antacids, cimetidine, penicillamine, phenytoin, quinidine, quinolones, ranitidine

REACTIONS

SKIN
- Angioedema
- Exanthems
- Facial edema
- Pruritus (<0.5%)
- Rash (sic) (<0.5%)
- Urticaria

SULFADOXINE

Trade name: Fansidar (Roche)
Other common trade names: Cryodoxin; Malocide; Methipox
Category: Sulfonamide antimalarial; folic acid antagonist
Clinically important, potentially serious interactions with: cotrimoxazole, methotrexate, other sulfonamides

Fansidar is sulfadoxine & pyrimethamine

REACTIONS

SKIN
- Bullous eruption
- Erythema multiforme (<1%)
- Exanthems
- Exfoliative dermatitis
- Lupus erythematosus
- Periorbital edema
- Photosensitivity (>10%)
- Pruritus
- Purpura
- Pustular eruption
- Rash (sic) (<1%)
- Stevens-Johnson syndrome (1–10%)
- Toxic epidermal necrolysis (<1%)
- Urticaria

OTHER
- Ageusia
- Anaphylactoid reaction
- Glossitis (>10%)
- Hypersensitivity (>10%)
- Oral lichenoid eruption
- Oral ulceration
- Stomatitis
- Urogenital ulceration

SULFAMETHOXAZOLE

Trade name: Gantanol (Roche)
Other common trade name: Sinomin
Category: Antibacterial & antiprotozoal sulfonamide
Clinically important, potentially serious interactions with: anticoagulants, hypoglycemics, MAO inhibitors, methotrexate

Note: Sulfamethoxazole is commonly used in conjunction with trimethoprim (See cotrimoxazole).

REACTIONS

SKIN
- Acute febrile neutrophilic dermatosis (Sweet's syndrome)
- Acute generalized exanthematous pustulosis (AGEP)
- Angioedema
- Aphthous stomatitis
- Bullous eruption
- Cutaneous side effects (sic)
- Dermatitis (sic)

Erythema multiforme
Erythema nodosum
Erythroderma
Exanthems
Exfoliative dermatitis
Fixed eruption
Flushing
Lichenoid eruption
Lupus erythematosus
Mucocutaneous syndrome
Photosensitivity
Pruritus
Pruritus vulvae
Psoriasis
Purpura
Pustular eruption
Radiation recall
Rash (sic)
Stevens-Johnson syndrome
Toxic epidermal necrolysis
Urticaria
Vasculitis

OTHER
Anaphylactoid reaction
Black hairy tongue
Dysgeusia
Glossitis
Hypersensitivity
Oral mucosal eruption
Oral ulceration
Pseudolymphoma
Serum sickness
Stomatitis
Tongue ulceration
Vulvovaginitis

SULFASALAZINE

Trade name: Azulfidine (Pharmacia & Upjohn)
Other common trade names: Colo-Pleon; Salazopyrin; Salisulf; Saridine; Sulfazine; Ulcol
Category: Inflammatory bowel disease agent
Clinically important, potentially serious interactions with: anticoagulants, digitalis, hypoglycemics, methotrexate

REACTIONS

SKIN
Acute generalized exanthematous pustulosis (AGEP)
Angioedema
Aphthous stomatitis
Bullous eruption
Bullous pemphigoid
Cheilitis
Cutaneous side effects (sic)
Dermatitis (sic)
Eczematous eruption (sic)
Erythema multiforme
Erythema nodosum
Erythroderma
Exanthems
Exfoliative dermatitis
Fixed eruption
Flushing
Hyperhidrosis
Lichen planus
Lupus erythematosus
Necrosis
Photosensitivity (>10%)
Pigmentation
Pruritus (>10%)
Pruritus vulvae
Psoriasis
Purpura
Pustular eruption
Rash (sic) (>10%)
Raynaud's phenomenon
Skin reactions (sic)
Stevens-Johnson syndrome (1–10%)
Toxic epidermal necrolysis (1–10%)
Urticaria
Vasculitis
Vulvovaginitis
Xerosis

HAIR
Hair – alopecia

OTHER
Anaphylactoid reaction
Dysgeusia
Glossitis
Hypersensitivity
Hypogeusia
Lymphoproliferative disease
Mononucleosis
Mucocutaneous side effects (sic)
Myopathy

Oral mucosal eruption
Oral ulceration
Pseudolymphoma
Serum sickness (<1%)
Stomatitis
Tongue ulceration
Xerostomia

SULFINPYRAZONE

Trade name: Anturane (Novartis)
Other common trade names: Antazone; Antiran; Anturano; Enturen; Falizal; Novopyrazone
Category: Antigout; antihyperuricemic
Clinically important, potentially serious interactions with: acetaminophen, anticoagulants, beta-blockers, hypoglycemics, salicylates

REACTIONS

SKIN
Dermatitis (sic) (1–10%)
Edema
Exanthems (<3%)
Flushing (<1%)
Purpura
Rash (sic) (1–10%)

SULFISOXAZOLE

Trade names: Azo-Gantrisin (Roche); Gantrisin (Roche)
Other common trade names: Isoxazine; Oxazole; Sulfazin; Sulfazole; Thiazin; Urazole
Category: Urinary tract antibacterial & antiprotozoal
Clinically important, potentially serious interactions with: anticoagulants, cyclosporine, hypoglycemics, MAO inhibitors, methotrexate

REACTIONS

SKIN
Allergic reactions (sic)
Angioedema (<1%)
Aphthous stomatitis
Bullous eruption (<1%)
Cutaneous side effects (sic)
Eczematous eruption (sic)
Erythema multiforme (<1%)
Erythema nodosum
Exanthems (1–5%)
Exfoliative dermatitis
Fixed eruption (<1%)
Flushing
Linear IgA bullous dermatosis
Lupus erythematosus
Photoallergic reaction
Photosensitivity (>10%)
Phototoxic reaction
Pruritus (>10%)
Pruritus vulvae
Purpura
Pustular eruption
Rash (sic) (>10%)
Stevens-Johnson syndrome (1–10%)
Toxic epidermal necrolysis (1–10%)
Urticaria
Vasculitis
Vulvovaginitis

HAIR
Hair – alopecia

OTHER
Anaphylactoid reaction
Dysgeusia
Glossitis
Oral psoriasis (sic)
Oral ulceration
Stomatitis
Serum sickness (<1%)
Temporal arteritis
Tongue ulceration

SULINDAC

Trade name: Clinoril (Merck)
Other common trade names: Aflodac; Algocetil; Arthrocine; Mobilin; Sulene; Sulic; Suloril
Category: Nonsteroidal anti-inflammatory (NSAID)
Clinically important, potentially serious interactions with: aminoglycosides, anticoagulants, cyclosporine, digoxin, diuretics, lithium, methotrexate, NSAIDs, probenecid

REACTIONS

SKIN
Angioedema (<1%)
Aphthous stomatitis (rare)
Dermatitis (sic)
Ecchymoses (<1%)
Erythema
Erythema multiforme (<1%)
Exanthems (1–5%)
Exfoliative dermatitis (<1%)
Exfoliative erythroderma
Facial erythema
Fixed eruption (<1%)
Hyperhidrosis
Jaundice
Lichen planus
Pernio
Photosensitivity (<1%)
Phototoxic reaction
Pruritus (1–10%)
Purpura (<1%)
Rash (sic) (>10%)
Raynaud's phenomenon
Skin pain (sic)
Stevens-Johnson syndrome
Toxic epidermal necrolysis
Urticaria
Vasculitis (<1%)

HAIR
Hair – alopecia (<1%)

OTHER
Ageusia (<1%)
Anaphylactoid reaction (<1%)
Dysesthesia
Dysgeusia (<1%)
Glossitis (<1%)
Gynecomastia
Hypersensitivity (<1%) (potentially fatal)
Oral lichenoid eruption
Oral mucosal eruption
Oral mucosal erythema
Oral ulceration
Paresthesias (<1%)
Serum sickness
Stomatitis (<1%)
Xerostomia

SUMATRIPTAN

Trade name: Imitrex (Glaxo Wellcome)
Other common trade name: Imigrane
Category: Antimigraine; serotonin antagonist
Clinically important, potentially serious interactions with: ergot-containing drugs, MAO inhibitors

REACTIONS

SKIN
Angioedema
Erythema (<1%)
Exanthems
Flushing (6.6%)
Hot sensations (sic)
Hyperhidrosis (1.6%)
Photosensitivity (<1%)
Pruritus (<1%)
Rash (sic) (<1%)
Raynaud's syndrome (<1%)
Sensitivity (sic)
Urticaria

OTHER
Anaphylactoid reaction
Dysesthesia (<1%)
Dysgeusia (<1%)
Hyperesthesia (<1%)
Injection-site reactions (sic) (58%)
Myalgia (1.8%)
Parageusia (<1%)

Paresthesias (13.5%)
Parosmia (<1%)
Xerostomia

TACRINE

Trade name: Cognex (Parke-Davis)
Category: Anticholinesterase
Clinically important, potentially serious interactions with: beta-blockers, cholinesterase inhibitors, cimetidine, succinylcholine, theophylline

REACTIONS

SKIN
Acne (<1%)
Basal cell carcinoma
Bullous eruption
Cellulitis
Cyst (sic)
Dermatitis (sic) (<1%)
Desquamation (sic)
Eczema (sic)
Edema (<1%)
Exanthems (7%)
Facial edema (<1%)
Flushing (3%)
Furunculosis (<1%)
Herpes simplex (<1%)
Herpes zoster (<1%)
Hyperhidrosis
Melanoma (<1%)
Necrosis (<1%)
Peripheral edema (<1%)
Petechiae
Pruritus (7%)
Psoriasis (<1%)
Purpura (2%)
Rash (sic) (7%)
Seborrhea
Squamous cell carcinoma
Ulceration (<1%)
Urticaria (7%)
Xerosis (<1%)

HAIR
Hair – alopecia (<1%)

OTHER
Dysgeusia (<1%)
Gingivitis (<1%)
Glossitis (<1%)
Myalgia (9%)
Paresthesias (<1%)
Sialorrhea (<1%)
Stomatitis (<1%)
Xerostomia (<1%)

TACROLIMUS

Trade name: Prograf (Fujisawa)
Category: Immunosuppressant
Clinically important, potentially serious interactions with: amphotericin B, bromocriptine, cimetidine, clarithromycin, clotrimazole, cyclosporine, danazol, diltiazem, erythromycin, fluconazole, itraconazole, ketoconazole, methylprednisolone, metoclopramide, nicardipine, phenobarbital, phenytoin, rifampin, vaccines, verapamil

REACTIONS

SKIN
Burning at application site
Ecchymoses (>3%)
Edema (>10%)
Flushing
Hyperhidrosis (>3%)
Peripheral edema (26%)
Photosensitivity (>3%)
Pruritus (36%)
Purpura
Rash (sic) (24%)

HAIR
Hair – alopecia (>3%)
Hair – growth (sic)

OTHER
Dysphagia (>3%)
Myalgia (>3%)
Oral candidiasis (>3%)
Paresthesias (40%)

TAMOXIFEN

Trade name: Nolvadex (Zeneca)
Other common trade names: Istubol; Kessar; Mamofen; Novofen; Tamaxin; Tamofen; Valodex
Category: Antiestrogen antineoplastic estrogen receptor
Clinically important, potentially serious interactions with: allopurinol, aminoglutethimide, anticoagulants, cyclosporine, warfarin

REACTIONS

SKIN
- Dermatomyositis
- Edema (3.8%)
- Exanthems
- Flushing (>10%)
- Hyperhidrosis
- Peripheral edema
- Pruritus
- Pruritus vulvae
- Purpura
- Radiation recall
- Rash (sic) (1–10%)
- Urticaria
- Vaginal pruritus
- Vasculitis
- Xerosis

HAIR
- Hair – alopecia
- Hair – color change
- Hair – hirsutism
- Hair – hypertrichosis

OTHER
- Dysgeusia
- Galactorrhea (1–10%)
- Myopathy
- Thrombophlebitis
- Xerostomia

TEMAZEPAM

Trade names: Razepam (Major); Restoril (Novartis)
Other common trade names: Cerepax; Euhypnos; Lenal; Levanxene; Normison; Planum
Category: Benzodiazepine sedative & hypnotic
Clinically important, potentially serious interactions with: CNS depressants, cimetidine, clarithromycin, diltiazem, levodopa, verapamil

REACTIONS

SKIN
- Dermatitis (sic) (1–10%)
- Exanthems
- Fixed eruption
- Hyperhidrosis (>1%)
- Lichenoid eruption
- Pruritus
- Purpura
- Rash (sic) (>10%)
- Skin disorders (sic)
- Urticaria

OTHER
- Anaphylactoid reaction
- Dysgeusia
- Paresthesias
- Sialopenia (>10%)
- Sialorrhea (1–10%)
- Xerostomia (1.7%)

TERAZOSIN

Trade name: Hytrin (Abbott)
Other common trade names: Heitrin; Hitrin; Hytrine; Hytrinex; Itrin; Vicard
Category: Alpha$_1$-adrenergic blocking agent; antihypertensive
Clinically important, potentially serious interactions with: beta-blockers, diuretics, verapamil

REACTIONS

SKIN
Edema (1–10%)
Exanthems
Facial edema (>1%)
Hyperhidrosis (>1%)
Lichenoid eruption
Peripheral edema (5.5%)
Phototoxic reaction
Pruritus (>1%)
Rash (sic) (>1%)

OTHER
Anaphylactoid reaction
Myalgia (>1%)
Paresthesias (2.9%)
Priapism (<1%)
Xerostomia (1–10%)

TERBINAFINE

Trade name: Lamisil (Novartis)
Category: Antifungal
Clinically important, potentially serious interactions with: warfarin

REACTIONS

SKIN
Acute generalized exanthematous pustulosis (AGEP)
Allergic reactions (sic)
Angioedema
Aphthous stomatitis
Cutaneous side effects (sic) (2.7%)
Desquamation (sic)
Eczema (sic)
Erythema multiforme
Erythroderma
Exanthems
Fixed eruption
Peripheral edema
Photosensitivity
Pityriasis rosea
Pruritus (2.8%)
Psoriasis
Pustular psoriasis
Rash (sic) (5.6%)
Stevens-Johnson syndrome
Toxic epidermal necrolysis
Toxicoderma
Urticaria (1.1%)

HAIR
Hair – alopecia areata

OTHER
Ageusia
Anaphylactoid reaction
Anosmia
Dyschromatopsia (green vision)
Dysgeusia (metallic taste) (2.8)
Gingivitis
Hypersensitivity
Hypogeusia
Parosmia
Parotid gland swelling
Serum sickness
Stomatitis
Tongue pigmentation

TERBUTALINE

Trade names: Brethaire (Novartis); Brethine (Novartis); Bricanyl (Hoechst Marion Roussel)
Other common trade names: Ataline; Brothine; Bucaril; Butaline; Convon; Respirol; Vacanyl
Category: Adrenergic bronchodilator; sympathomimetic; tocolytic
Clinically important, potentially serious interactions with: MAO inhibitors, sympathomimetics, tricyclic antidepressants

REACTIONS

SKIN
- Contact dermatitis (irritant)
- Exanthems
- Hyperhidrosis (1–10%)
- Pruritus
- Urticaria
- Vasculitis

OTHER
- Dysgeusia (1–10%)
- Oral ulceration
- Xerostomia (1–10%)

TERFENADINE

Trade name: Seldane (Hoechst Marion Roussel)
Other common trade names: Alergist; Allerplus; Cyater; Ferdin; Teldane; Teldanex; Triludan
Category: H_1-receptor antihistamine
Clinically important, potentially serious interactions with: amiodarone, astemizole, azithromycin, bepridil, carbamazepine, cimetidine, clarithromycin, disopyramide, erythromycin, fluconazole, fluoxetine, fluvoxamine, hydrochlorothiazide, itraconazole, ketoconazole, metronidazole, miconazole, nefazodone, nifedipine, omeprazole, procainamide, pseudoephedrine, quinidine, ritonavir, saquinavir, sotalol, troleandomycin, verapamil. Also with grapefruit

REACTIONS

SKIN
- Angioedema (<1%)
- Atopic dermatitis (exacerbation)
- Cutaneous side effects (sic)
- Exanthems
- Fixed eruption
- Flushing
- Hyperhidrosis
- Lupus erythematosus
- Peeling skin (sic)
- Photosensitivity (<1%)
- Pruritus
- Psoriasis (exacerbation)
- Purpura
- Rash (sic) (<1%)
- Urticaria

HAIR
- Hair – alopecia

OTHER
- Anaphylactoid reaction
- Galactorrhea
- Gynecomastia
- Myalgia (<1%)
- Oral mucosal eruption
- Paresthesias (<1%)
- Pseudolymphoma
- Stomatitis
- Xerostomia (1–10%)

TESTOSTERONE

Trade names: Androderm (SmithKline Beecham); Testoderm (Alza)
Other common trade name: Malogen
Category: Androgen
Clinically important, potentially serious interactions with: anticoagulants, cyclosporine, tricyclic antidepressants

Reactions

SKIN
- Acne (<1%)
- Contact dermatitis (4%)
- Edema (1–10%)
- Exanthems
- Flushing (1–10%)
- Folliculitis
- Furunculosis
- Lichenoid eruption
- Lupus erythematosus
- Pruritus
- Psoriasis
- Rash (sic) (2%)
- Seborrhea (sic) (<1%)
- Seborrheic dermatitis
- Striae
- Urticaria

HAIR
- Hair – alopecia (<1%)
- Hair – hirsutism (1–10%)

OTHER
- Anaphylactoid reaction (<1%)
- Application-site bullae (12%)
- Application-site burning (3%)
- Application-site erythema (7%)
- Application-site induration (3%)
- Application-site pruritus (37%)
- Application-site vesicles (6%)
- Gynecomastia (<1%)
- Hypersensitivity (<1%)
- Injection-site pain
- Mastodynia (>10%)
- Paresthesias (<1%)
- Priapism (>10%)
- Stomatitis

TETRACYCLINE

Trade names: Achromycin V (Lederle); Ala-Tet (Del-Ray); Panmycin (Pharmacia & Upjohn); Robitet (Robins); Sumycin (Bristol-Myers Squibb)
Other common trade names: Apo-Tetra; Economycin; Florocycline; Steclin; Teflin; Tetramig
Category: Antibiotic
Clinically important, potentially serious interactions with: amoxicillin, ampicillin, antacids, cholestyramine, didanosine, etretinate, iron, isotretinoin, sucralfate, vitamin A, warfarin. Also dairy products

Reactions

SKIN
- Acne
- Angioedema
- Bullous eruption
- Candidiasis
- Dermatitis (sic)
- Eczematous eruption (sic)
- Erythema multiforme
- Exanthems
- Exfoliative dermatitis (<1%)
- Fixed eruption
- Granulomas
- Hyperhidrosis
- Lichenoid eruption
- Lupus erythematosus
- Lymphoepithelioma
- Photosensitivity (1–10%)
- Phototoxic reaction
- Pigmentation
- Pruritus (<1%)
- Pruritus ani
- Psoriasis (exacerbation)
- Purpura
- Pustular eruption
- Rash (sic)
- Stevens-Johnson syndrome
- Sunburn (exaggerated)
- Toxic epidermal necrolysis

Urticaria
Vasculitis
Warts (flat)

NAILS
Nails – discoloration (<1%)
Nails – onycholysis
Nails – photo-onycholysis

OTHER
Anaphylactoid reaction (<1%)
Black hairy tongue
Cheilitis
Fixed intraoral eruption
Glossitis
Hypersensitivity (<1%)
Mucocutaneous febrile syndrome
Mucous membrane pigmentation
Oral ulceration
Paresthesias (<1%)
Porphyria cutanea tarda
Pseudoporphyria
Pseudotumor cerebri
Serum sickness
Tongue pigmentation
Tooth discoloration (commonly in under 8-year-olds) (>10%)
Vaginitis

THALIDOMIDE

Trade name: Thalidomide
Category: Treatment for graft-versus-host disease & nodose leprosy
Clinically important, potentially serious interactions with: no data

REACTIONS

SKIN
Bullous eruption
Burning
Dermatitis (sic)
Edema
Erythema
Erythema nodosum
Erythroderma
Exanthems
Exfoliative dermatitis
Facial erythema
Hyperhidrosis
Pruritus
Purpura
Rash (sic)
Red palms
Toxic pustuloderma
Urticaria
Xerosis
Vasculitis

HAIR
Hair – alopecia

NAILS
Nails – brittle

OTHER
Dysesthesia
Galactorrhea
Xerostomia

THIABENDAZOLE

Trade name: Mintezol (Merck)
Other common trade name: Triasox
Category: Anthelmintic
Clinically important, potentially serious interactions with: theophylline

REACTIONS

SKIN
Angioedema
Contact dermatitis
Erythema multiforme (<1%)
Exanthems (>5%)
Fixed eruption (<1%)
Flushing
Jarisch-Herxheimer reaction
Perianal rash
Pruritus (<1%)
Psoriasis (exacerbation)
Rash (sic) (1–10%)
Sjøgren's syndrome
Stevens-Johnson syndrome (1–10%)

Toxic epidermal necrolysis (<1%)
Urticaria (1–5%)

OTHER
Anaphylactoid reaction
Dry mucous membranes (sic)
Hypersensitivity (<1%)
Paresthesias
Xanthopsia
Xerostomia

THIAMINE

Trade names: Betalin S (Lilly); Vitamin B_1
Other common trade names: Actamin; Beneuril; Betabion; Betamin; Bewon; Tiamina; Vitantial
Category: Water-soluble nutritional supplement
Clinically important, potentially serious interactions with: none

REACTIONS

SKIN
Allergic reactions (sic)
Angioedema (<1%)
Contact dermatitis
Eczematous eruption (sic)
Exanthems
Hyperhidrosis
Pruritus (<1%)
Purpura
Rash (sic) (<1%)
Systemic eczematous contact dermatitis
Urticaria
Vasculitis

OTHER
Anaphylactoid reaction
Foetor ex ore (halitosis)
Paresthesias (<1%)

THIOGUANINE

Trade name: Thioguanine (Glaxo Wellcome)
Other common trade name: Lanvis
Category: Antineoplastic
Clinically important, potentially serious interactions with: busulfan

REACTIONS

SKIN
Exanthems
Painful red hands
Petechiae
Photosensitivity (<1%)
Pruritus
Purpura
Rash (sic) (1–10%)

HAIR
Hair – alopecia

OTHER
Oral mucosal lesions
Stomatitis (1–10%)

THIOPENTAL

Trade name: Pentothal Sodium
Other common trade names: Anesthal; Hypnostan; Intraval; Nesdonal; Sodipental; Trapanal
Category: Barbiturate anesthetic
Clinically important, potentially serious interactions with: codeine, fentanyl, meperidine, methadone, narcotic analgesics, pentazocine

REACTIONS

SKIN
Angioedema
Bullous eruption
Erythema (<1%)
Erythema multiforme
Exanthems

Fixed eruption
Hypopigmentation
Pruritus
Purpura
Stevens-Johnson syndrome
Toxic epidermal necrolysis
Urticaria

OTHER
Anaphylactoid reaction
Injection-site necrosis
Injection-site pain (>10%)
Injection-site phlebitis
Porphyria
Shivering
Thrombophlebitis (<1%)
Twitching (<1%)

THIORIDAZINE

Trade name: Mellaril (Novartis)
Other common trade names: Aldazine; Calmaril; Dazine; Melleril; Ridazin; Thinin; Thioril
Category: Phenothiazine antipsychotic
Clinically important, potentially serious interactions with: CNS depressants, epinephrine, levodopa, pindolol, propranolol, tricyclic antidepressants

REACTIONS

SKIN
Acanthosis nigricans
Angioedema (<1%)
Dermatitis (sic)
Erythema multiforme
Exanthems
Hypohidrosis (>10%)
Lupus erythematosus
Photoallergic reaction
Phototoxic reaction
Pigmentation (blue-gray) (<1%)
Purpura
Rash (sic) (1–10%)
Toxic epidermal necrolysis
Urticaria

HAIR
Hair – alopecia
Hair – hypertrichosis

OTHER
Anaphylactoid reaction
Galactorrhea (<1%)
Gynecomastia
Lymphoproliferative disease
Mastodynia (1–10%)
Oral mucosal eruption
Paresthesias
Parotitis
Porphyria
Priapism (<1%)
Pseudolymphoma
Xerostomia

THIOTEPA

Trade name: Thioplex (Immunex)
Category: Antineoplastic
Clinically important, potentially serious interactions with: neuromuscular blocking agents, succinylcholine

REACTIONS

SKIN
Allergic reactions (sic) (1–10%)
Angioedema
Bruising
Ecchymoses
Eccrine squamous syringometaplasia
Hyperpigmentation
Leucoderma
Pruritus (1–10%)
Rash (sic) (1–10%)
Urticaria

HAIR
Hair – alopecia (1–10%)

OTHER
Anaphylactoid reaction (<1%)
Injection-site pain (>10%)
Stomatitis (<1%)

THIOTHIXENE

Trade name: Navane (Roerig)
Other common trade name: Orbinamon
Category: Antipsychotic
Clinically important, potentially serious interactions with: alcohol, anticholinergics, bromocriptine, CNS depressants

REACTIONS

SKIN
- Exanthems
- Hyperhidrosis
- Hypohidrosis (>10%)
- Palmar erythema
- Peripheral edema
- Photosensitivity
- Pigmentation (blue-gray) (<1%)
- Pruritus
- Rash (sic) (1–10%)
- Raynaud's phenomenon
- Seborrheic dermatitis
- Sensitivity (sic)
- Telangiectases
- Urticaria

HAIR
- Hair – alopecia

OTHER
- Anaphylactoid reaction
- Gynecomastia
- Paresthesias
- Priapism (<1%)
- Sialorrhea
- Xerostomia

TIAGABINE

Trade name: Gabitril (Abbott)
Category: Anticonvulsant
Clinically important, potentially serious interactions with: carbamazepine, phenobarbital, phenytoin, primidone, valproic acid

REACTIONS

SKIN
- Acne (>1%)
- Allergic reaction (sic) (<1%)
- Carcinoma (sic) (<1%)
- Contact dermatitis (<1%)
- Ecchymoses (>1%)
- Eczema (sic) (<1%)
- Edema (<1%)
- Exanthems (<1%)
- Exfoliative dermatitis (<1%)
- Facial edema (<1%)
- Furunculosis (<1%)
- Herpes simplex (<1%)
- Herpes zoster (<1%)
- Hyperhidrosis (<1%)
- Neoplasms, benign (<1%)
- Nodules (<1%)
- Peripheral edema (<1%)
- Petechiae (<1%)
- Photosensitivity (<1%)
- Pigmentation (<1%)
- Pruritus (2%)
- Psoriasis (<1%)
- Rash (sic) (5%)
- Ulcerations (<1%)
- Urticaria (<1%)
- Vesiculobullous eruption (<1%)
- Xerosis (<1%)

HAIR
- Alopecia (<1%)
- Hirsutism (<1%)

OTHER
- Ageusia (<1%)
- Dysgeusia (<1%)
- Gingival hyperplasia (<1%)
- Gingivitis (<1%)
- Glossitis (<1%)
- Gynecomastia (<1%)
- Halitosis (<1%)
- Mastodynia (<1%)
- Myalgia (>1%)
- Oral ulceration (2%)
- Paresthesias (4%)
- Parosmia (<1%)

Sialorrhea (<1%)
Stomatitis (<1%)
Thrombophlebitis (<1%)
Ulcerative stomatitis (<1%)
Vaginitis (<1%)
Xerostomia (>1%)

TICARCILLIN

Trade name: Ticar (SmithKline Beecham)
Category: Penicillinase-sensitive penicillin
Clinically important, potentially serious interactions with: aminoglycosides, anticoagulants, cyclosporine, methotrexate, neuromuscular blockers, probenecid, tetracycline

REACTIONS

SKIN
Allergic reactions (sic)
Angioedema
Ecchymoses
Erythema multiforme
Exanthems
Exfoliative dermatitis
Hematomas
Jarisch-Herxheimer reaction (<1%)
Pruritus
Rash (sic) (<1%)
Stevens-Johnson syndrome
Urticaria

OTHER
Anaphylactoid reaction (<1%)
Black tongue
Dysgeusia
Glossitis
Glossodynia
Hypersensitivity (<1%)
Injection-site pain
Injection-site phlebitis
Oral candidiasis
Serum sickness
Stomatitis
Stomatodynia
Thrombophlebitis (<1%)
Vaginitis
Xerostomia

TICLOPIDINE

Trade name: Ticlid (Syntex)
Other common trade names: Anagregal; Panaldine; Ticlidil; Ticlodix; Ticlodone; Tiklid; Tiklyd
Category: Antithrombotic; platelet aggregation inhibitor
Clinically important, potentially serious interactions with: anticoagulants, antipyrine, aspirin, cimetidine, cyclosporine, NSAIDs, theophylline

REACTIONS

SKIN
Angioedema
Cutaneous bleeding (sic)
Cutaneous side effects (sic)
Ecchymoses (<1%)
Erythema
Erythema multiforme
Exanthems
Exfoliative dermatitis
Hematomas
Hyperhidrosis
Lupus erythematosus (positive ANA)
Petechiae
Pruritus (1.3%)
Purpura (2.2%)
Rash (sic) (5.1%)
Stevens-Johnson syndrome
Urticaria (<1%)
Vasculitis

OTHER
Serum sickness

TIMOLOL

Trade names: Betimol (Ciba); Blocadren (Merck); Timoptic (ophthalmic) (Merck)
Other common trade names: Aquanil; Blocadren; Dispatim; Tenopt; Tiloptic; Timacor; Timoptic
Category: Beta-adrenergic blocking agent; antihypertensive
Clinically important, potentially serious interactions with: calcium channel blockers, clonidine, epinephrine, flecainide, insulin, nifedipine, oral contraceptives, salicylates, verapamil

REACTIONS

SKIN
Angioedema
Contact dermatitis (eyedrops)
Eczematous eruption (sic)
Edema (0.6%)
Erythema multiforme
Erythroderma
Exanthems
Exfoliative dermatitis
Hyperhidrosis
Hyperkeratosis (palms & soles)
Lichenoid eruption
Lupus erythematosus
Pemphigoid
Photosensitivity
Pigmentation
Pityriasis rubra pilaris
Pruritus (1–5%)
Psoriasis
Purpura
Rash (sic) (1–10%)
Raynaud's phenomenon
Toxic epidermal necrolysis
Urticaria
Xerosis

HAIR
Hair – alopecia (also from Timoptic eye drops) (1–10%)

NAILS
Nails – dystrophy
Nails – onycholysis
Nails – pigmentation

OTHER
Anaphylactoid reaction
Digital necrosis
Ocular pemphigoid
Oculo-mucocutaneous syndrome
Oral lichenoid eruption
Paresthesias
Peyronie's disease

TIOPRONIN

Trade name: Thiola (Mission)
Other common trade names: Acadione; Captimer
Category: Antiurolithic
Clinically important, potentially serious interactions with: no data

REACTIONS

SKIN
Angioedema
Bullous pemphigoid
Contact dermatitis
Cutaneous side effects (sic)
Ecchymoses
Edema
Elastosis perforans serpiginosa
Erythema
Erythema multiforme
Exanthems
Lichenoid eruption
Lupus erythematosus
Pemphigus
Pemphigus erythematosus
Pemphigus foliaceus
Photosensitivity
Pityriasis rosea
Pruritus
Rash (sic)
Toxic epidermal necrolysis
Urticaria
Wrinkling (sic)

HAIR
Hair – alopecia

Hair – hypertrichosis

OTHER
Mucocutaneous side effects (sic)
Myopathy
Oral mucosal lesions
Oral ulceration
Parageusia
Parosmia
Stomatitis
Xerostomia

TIZANIDINE

Trade name: Zanaflex (Athena)
Other common trade names: Sirdalud; Ternalax; Ternelin
Category: Alpha-adrenergic agonist
Clinically important, potentially serious interactions with: none

REACTIONS

SKIN
Acne (<1%)
Allergic reactions (sic) (<1%)
Candidiasis (<1%)
Cellulitis (<1%)
Ecchymoses (<1%)
Edema (<1%)
Exanthems (<1%)
Exfoliative dermatitis (<1%)
Herpes simplex (<1%)
Herpes zoster (<1%)
Hyperhidrosis (>1%)
Petechiae (<1%)
Pruritus (<1%)
Purpura (<1%)
Rash (sic) (>1%)
Ulceration (>1%)
Urticaria (<1%)
Xerosis (<1%)

HAIR
Hair – alopecia (<1%)

OTHER
Paresthesias (>1%)
Vaginal candidiasis (<1%)
Xerostomia (49%)

TOBRAMYCIN

Trade names: Nebcin (Lilly); Tobrex (Alcon)
Other common trade name: Oftalmotrisol-T
Category: Aminoglycoside antibiotic
Clinically important, potentially serious interactions with: aminoglycosides, amphotericin B, cephalosporins, furosemide, loop diuretics, neuromuscular blockers, torsemide

REACTIONS

SKIN
Contact dermatitis
Cutaneous side effects (sic)
Eczematous eruption (sic)
Erythema multiforme
Exanthems
Exfoliative dermatitis
Pruritus (<1%)
Purpura
Rash (sic) (<1%)
Urticaria

OTHER
Hypersensitivity
Injection-site pain
Paresthesias (<1%)
Sialorrhea

TOLAZAMIDE

Trade name: Tolinase (Pharmacia & Upjohn)
Other common trade names: Diabewas; Diadutos; Norglycin; Tolanase; Tolisan
Category: First generation sulfonylurea antidiabetic
Clinically important, potentially serious interactions with: anticoagulants, beta-blockers, MAO inhibitors, phenylbutazones, salicylates, thiazides, tricyclic antidepressants

REACTIONS

SKIN
- Dermatitis (sic)
- Eczematous eruption (sic)
- Erythema (0.4%)
- Exanthems (0.4%)
- Hyperhidrosis
- Lichenoid eruption
- Lupus erythematosus
- Photosensitivity (1–10%)
- Pruritus (0.4%)
- Purpura
- Rash (sic) (1–10%)
- Urticaria (1–10%)

OTHER
- Acute intermittent porphyria
- Dysgeusia
- Paresthesias
- Porphyria cutanea tarda
- Tongue ulceration

TOLAZOLINE

Trade name: Priscoline (Novartis)
Category: Alpha-adrenergic blocking agent; peripheral vasodilator antihypertensive (of the newborn)
Clinically important, potentially serious interactions with: none

REACTIONS

SKIN
- Contact dermatitis
- Edema
- Exanthems
- Flushing
- Rash (sic)
- Urticaria

OTHER
- Injection-site burning (>10%)

TOLBUTAMIDE

Trade name: Orinase (Pharmacia & Upjohn)
Other common trade names: Abemin; Aglycid; Diaben; Diatol; Dolipol; Mobenol; Orabet
Category: First generation sulfonylurea antidiabetic
Clinically important, potentially serious interactions with: beta-blockers, chloramphenicol, phenylbutazone

REACTIONS

SKIN
- Allergic reactions (sic)
- Bullous eruption (<1%)
- Bullous pemphigoid
- Contact dermatitis
- Cutaneous side effects (sic)
- Erythema (1.1%)
- Erythema multiforme (<1%)
- Exanthems (1–5%)
- Fixed eruption (<1%)
- Flushing
- Lichenoid eruption
- Photoallergic reaction
- Photosensitivity (1–10%)
- Poikiloderma
- Pruritus (1.1%)
- Purpura
- Rash (sic) (1–10%)
- Toxic epidermal necrolysis (<1%)
- Urticaria (1–10%)

OTHER
- Acute intermittent porphyria
- Dysgeusia
- Hypersensitivity (<1%)
- Oral lichenoid eruption
- Paresthesias
- Porphyria
- Porphyria cutanea tarda
- Thrombophlebitis (<1%)

TOLCAPONE

Trade name: Tasmar (Roche)
Category: Anti-parkinsonian adjunct
Clinically important, potentially serious interactions with: none

REACTIONS

SKIN
- Allergic reaction (sic) (<1%)
- Burning (sic) (2%)
- Eczema (<1%)
- Edema (<1%)
- Erythema multiforme (<1%)
- Facial edema (<1%)
- Fungal infection (<1%)
- Furunculosis (<1%)
- Herpes simplex (<1%)
- Herpes zoster (<1%)
- Hyperhidrosis (7%)
- Pigmentation (<1%)
- Pruritus (<1%)
- Rash (sic) (<1%)
- Seborrhea (<1%)
- Tumor (sic) (1%)
- Urticaria (<1%)

HAIR
- Hair – alopecia (1%)

OTHER
- Hypesthesia (<1%)
- Myalgia (<1%)
- Oral ulceration (<1%)
- Paresthesias (3%)
- Parosmia (<1%)
- Sialorrhea (<1%)
- Tongue disorder (<1%)
- Tooth disorder (<1%)
- Twitching (<1%)
- Vaginitis (<1%)
- Xerostomia (5%)

TOLMETIN

Trade name: Tolectin (McNeil)
Other common trade names: Donison; Midocil; Reutol; Safitex
Category: Nonsteroidal anti-inflammatory (NSAID)
Clinically important, potentially serious interactions with: aminoglycosides, anticoagulants, aspirin, cyclosporine, digoxin, diuretics, insulin, lithium, methotrexate, sulfonylureas

REACTIONS

SKIN
- Angioedema (<1%)
- Aphthous stomatitis (rare)
- Edema (3–9%)
- Erythema multiforme (<1%)
- Exanthems
- Photodermatitis
- Pruritus (<1%)
- Purpura
- Rash (sic) (>10%)
- Stevens-Johnson syndrome (<1%)
- Toxic epidermal necrolysis (<1%)
- Urticaria (1–5%)

OTHER
- Anaphylactoid reaction
- Dysgeusia
- Gingival ulceration
- Glossitis
- Gynecomastia
- Oral ulceration
- Serum sickness (<1%)
- Stomatitis
- Xerostomia

TOLTERODINE

Trade name: Detrol (Pharmacia & Upjohn)
Category: Muscarinic antagonist for overactive bladder
Clinically important, potentially serious interactions with: erythromycin

REACTIONS

SKIN
- Erythema (1.9%)
- Fungal infection (sic) (1.1%)
- Pruritus (1.3%)
- Rash (sic) (1.9%)
- Xerosis (1.7%)

OTHER
- Paresthesias (1.1%)
- Xerostomia

TOPIRAMATE

Trade name: Topamax (McNeil)
Category: Anticonvulsant
Clinically important, potentially serious interactions with: acetazolamide, carbamazepine, oral contraceptives, phenytoin

REACTIONS

SKIN
- Acne (>1%)
- Basal cell carcinoma (<1%)
- Dermatitis (sic) (<1%)
- Eczema (sic) (<1%)
- Edema (1.8%)
- Exanthems (<1%)
- Facial edema (<1%)
- Flushing (<1%)
- Folliculitis (<1%)
- Hyperhidrosis (1.8%)
- Hypohidrosis (<1%)
- Photosensitivity (<1%)
- Pigmentation (<1%)
- Pruritus (1.8%)
- Purpura (<1%)
- Rash (sic) (4.4%)
- Seborrhea (<1%)
- Urticaria (<1%)
- Xerosis (<1%)

HAIR
- Hair – abnormal texture (<1%)
- Hair – alopecia (>1%)

NAILS
- Nails – disorder (sic) (<1%)

OTHER
- Ageusia (<1%)
- Bromhidrosis (1.8%)
- Dysgeusia (>1%)
- Gingival hyperplasia (<1%)
- Gingivitis (1.8%)
- Gynecomastia (8.3%)
- Hyperesthesia (<1%)
- Hypesthesia (2.7%)
- Myalgia (1.8%)
- Paresthesias (15%)
- Parosmia (<1%)
- Stomatitis (<1%)
- Tongue edema (<1%)
- Xerostomia (2.7%)

TOPOTECAN

Trade name: Hycamtin (SmithKline Beecham)
Category: Antineoplastic
Clinically important, potentially serious interactions with: cisplatin, filgrastim

REACTIONS

SKIN
- Erythema (<1%)
- Purpura (<1%)

HAIR
- Hair – alopecia (59%)

OTHER
- Paresthesias (9%)
- Stomatitis (24%)

TOREMIFENE

Trade name: Fareston (Schering)
Category: Antiestrogen (for metastatic breast cancer)
Clinically important, potentially serious interactions with: thiazides, warfarin

REACTIONS

SKIN
- Dermatitis (sic)
- Edema (5%)
- Hot flashes (35%)
- Hyperhidrosis (20%)
- Pigmentation
- Pruritus

OTHER
- Thrombophlebitis (1%)
- Vaginal discharge (13%)

TORSEMIDE

Trade name: Demadex (Boehringer Mannheim)
Other common trade name: Unat
Category: Loop diuretic; antihypertensive
Clinically important, potentially serious interactions with: ACE-inhibitors, aminoglycosides, anticoagulants, beta-blockers, cisplatin, digitalis, lithium, sulfonylureas, thiazides

REACTIONS

SKIN
- Angioedema
- Edema (1.1%)
- Exanthems
- Lichenoid eruption
- Photosensitivity (1–10%)
- Purpura
- Rash (sic) (<1%)
- Stevens-Johnson syndrome
- Urticaria (1–10%)
- Vasculitis

OTHER
- Injection-site erythema (<1%)
- Myalgia (1.6%)

TRAMADOL

Trade name: Ultram (McNeil)
Other common trade names: Contramal; Tadol; Tradol; Tramal; Tramed; Tramol; Tridol; Zipan
Category: Centrally-acting synthetic analgesic
Clinically important, potentially serious interactions with: cimetidine, MAO inhibitors, quinidine, ritonavir

REACTIONS

SKIN
- Allergic reactions (sic) (<1%)
- Angioedema
- Exanthems
- Hyperhidrosis (9%)
- Pruritus (10%)
- Rash (sic) (1–5%)
- Urticaria (<1%)

OTHER
- Dysgeusia (<1%)
- Paresthesias (<1%)
- Stomatitis
- Xerostomia (10%)

TRANDOLAPRIL

Trade names: Mavik (Knoll); Tarka (Knoll)
Other common trade names: Gopten; Odrik; Udrik
Category: ACE inhibitor & calcium channel blocker
Clinically important, potentially serious interactions with: beta-blockers, bumetanide, carbamazepine, cyclosporine, digitalis, fentanyl, lithium, quinidine, salicylates, theophylline

Tarka is trandolapril & verapamil

REACTIONS

SKIN
- Angioedema (0.15%)
- Edema (>3%)
- Flushing (>3%)
- Pruritus (>3%)
- Rash (sic) (>10%)

OTHER
- Hypesthesia (>3%)
- Myalgia (>3%)
- Paresthesias (>3%)
- Xerostomia (>3%)

TRANYLCYPROMINE

Trade name: Parnate (SmithKline Beecham)
Other common trade name: Siciton
Category: Monoamine oxidase (MAO) inhibitor; antidepressant & antimanic
Clinically important, potentially serious interactions with: CNS depressants, dextroamphetamine, disulfiram, fluoxetine, levodopa, meperidine, phenothiazines, sumatriptan, sympathomimetics, tricyclic antidepressants. Also tyramine-containing foods

REACTIONS

SKIN
- Edema (<1%)
- Exanthems
- Flushing
- Hyperhidrosis
- Photosensitivity (<1%)
- Pruritus
- Rash (sic) (<1%)
- Urticaria

OTHER
- Acute intermittent porphyria
- Black tongue
- Paresthesias
- Xerostomia (<1%)

TRAZODONE

Trade name: Desyrel (Bristol-Myers Squibb)
Other common trade names: Bimaran; Deprax; Desirel; Molipaxin; Sideril; Taxagon; Trazalon
Category: Heterocyclic antidepressant & antineuralgic
Clinically important, potentially serious interactions with: CNS depressants, digoxin, fluoxetine, fluvoxamine, MAO inhibitors, paroxetine, sertraline, tricyclic antidepressants, venlafaxine

REACTIONS

SKIN
- Edema
- Erythema multiforme
- Exanthems
- Exfoliative dermatitis
- Hyperhidrosis (>1%)
- Photosensitivity
- Pruritus (<1%)
- Psoriasis (exacerbation)
- Purpura
- Rash (sic) (<1%)
- Urticaria
- Vasculitis

HAIR
Hair – alopecia

NAILS
Nails – leukonychia

OTHER
Dysgeusia (>10%)
Formication
Galactorrhea
Gynecomastia
Paresthesias (>1%)
Priapism (<1%)
Sialorrhea
Xerostomia (>10%)

TRIAMTERENE

Trade names: Dyazide (SmithKline Beecham); Dyrenium (SmithKline Beecham); Maxzide (SmithKline Beecham)
Other common trade names: Amterene; Diarrol; Diuteren; Dytac; Reviten; Suloton; Trian
Category: Potassium-sparing diuretic
Clinically important, potentially serious interactions with: ACE inhibitors, amantadine, amiloride, diclofenac, ibuprofen, indomethacin, spironolactone

Dyazide is triamterene & hydrochlorothiazide; Maxzide is triamterene & hydrochlorothiazide

REACTIONS

SKIN
Edema (1–10%)
Exanthems
Flushing (<1%)
Hyperhidrosis
Lupus erythematosus (in combination with hydrochlorothiazide)
Perleche
Photosensitivity
Pruritus
Purpura
Rash (sic) (1–10%)
Urticaria
Vasculitis

OTHER
Anaphylactoid reaction
Dysgeusia
Glossitis
Gynecomastia (<1%)
Paresthesias
Pseudoporphyria
Xerostomia

TRIAZOLAM

Trade name: Halcion (Pharmacia & Upjohn)
Other common trade names: Dumozolam; Nuctane; Somese; Somniton; Songar; Trialam
Category: Benzodiazepine sedative-hypnotic
Clinically important, potentially serious interactions with: CNS depressants, cimetidine, clarithromycin, diltiazem, erythromycin, verapamil

REACTIONS

SKIN
Dermatitis (sic) (1–10%)
Exanthems
Hyperhidrosis (>10%)
Photosensitivity
Pruritus
Purpura
Rash (sic) (>10%)
Urticaria

HAIR
Hair – alopecia
Hair – hirsutism

OTHER
Dysesthesia (<1%)
Dysgeusia (<1%)
Gingivitis
Glossitis (<1%)
Glossodynia (<1%)
Paresthesias (<1%)

Sialopenia (>10%)
Sialorrhea (1–10%)
Stomatitis (<1%)
Xerostomia (>10%)

TRICHLORMETHIAZIDE

Trade names: Metahydrin (Hoechst Marion Roussel); Naqua (Schering)
Other common trade names: Anatran; Carvacron; Doqua; Esmarin; Flute; Iopran; Trichlon
Category: Thiazide diuretic; antihypertensive
Clinically important, potentially serious interactions with: antidiabetics, digitalis, furosemide, lithium, loop diuretics, methotrexate

Reactions

SKIN
Exanthems
Lupus erythematosus
Photosensitivity (<1%)
Purpura
Rash (sic)
Urticaria
Vasculitis

OTHER
Anaphylactoid reaction
Paresthesias
Xerostomia

TRIENTINE

Trade name: Syprine (Merck)
Category: Chelating agent; antidote (copper toxicity)
Clinically important, potentially serious interactions with: none

Reactions

SKIN
Aphthous stomatitis
Dermatitis (sic)
Desquamation
Lupus erythematosus (<1%)
Thickening (sic) (<1%)

OTHER
Oral mucosal lesions

TRIFLUOPERAZINE

Trade name: Stelazine (Beecham)
Other common trade names: Calmazine; Domilium; Fluzine; Nerolet; Psyrazine; Sedizine; Tfp
Category: Phenothiazine tranquilizer; anxiolytic; antipsychotic
Clinically important, potentially serious interactions with: barbiturates, CNS depressants, levodopa, lithium, piperazine, propranolol

Reactions

SKIN
Angioedema
Eczema (sic)
Erythema
Exanthems
Exfoliative dermatitis
Fixed eruption
Hypohidrosis
Lupus erythematosus
Peripheral edema
Photosensitivity
Pigmentation (blue-gray) (<1%)
Pruritus
Purpura
Rash (sic) (1–10%)
Urticaria

OTHER
Anaphylactoid reaction
Galactorrhea (<1%)

Gynecomastia
Mastodynia (1–10%)
Oral mucosal eruption
Priapism (<1%)
Tongue edema
Xerostomia

TRIHEXYPHENIDYL

Trade name: Artane (Lederle)
Other common trade names: Acamed; Aparkane; Bentex; Hexinal; Parkines; Partane; Tridyl
Category: Antidyskinetic; anti-parkinsonian; anticholinergic
Clinically important, potentially serious interactions with: anticholinergics, digitalis, levodopa, phenothiazines, quinidine, tacrine, tricyclic antidepressants

REACTIONS

SKIN
Flushing
Hypohidrosis (>10%)
Rash (sic) (<1%)
Spider angiomas
Urticaria
Xerosis (>10%)

OTHER
Glossitis
Glossodynia
Paresthesias
Xerostomia (30–50%)

TRIMEPRAZINE

Trade name: Temaril (Allergan)
Other common trade names: Nedeltran; Panectyl; Theralene; Vallergan; Variargil
Category: Phenothiazine H_1-receptor antihistamine & sedative-hypnotic
Clinically important, potentially serious interactions with: alcohol, CNS depressants, MAO inhibitors, oral contraceptives, progesterone, reserpine

REACTIONS

SKIN
Angioedema (<1%)
Dermatitis (sic)
Edema (<1%)
Exanthems
Hyperhidrosis
Lupus erythematosus
Peripheral edema
Photosensitivity (<1%)
Pruritus
Purpura
Rash (sic) (<1%)
Urticaria

OTHER
Anaphylactoid reaction
Gynecomastia
Myalgia (<1%)
Paresthesias (<1%)
Stomatitis
Xerostomia (1–10%)

TRIMETHADIONE

Trade name: Tridione (Abbott)
Other common trade name: Mino Aleviatin
Category: Anticonvulsant
Clinically important, potentially serious interactions with: phenytoin, valproic acid

REACTIONS

SKIN
Acne
Bullous eruption
Erythema multiforme
Exanthems
Exfoliative dermatitis
Fixed eruption
Lupus erythematosus

Petechiae
Photosensitivity
Pruritus
Purpura
Stevens-Johnson syndrome
Urticaria
Vasculitis

HAIR
Hair – alopecia

OTHER
Acute intermittent porphyria
Gingivitis
Paresthesias

TRIMETHOPRIM

Trade names: Proloprim (Glaxo Wellcome); Trimpex (Roche)
Other common trade names: Alprim; Bactin; Ipral; Monotrim; Primsol; Tiempe; Triprim; Unitrim
Category: Antibacterial
Clinically important, potentially serious interactions with: amantadine, cyclosporine, methotrexate, phenytoin

Trimethoprim is commonly used in conjunction with sulfamethoxazole (cotrimoxazole). The trade names for this combination are: Bactrim; Cotrim; Septra

REACTIONS

Please see cotrimoxazole for the specific reactions and references

TRIMETREXATE

Trade name: Neutrexin (US Bioscience)
Category: Antineoplastic, folate antagonist
Clinically important, potentially serious interactions with: none

REACTIONS

SKIN
Angioedema
Exanthems
Fixed eruption
Flushing
Photosensitivity
Pruritus (5.5%)
Rash (1–10%)

OTHER
Hypersensitivity (1–10%)
Oral mucosal lesions
Stomatitis (1–10%)

TRIMIPRAMINE

Trade name: Surmontil (Wyeth)
Other common trade names: Rhotrimine; Stangyl; Sumontil
Category: Tricyclic antidepressant, antineuralgic & antiulcer
Clinically important, potentially serious interactions with: alcohol, anticholinergics, CNS depressants, cimetidine, clonidine, epinephrine, guanethidine, MAO inhibitors, methylphenidate

REACTIONS

SKIN
Allergic reactions (sic) (<1%)
Exanthems
Hyperhidrosis (1–10%)
Petechiae
Photosensitivity (<1%)
Pruritus
Purpura
Rash (sic)
Urticaria

HAIR
Hair – alopecia (<1%)

OTHER
Dysgeusia (>10%)
Galactorrhea (<1%)
Glossitis
Gynecomastia (<1%)
Paresthesias
Stomatitis
Xerostomia (>10%)

TRIOXSALEN

Trade name: Trisoralen (ICN)
Other common trade names: Neosoralen; Puvadin
Category: Repigmenting agent & antipsoriatic
Clinically important, potentially serious interactions with: no data

REACTIONS

SKIN
Acne
Bullous eruption (with UVA)
Eczematous eruption (sic)
Freckles
Granuloma annulare
Herpes simplex
Herpes zoster
Lupus erythematosus
Melanoma
Pemphigoid
Photoallergic reaction
Photosensitivity
Phototoxic reaction
Pigmentation
Porokeratosis (actinic)
Pruritus (>10%)
Scleroderma
Seborrheic dermatitis
Skin pain (sic)
Tumors (sic)
Vasculitis
Vitiligo

HAIR
Hair – hypertrichosis

NAILS
Nails – photo-onycholysis
Nails – pigmentation

OTHER
Lymphoproliferative disease

TRIPELENNAMINE

Trade name: PBZ (Novartis)
Other common trade name: Azaron
Category: H_1-receptor antihistamine
Clinically important, potentially serious interactions with: alcohol, CNS depressants, MAO inhibitors

REACTIONS

SKIN
Angioedema (<1%)
Edema (<1%)
Fixed eruption
Flushing
Hyperhidrosis
Lichenoid eruption
Lupus erythematosus
Peripheral edema
Photosensitivity (<1%)
Pityriasis rosea
Purpura
Rash (sic)
Systemic eczematous contact dermatitis
Urticaria

OTHER
Anaphylactoid reaction
Myalgia (<1%)
Paresthesias (<1%)
Stomatitis
Xerostomia (1–10%)

TRIPROLIDINE

Trade names: Actagen; Actidil; Actifed; Allerphed; Cenafed; Genac; Myidil; Trifed; Triofed; Triposed. (Various pharmaceutical companies.)
Other common trade name: Actidilon
Category: H_1-receptor antihistamine; sympathomimetic
Clinically important, potentially serious interactions with: alcohol, CNS depressants, MAO inhibitors, sympathomimetics

REACTIONS

SKIN
- Angioedema (<1%)
- Edema (<1%)
- Exanthems
- Fixed eruption
- Flushing
- Hyperhidrosis (1–10%)
- Lichenoid eruption
- Photosensitivity (<1%)
- Purpura
- Rash (sic) (<1%)
- Urticaria

OTHER
- Myalgia (<1%)
- Paresthesias (<1%)
- Xerostomia (1–10%)

TROGLITAZONE

Trade name: Rezulin (Parke-Davis)
Category: Oral antihyperglycemic (antidiabetic)
Clinically important, potentially serious interactions with: cholestyramine, cyclosporine, HMG-CoA reductase inhibitors, oral contraceptives, tacrolimus, terfenadine

REACTIONS

SKIN
- Peripheral edema (5%)

TROLEANDOMYCIN

Trade name: TAO (Roerig)
Category: Macrolide antibiotic
Clinically important, potentially serious interactions with: astemizole, carbamazepine, cisapride, cyclosporine, ergot alkaloids, terfenadine, theophylline, triazolam

REACTIONS

SKIN
- Angioedema
- Erythema multiforme
- Exanthems
- Pruritus
- Rash (sic) (1–10%)
- Urticaria (1–10%)

OTHER
- Anaphylactoid reaction
- Oral mucosal lesions

TROVAFLOXACIN

Trade name: Trovan (Pfizer)
Category: Fourth generation fluoroquinoline antibiotic
Clinically important, potentially serious interactions with: antacids, iron, morphine, sucralfate

REACTIONS

SKIN
- Acne
- Allergic reactions (sic) (<1%)
- Angioedema (<1%)
- Balanoposthitis (<1%)
- Candidiasis (<1%)
- Cheilitis (<1%)
- Dermatitis (sic) (<1%)
- Edema (<1%)
- Exfoliation (<1%)
- Facial edema (<1%)
- Flushing (<1%)
- Hyperhidrosis (<1%)
- Periorbital edema (<1%)
- Peripheral edema (<1%)
- Photosensitivity (0.03%)
- Pruritus (2%)
- Pruritus ani (<1%)
- Rash (sic) (2%)
- Seborrhea (<1%)
- Ulceration (<1%)
- Urticaria (<1%)

OTHER
- Anaphylactoid reaction (<1%)
- Dysgeusia (<1%)
- Foetor ex ore (halitosis) (<1%)
- Injection-site edema (<1%)
- Injection-site inflammation (<1%)
- Injection-site pain (<1%)
- Gingivitis (<1%)
- Myalgia (<1%)
- Sialorrhea (<1%)
- Paresthesias (<1%)
- Stomatitis (<1%)
- Thrombophlebitis (<1%)
- Tongue disorder (<1%)
- Tongue edema (<1%)
- Vaginitis (<1%)
- Xerostomia (<1%)

UROKINASE

Trade name: Abbokinase (Abbott)
Category: Thrombolytic enzyme
Clinically important, potentially serious interactions with: anticoagulants, antiplatelet drugs, aspirin, dextran, indomethacin

REACTIONS

SKIN
- Angioedema (>10%)
- Bleeding (44%)
- Bullous eruption (hemorrhagic)
- Exanthems
- Flushing
- Hyperhidrosis (<1%)
- Periorbital edema (>10%)
- Pruritus
- Purpura
- Rash (sic) (<1%)
- Urticaria

OTHER
- Anaphylactoid reaction (>10%)
- Injection-site phlebitis

URSODIOL

Trade name: Actigall (Novartis)
Other common trade names: Arsacol; Cholit-Ursan; Destolit; Litanin; Ursochol; Ursolvan
Category: Gallstone dissolution agent
Clinically important, potentially serious interactions with: none

REACTIONS

SKIN
- Hyperhidrosis
- Lichen planus
- Pruritus (<1%)
- Rash (sic) (<1%)
- Urticaria
- Xerosis

HAIR
- Hair – alopecia

OTHER
- Dysgeusia (<1%)
- Myalgia
- Stomatitis

VALPROIC ACID

Trade name: Depakene (Abbott)
Other common trade names: Convulex; Depakin; Leptilan; Orfiril; Valporal; Valprosid
Category: Anticonvulsant
Clinically important, potentially serious interactions with: alcohol, aspirin, CNS depressants, phenytoin, salicylates, warfarin

REACTIONS

SKIN
- Acne
- Contact dermatitis
- Edema
- Erythema multiforme (<1%)
- Exanthems
- Facial edema
- Fixed eruption
- Lupus erythematosus
- Morphea
- Petechiae
- Photosensitivity
- Pruritus
- Psoriasis
- Purpura
- Rash (sic)
- Scleroderma
- Stevens-Johnson syndrome
- Toxic epidermal necrolysis
- Urticaria
- Vasculitis

HAIR
- Hair – alopecia (1–2%)
- Hair – curly
- Hair – depigmentation
- Hair – perming effect (sic)

OTHER
- Acute intermittent porphyria
- Aplasia cutis congenita
- Galactorrhea
- Gingival hyperplasia
- Gynecomastia
- Hypersensitivity
- Paresthesias
- Porphyria
- Sialorrhea
- Stomatitis

VALSARTAN

Trade name: Diovan (Novartis)
Category: Angiotensin II antagonist; antihypertensive
Clinically important, potentially serious interactions with: none

REACTIONS

SKIN
- Allergic reactions (sic) (>2%)
- Angioedema (>2%)
- Edema (>1%)
- Pruritus (>2%)
- Rash (sic) (>2%)

OTHER
- Myalgia (>2%)
- Paresthesias (>2%)
- Xerostomia (>2%)

VANCOMYCIN

Trade names: Lymphocin (Fujisawa); Vancocin (Lilly); Vancoled (Lederle)
Other common trade name: Diatracin
Category: Narrow-spectrum antibacterial
Clinically important, potentially serious interactions with: aminoglycosides, anesthetics, succinylcholine

REACTIONS

SKIN
- Acute generalized exanthematous pustulosis (AGEP)
- Allergic reactions (sic) (<5%)
- Angioedema
- Bullous eruption
- Cutaneous reactions (sic)
- Erythema multiforme
- Exanthems
- Exfoliative dermatitis
- Flushing (1–10%)
- Linear IgA bullous dermatosis
- Lupus erythematosus
- Pruritus
- Purpura
- Rash (sic)
- Red man syndrome* (1–10%)
- Red neck syndrome (sic)
- Stevens-Johnson syndrome
- Toxic epidermal necrolysis
- Urticaria
- Vasculitis (<1%)

OTHER
- Anaphylactoid reaction
- Dysgeusia
- Hypersensitivity
- Injection-site thrombophlebitis
- Paresthesias
- Priapism

*Note: The vancomycin-induced red man syndrome is characterized by pruritus, erythema, and, in severe cases, angioedema, hypotension, and cardiovascular collapse.

VASOPRESSIN

Trade name: Pitressin (Parke-Davis)
Category: Vasoconstrictor & antidiuretic pituitary hormone
Clinically important, potentially serious interactions with: chlorpropamide, phenformin, urea

REACTIONS

SKIN
- Allergic reactions (sic) (<1%)
- Angioedema
- Bullous eruption
- Ecchymoses
- Exanthems
- Gangrene
- Hyperhidrosis (1–10%)

Purpura
Rash (sic)
Urticaria (1–10%)

HAIR
Hair – alopecia

OTHER
Anaphylactoid reaction
Infusion-site necrosis

VENLAFAXINE

Trade name: Effexor (Wyeth)
Category: Heterocyclic antidepressant; selective serotonin reuptake inhibitor (SSRI)
Clinically important, potentially serious interactions with: antiarrhythmics, beta-blockers, cimetidine, fluoxetine, MAO inhibitors, phenothiazines, sertraline, trazodone, tricyclic antidepressants, warfarin

REACTIONS

SKIN
Acne (<1%)
Allergic reactions (sic) (<1%)
Candidiasis
Contact dermatitis
Ecchymoses (<1%)
Eczema (sic) (<1%)
Edema (<1%)
Exanthems (<1%)
Exfoliative dermatitis (<1%)
Facial edema (<1%)
Furunculosis (<1%)
Herpes simplex (<1%)
Herpes zoster (<1%)
Hyperhidrosis (12%)
Lichenoid eruption (<1%)
Photosensitivity (<1%)
Pruritus (1%)
Psoriasis (<1%)
Pustular eruption (<1%)
Rash (sic) (3%)
Urticaria (<1%)
Vesiculobullous eruption (<1%)
Xerosis (<1%)

HAIR
Hair – alopecia (<1%)
Hair – discoloration (<1%)
Hair – hirsutism (<1%)

OTHER
Ageusia (<1%)
Bromhidrosis (<1%)
Dysgeusia (2%)
Gingivitis (<1%)
Glossitis (<1%)
Gynecomastia (<1%)
Hyperesthesia (<1%)
Hypesthesia (>1%)
Mastodynia
Myalgia (>1%)
Oral ulceration (<1%)
Paresthesias (3%)
Parosmia (<1%)
Sialorrhea (<1%)
Stomatitis (<1%)
Thrombophlebitis (<1%)
Tongue pigmentation (<1%)
Tongue edema (<1%)
Vaginal candidiasis (<1%)
Vaginitis
Xerostomia (22%)

VERAPAMIL

Trade names: Calan (Searle); Isoptin (Knoll); Tarka (Knoll); Verelan (Knoll)
Other common trade names: Arpamyl LP; Azupamil; Berkatens; Cordilox; Geangin; Isoptine
Category: Calcium channel blocker; antianginal, antihypertensive & antiarrhythmic
Clinically important, potentially serious interactions with: beta-blockers, carbamazepine, clonidine, cyclosporine, dantrolene, digitalis, fentanyl, phenytoin, quinidine, theophylline

Tarka is trandolapril & verapamil

REACTIONS

SKIN
- Acne
- Acute febrile neutrophilic dermatosis (Sweet's syndrome)
- Angioedema
- Ankle edema
- Cutaneous side effects (sic)
- Ecchymoses (<1%)
- Edema (1.9%)
- Erythema multiforme (<1%)
- Erythema nodosum
- Exanthems
- Exfoliative dermatitis
- Flushing (0.6%)
- Hyperhidrosis (<1%)
- Hyperkeratosis (palms) (<1%)
- Lichenoid eruption
- Peripheral edema (1–10%)
- Photosensitivity
- Prurigo (sic)
- Pruritus
- Purpura (<1%)
- Rash (sic) (1–10%)
- Stevens-Johnson syndrome (<1%)
- Urticaria (<1%)
- Vasculitis (<1%)

HAIR
- Hair – alopecia (<1%)
- Hair – hypertrichosis
- Hair – pigmentation

NAILS
- Nails – dystrophy

OTHER
- Erythermalgia
- Galactorrhea (<1%)
- Gingival hyperplasia (<1%)
- Gynecomastia (<1%)
- Paresthesias (<1%)
- Serum sickness
- Xerostomia (<1%)

VINBLASTINE

Trade name: Velban (Lilly)
Category: Antineoplastic
Clinically important, potentially serious interactions with: interferon, mitomycin, phenytoin

REACTIONS

SKIN
- Acne
- Acral gangrene
- Bullous eruption (<1%)
- Cellulitis
- Dermatitis (sic) (1–10%)
- Erythema
- Erythema multiforme
- Exanthems
- Hyperpigmentation
- Photosensitivity (1–10%)
- Phototoxic reaction
- Purpura
- Radiation recall
- Radiodermatitis (reactivation)
- Rash (sic) (1–10%)
- Raynaud's phenomenon
- Urticaria

HAIR
- Hair – alopecia (>10%)
- Hair – changes

OTHER
- Dysgeusia (metallic taste) (>10%)
- Injection-site necrosis

Injection-site pain
Oral mucosal lesions
Paresthesias (1–10%)
Phlebitis
Stomatitis (>10%)
Ulceration due to extravasation
Vesiculation of mouth (sic)

VINCRISTINE

Trade names: Oncovin (Lilly); Vincasar (Pharmacia & Upjohn)
Category: Antineoplastic mitotic inhibitor
Clinically important, potentially serious interactions with: digoxin, mitomycin, nifedipine, quinolones

REACTIONS

SKIN
Angioedema
Dermatitis herpetiformis
Edema
Erythroderma
Exanthems
Palmar-plantar erythema
Pruritus
Rash (sic) (1–10%)
Raynaud's phenomenon
Sjøgren's syndrome
Urticaria

HAIR
Hair – alopecia (20–70%)

NAILS
Nails – Beau's lines (transverse nail ridging)
Nails – leukonychia
Nails – Mees' lines
Nails – onychodermal band

OTHER
Anaphylactoid reaction
Dysgeusia (metallic taste) (1–10%)
Injection-site cellulitis (>10%)
Injection-site necrosis (>10%)
Oral mucosal lesions (1–10%)
Paresthesias (1–10%)
Phlebitis (1–10%)

VINORELBINE

Trade name: Navelbine (Glaxo Wellcome)
Category: Antineoplastic
Clinically important, potentially serious interactions with: cisplatin, mitomycin

REACTIONS

SKIN
Hand-foot syndrome
Pigmentation
Rash (sic) (<5%)
Toxic epidermal necrolysis

HAIR
Hair – alopecia (12%)

OTHER
Dysgeusia (metallic taste) (>10%)
Hypesthesia
Injection-site irritation (1–10%)
Injection-site necrosis (1–10%)
Injection-site pain (1.6%)
Injection-site phlebitis
Myalgia (<5%)
Paresthesias (1–10%)
Phlebitis (7%)
Stomatitis (>10%)

VITAMIN A

Trade names: Aquasol A (Astra); Del-Vi-A (DelRay); Palmitate A
Other common trade names: Acaren; Acon; Afaxin; Arovit; Avipur; Avitin; Axerol; Dolce; Vogan
Category: Nutritional fat-soluble vitamin supplement
Clinically important, potentially serious interactions with: retinoids

REACTIONS

SKIN
- Cheilitis
- Contact dermatitis
- Dermatitis (dry, scaly, keratotic – mainly palms & soles)
- Eczematous eruption (pellagra-like)
- Erythema
- Erythema multiforme (<1%)
- Exanthems
- Exfoliative dermatitis
- Fissuring
- Generalized peeling (sic)
- Hyperkeratosis
- Perleche
- Photosensitivity
- Pigmentation (yellow-orange)
- Pruritus (<1%)
- Shedding
- Stevens-Johnson syndrome
- Xerosis (1–10%)

HAIR
- Hair – alopecia

OTHER
- Anaphylactoid reaction
- Gingivitis
- Hypersensitivity
- Oral mucosal eruption
- Pseudotumor cerebri
- Stomatodynia
- Xerostomia

VITAMIN B_1 (See THIAMINE)

VITAMIN B_2 (See RIBOFLAVIN)

VITAMIN B_3 (See NIACIN; NIACINAMIDE)

VITAMIN B_6 (See PYRIDOXINE)

VITAMIN B_{12} (See CYANOCOBALAMIN)

VITAMIN C (See ASCORBIC ACID)

VITAMIN D (See ERGOCALCIFEROL)

VITAMIN E (alpha TOCOPHEROL)

Trade names: Aquasol E; Eprolin; E-Vitamin Succinate; Pheryl-E; Vita Plus E; Vitec. (Various pharmaceutical companies)
Other common trade names: Bio E; Davitamon E; Detulin; E Perle; Ephynal; Optovit-E; Vita-E
Category: Fat-soluble vitamin
Clinically important, potentially serious interactions with: anticoagulants

REACTIONS

SKIN
- Contact dermatitis (<1%)
- Dermatitis
- Erythema multiforme
- Exanthems
- Lupus erythematosus
- Urticaria

HAIR
- Hair – depigmentation (at injection sites)

OTHER
- Gynecomastia
- Sclerosing lipogranuloma
- Thrombophlebitis
- Yellow spots on dental enamel

VITAMIN K (See PHYTONADIONE)

WARFARIN

Trade name: Coumadin (Dupont)
Other common trade names: Aldocumar; Coumadine; Marevan; Waran; Warfilone
Category: Oral anticoagulant
Clinically important, potentially serious interactions with: scores of drugs. Too extensive a list for review here

REACTIONS

SKIN
- Abscess
- Acral purpura
- Angioedema (<1%)
- Bullous eruption
- Dermatitis (sic)
- Ecchymoses
- Exanthems
- Exfoliative dermatitis
- Hemorrhagic skin infarcts
- Livedo reticularis
- Necrosis (>10%)
- Pruritus (<1%)
- Purplish erythema (feet & toes) (sic) (<1%)
- Purpura
- Urticaria
- Vasculitis
- Vesicular eruption

HAIR
- Hair – alopecia (>10%)

OTHER
- Gangrene
- Hematoma
- Hypersensitivity
- Oral ulceration (<1%)
- Priapism

YOHIMBINE

Trade names: Actibine (Consolidated Midland); Aphrodyne (Star); Yocon (Palisades); Yohimex (Kramer)
Category: Impotence therapy agent; alpha$_2$-adrenergic blocking agent
Clinically important, potentially serious interactions with: none

REACTIONS

SKIN
- Exfoliative dermatitis
- Flushing
- Hyperhidrosis
- Lupus erythematosus

ZAFIRLUKAST

Trade name: Accolate (Zeneca)
Category: Antiasthmatic
Clinically important, potentially serious interactions with: aspirin, erythromycin, terfenadine, theophylline, warfarin

REACTIONS

SKIN
- Allergic granulomatous angiitis (Churg-Strauss syndrome)

OTHER
- Myalgia (1.6%)

ZALCITABINE (ddC)

Trade name: Hivid (Roche)
Category: Antiviral – used in treatment of acquired immunodeficiency syndrome (AIDS)
Clinically important, potentially serious interactions with: aminoglycosides, amphotericin, didanosine, foscarnet

REACTIONS

SKIN
- Acne (<1%)
- Angioedema
- Ankle edema
- Aphthous stomatitis
- Bullous eruption (<1%)
- Cutaneous side effects (sic)
- Dermatitis (sic) (<1%)
- Edema (<1%)
- Erythema multiforme
- Erythroderma
- Exanthems (<1%)
- Exfoliative dermatitis (<1%)
- Flushing (<1%)
- Hyperhidrosis (<1%)
- Photosensitivity (<1%)
- Pruritus (3.4%)
- Rash (sic) (3.4%)
- Urticaria (3.4%)
- Xerosis (<1%)

HAIR
- Hair – alopecia

NAILS
- Nails – changes

OTHER
- Ageusia (<1%)
- Anaphylactoid reaction
- Dysgeusia (<1%)
- Gingivitis (<1%)
- Glossitis (<1%)
- Glossodynia (<1%)
- Myalgia (<1%)
- Myopathy (<1%)
- Oral mucosal lesions (3%)
- Oral ulceration (>10%)
- Paresthesias
- Parosmia (<1%)
- Penile edema (<1%)
- Stomatitis (3%)
- Tongue disorder (sic) (<1%)
- Xerostomia (<1%)

ZIDOVUDINE

Trade name: AZT, Retrovir (Glaxo Wellcome)
Other common trade names: Retrovis
Category: Reverse transcriptase inhibitor; antiviral
Clinically important, potentially serious interactions with: acetaminophen, acyclovir, amphotericin B, aspirin, cimetidine, dapsone, ganciclovir, indomethacin, lorazepam, pentamidine, probenecid, valproic acid

REACTIONS

SKIN
- Acne (<5%)
- Blue vitiligo (sic)
- Bullous eruption
- Ecchymoses
- Erythema multiforme
- Erythroderma
- Exanthems
- Heightened cutaneous reactions to mosquito bites (sic)
- Hyperhidrosis (5–19%)
- Neutrophilic eccrine hidradenitis
- Pigmentation
- Pruritus
- Purpura
- Rash (sic) (1–10%)
- Stevens-Johnson syndrome
- Toxic epidermal necrolysis
- Urticaria (<5%)
- Vasculitis

HAIR
- Hair – alopecia
- Hair – hypertrichosis (eyelashes)

NAILS
- Nails – blue lunulae
- Nails – pigmentation (1–10%)
- Nails – pigmented bands

OTHER
- Bromhidrosis (<5%)
- Dysgeusia (5–19%)
- Edema of lip (<5%)
- Myopathy (<1%)
- Oral lichenoid eruption
- Oral mucosal eruption
- Oral mucosal pigmentation
- Oral ulceration (<5%)
- Paresthesias (<8%)
- Polymyositis
- Porphyria cutanea tarda
- Tongue edema (<5%)
- Tongue pigmentation
- Tongue ulceration

ZILEUTON

Trade name: Zyflo (Abbott)
Category: Antiasthmatic bronchodilator
Clinically important, potentially serious interactions with: anticoagulants, propranolol, terfenadine, xanthines

REACTIONS

SKIN
- Pruritus (>1%)

OTHER
- Myalgia (3.2%)
- Vaginitis (>1%)

ZOLMITRIPTAN

Trade name: Zomig (Zeneca)
Category: Antimigraine
Clinically important, potentially serious interactions with: cimetidine, ergot, estrogens, MAO inhibitors

REACTIONS

SKIN
- Allergic reactions (sic) (<1%)
- Ecchymoses (<1%)
- Edema (<1%)
- Facial edema (<1%)
- Hyperhidrosis (2%)
- Photosensitivity (<1%)
- Pruritus (<1%)
- Rash (sic) (<1%)
- Urticaria (<1%)

OTHER
- Hyperesthesia (<1%)
- Hypesthesia (2%)
- Myalgia (2%)
- Paresthesias (9%)
- Parosmia (<1%)
- Thrombophlebitis (<1%)
- Tongue edema (<1%)
- Twitching (<1%)
- Xerostomia (3%)

ZOLPIDEM

Trade name: Ambien (Searle)
Other common trade names: Niotal; Stilnoct; Stilnox
Category: Non-benzodiazepine sedative-hypnotic
Clinically important, potentially serious interactions with: alcohol, CNS depressants, ritonavir

REACTIONS

SKIN
- Acne (<1%)
- Allergic reactions (sic) (4%)
- Bullous eruption (<1%)
- Dermatitis (sic) (<1%)
- Edema (<1%)

Facial edema (<1%)
Flushing (<1%)
Furunculosis (<1%)
Herpes simplex (<1%)
Herpes zoster (<1%)
Hot flashes (<1%)
Hyperhidrosis (<1%)
Periorbital edema (<1%)
Photosensitivity (<1%)
Pruritus
Purpura (<1%)
Rash (sic) (2%)
Urticaria (<1%)

OTHER

Anaphylactoid reaction (<1%)
Dysgeusia (<1%)
Hypesthesia (<1%)
Injection-site inflammation (<1%)
Mastodynia (<1%)
Myalgia (7%)
Paresthesias (<1%)
Vaginitis (<1%)
Xerostomia (3%)

Description of the 29 most common reaction patterns

Acanthosis nigricans

Acanthosis nigricans (AN) is a process characterized by a soft, velvety, brown or grayish-black thickening of the skin that is symmetrically distributed over the axillae, neck, inguinal areas and other body folds.

While most cases of AN are seen in obese and prepubertal children, it can occur as a marker for various endocrinopathies as well as in female patients with elevated testosterone levels, irregular menses, and hirsutism.

It is frequently a concomitant of an underlying malignant condition, principally an adenocarcinoma of the intestinal tract.

Acneform lesions

Acneform eruptions are inflammatory follicular reactions that resemble acne vulgaris and that are manifested clinically as papules or pustules. They are monomorphic reactions, have a monomorphic appearance, and are found primarily on the upper parts of the body. Unlike acne vulgaris, there are rarely comedones present. Consider a drug-induced acneform eruption if:

- The onset is sudden
- There is a worsening of existing acne lesions
- The extent is considerable from the outset
- The appearance is monomorphic
- The localization is unusual for acne as, for example, when the distal extremities are involved
- The patient's age is unusual for regular acne
- There is an exposure to a potentially responsible drug.

The most common drugs responsible for acneform eruptions are: ACTH, androgenic hormones, anticonvulsants (hydantoin derivatives, phenobarbital, trimethadione), corticosteroids, danazol, disulfiram, halogens (bromides, chlorides, iodides), lithium, oral contraceptives, tuberculostatics (ethionamide, isoniazid, rifampin), vitamins B_2, B_6, and B_{12}.

Acute generalized exanthematous pustulosis

Arising on the face or intertriginous areas, acute generalized exanthematous pustulosis (AGEP) is characterized by a rapidly evolving, widespread, scarlatiniform eruption covered with hundreds of small superficial pustules.

Often accompanied by a high fever, AGEP is most frequently associated with penicillin and macrolide antibiotics, and usually occurs within 24 hours of the drug exposure.

Alopecia

Many drugs have been reported to occasion hair loss. Commonly appearing as a diffuse alopecia, it affects women more frequently than men and is limited in most instances to the scalp. Axillary and pubic hairs are rarely affected except with anticoagulants.

The hair loss from cytostatic agents, which is dose-dependent and begins about 2 weeks after the onset of therapy, is a result of the interruption of the anagen (growing) cycle of hair. With other drugs the hair loss does not begin until 2–5 months after the medication has been begun. With cholesterol-lowering drugs, diffuse alopecia is a result of interference with normal keratinization.

The scalp is normal and the drug-induced alopecia is almost always reversible within 1–3 months after the therapy has been discontinued. The regrown hair is frequently depigmented and occasionally more curly.

The most frequent offenders are cytostatic agents and anticoagulants, but hair loss can occur with a variety of common drugs, including hormones, anticonvulsants, amantadine, amiodarone, captopril, cholesterol-lowering drugs, cimetidine, colchicine, etretinate, isotretinoin, ketoconazole, heavy metals, lithium, penicillamine, valproic acid, and propranolol.

Angioedema

Angioedema is a term applied to a variant of urticaria in which the subcutaneous tissues, rather than the dermis, are mainly involved.

Also known as Quincke's edema, giant urticaria, and angioneurotic edema, this acute, evanescent, skin-colored, circumscribed edema usually affects the most distensible tissues: the lips, eyelids, earlobes, and genitalia. It can also affect the mucous membranes of the tongue, mouth, and larynx.

Symptoms of angioedema, frequently unilateral, asymmetrical and non-pruritic, last for an hour or two but can persist for 2–5 days.

The etiological factors associated with angioedema are as varied as that of urticaria (which see).

Aphthous stomatitis

Aphthous stomatitis – also known as canker sores – is a common disease of the oral mucous membranes.

Arising as tiny, discrete or grouped, papules or vesicles, these painful lesions develop into small (2–5 mm in diameter), round, shallow ulcerations having a grayish, yellow base surrounded by a thin red border.

Located predominantly over the labial and buccal mucosae, these aphthae heal without scarring in 10–14 days. Recurrences are common.

Black hairy tongue (lingua villosa nigra)

Black hairy tongue (BHT) represents a benign hyperplasia of the filiform papillae of the anterior two-thirds of the tongue.

These papillary elongations, usually associated with black, brown, or yellow pigmentation attributed to the overgrowth of pigment-producing bacteria, may be as long as 2 cm.

Occurring only in adults, BHT has been associated with the administration of oral antibiotics, poor dental hygiene, and excessive smoking.

Bullous eruptions

Bullous and vesicular drug eruptions are diseases in which blisters and vesicles occur as a complication of the administration of drugs. Blisters are a well-known manifestation of cutaneous reactions to drugs.

In many types of drug reactions, bullae and vesicles may be found in addition to other manifestations. Bullae are usually noted in erythema multiforme, Stevens-Johnson syndrome, toxic epidermal necrolysis, fixed eruptions when very intense, urticaria, vasculitis, porphyria cutanea tarda, and phototoxic reactions (from furosemide and nalidixic acid). Tense, thick-walled bullae can be seen in bromoderma and iododerma as well as in barbiturate overdosage.

Common drugs that cause bullous eruptions and bullous pemphigoid are: nadalol, penicillamine, piroxicam, psoralens, rifampin, clonidine, furosemide, diclofenac, mefenamic acid, bleomycin, and others.

Erythema multiforme & Stevens-Johnson syndrome

Erythema multiforme is a relatively common, acute, self-limited, inflammatory reaction pattern that is often associated with a preceding herpes simplex or mycoplasma infection. Other causes are associated with connective tissue disease, physical agents, X-Ray therapy, pregnancy and internal malignancies, to mention a few. In 50 percent of the cases, no cause can be found. In a recent prospective study of erythema multiforme, only 10 percent were drug related.

The eruption rapidly occurs over a period of 12 to 24 hours. In about half the cases there are prodromal symptoms of an upper respiratory infection accompanied by fever, malaise, and varying degrees of muscular and joint pains.

Clinically, bluish-red, well-demarcated, macular, papular, or urticarial lesions, as well as the classical "iris" or "target lesions," sometimes with central vesicles, bullae, or purpura, are distributed preferentially over the distal extremities, especially over the dorsa of the hands and extensor aspects of the forearms. Lesions tend to spread peripherally and may involve the palms and trunk as well as the mucous membranes of the mouth and genitalia. Central healing and overlapping lesions often lead to arciform, annular and gyrate patterns. Lesions appear over the course of a week or 10 days and resolve over the next 2 weeks.

The Stevens-Johnson syndrome (erythema multiforme major), a severe and occasionally fatal variety of erythema multiforme, has an abrupt onset and is accompanied by any or all of the following: fever, myalgia, malaise, headache, arthralgia, ocular involvement, with occasional bullae and erosions covering less than 10 percent of the body surface. Painful stomatitis is an early and conspicuous symptom. Hemorrhagic bullae may appear over the lips, mouth and genital mucous membranes. Patients are often acutely ill with high fever. The course from eruption to the healing of the lesions may extend up to 6 weeks.

The following drugs have been most often associated with erythema multiforme and Stevens-Johnson syndrome: allopurinol, anticonvulsants (phenytoin), barbiturates, carbamazepine, estrogens/progestins, gold, NSAIDs, penicillamine, sulfonamides, tetracycline, and tolbutamide.

Erythema nodosum

Erythema nodosum is a cutaneous reaction pattern characterized by erythematous, tender or painful subcutaneous nodules commonly distributed over the anterior aspect of the lower legs, and occasionally elsewhere.

More common in young women, erythema nodosum is often associated with increased estrogen levels as occurs during pregnancy and with the ingestion of oral contraceptives. It is also an occasional manifestation of streptococcal infection, sarcoidosis, secondary syphilis, tuberculosis, certain deep fungal infections, Hodgkin's disease, leukemia, ulcerative colitis, and radiation therapy and is often preceded by fever, fatigue, arthralgia, vomiting, and diarrhea.

The incidence of erythema nodosum due to drugs is low and it is impossible to distinguish clinically between erythema nodosum due to drugs and that caused by other factors.

Some of the drugs that are known to occasion erythema nodosum are: antibiotics, estrogens, amiodarone, gold, NSAIDs, oral contraceptives, sulfonamides, and opiates.

Exanthems

Exanthems, commonly resembling viral rashes, represent the most common type of cutaneous drug eruption. Described as maculopapular or morbilliform eruptions, these flat, barely raised, erythematous patches, from one to several millimeters in diameter, are usually bilateral and symmetrical. They commonly begin on the head and neck or upper torso and progress downward to the limbs. They may present or develop into confluent areas and may be accompanied by pruritus and a mild fever.

The exanthems caused by drugs can be classified as either:

- Morbilliform eruptions: fingernail-sized erythematous patches.
- Scarlatiniform eruptions: punctate, pinpoint, or pinhead-sized lesions in erythematous areas that have a tendency to coalesce. Circumoral pallor and the subsequent appearance of scaling may also be noted.

Maculopapular drug eruptions usually fade with desquamation and, occasionally, post-inflammatory hyperpigmentation, in about 2 weeks. They invariably recur on rechallenge.

Exanthems often have a sudden onset during the first 2 weeks of administration, except for semisynthetic penicillins that frequently develop after the first 2 weeks following the initial dose.

The drugs most commonly associated with exanthems are: amoxicillin, ampicillin, bleomycin, captopril, carbamazepine, chlorpromazine, cotrimoxazole, gold, nalidixic acid, naproxen, phenytoin, penicillamine, and piroxicam.

Exfoliative dermatitis

Exfoliative dermatitis is a rare but serious reaction pattern that is characterized by erythema, pruritus and scaling over the entire body (erythroderma).

Drug-induced exfoliative dermatitis usually begins a few weeks or longer following the administration of a culpable drug. Beginning as erythematous, edematous patches, often on the face, it spreads to involve the entire integument. The skin becomes swollen and scarlet and may ooze a straw-colored fluid; this is followed in a few days by desquamation.

High fever, severe malaise and chills, along with enlargement of lymph nodes, often coexist with the cutaneous changes.

One of the most dangerous of all reaction patterns, exfoliative dermatitis can be accompanied by any or all of the following: hypothermia, fluid and electrolyte loss, cardiac failure, and gastrointestinal hemorrhage. Death may supervene if the drug is continued after the onset of the eruption. Secondary infection often complicates the course of the disease. Once the active dermatitis has receded, hyperpigmentation as well as loss of hair and nails may ensue. The following drugs, among others, can bring about exfoliative dermatitis: barbiturates, captopril, carbamazepine, cimetidine, furosemide, gold, isoniazid, lithium, nitrofurantoin, NSAIDs, penicillamine, phenytoin, pyrazolons, quinidine, streptomycin, sulfonamides, and thiazides.

Fixed eruptions

A fixed eruption is an unusual hypersensitivity reaction characterized by one or more well-demarcated erythematous plaques that recur at the same cutaneous (or mucosal) site or sites each time exposure to the offending agent occurs. The sizes of the lesions vary from a few millimeters to as much as 20 centimeters in diameter. Almost any drug that is ingested, injected, inhaled, or inserted into the body can trigger this skin reaction.

The eruption typically begins as a sharply marginated, solitary edematous papule or plaque – occasionally surmounted by a large bulla – which usually develops 30 minutes to 8 hours following the administration of a drug. If the offending agent is not promptly eliminated, the inflammation intensifies, producing a dusky red, violaceous or brown patch that may crust, desquamate, or blister within 7 to 10 days. The lesions are rarely pruritic. Favored sites are the hands, feet, face, and genitalia – especially the glans penis.

The reason for the specific localization of the skin lesions in a fixed drug eruption is unknown. The offending drug cannot be detected at the skin site. Certain drugs cause a fixed eruption at specific sites, for example, tetracycline and ampicillin often elicit a fixed eruption on the penis, whereas aspirin usually causes skin lesions on the face, limbs and trunk.

Common causes of fixed eruptions are: ampicillin, aspirin, barbiturates, dapsone, metronidazole, NSAIDs, oral contraceptives, phenolphthalein, phenytoin, quinine, sulfonamides, and tetracyclines.

Gingival hyperplasia

Gingival hyperplasia, a common, undesirable, non-allergic drug reaction begins as a diffuse swelling of the interdental papillae.

Particularly prevalent with phenytoin therapy, gingival hyperplasia begins about 3 months after the onset of therapy, and occurs in 30 to 70 percent of patients receiving it. The severity of the reaction is dose-dependent and children and young adults are more frequently affected. The most severe cases are noted in young women.

In many cases, gingival hyperplasia is accompanied by painful and bleeding gums. There is often superimposed secondary bacterial gingivitis. This can be so extensive that the teeth of the maxilla and mandible are completely overgrown.

While it is characteristically a side effect of hydantoin derivatives, it may occur during the administration of phenobarbital, nifedipine, diltiazem and other medications.

Lichenoid (lichen planus-like) eruptions

Lichenoid eruptions are so called because of their resemblance to lichen planus, a papulosquamous disorder that characteristically presents as multiple, discrete, violaceous, flat-topped papules, often polygonal in shape and which are extremely pruritic.

Not infrequently, lichenoid lesions appear weeks or months following exposure to the responsible drug. As a rule, the symptoms begin to recede a few weeks following the discontinuation of the drug.

Common drug causes of lichenoid eruptions are: antimalarials, beta-blockers, chlorpropamide, furosemide, gold, methyldopa, phenothiazines, quinidine, thiazides, and tolazamide.

Lupus erythematosus

A reaction, clinically and pathologically resembling idiopathic systemic lupus erythematosus (SLE), has been reported in association with a large variety of drugs. There is some evidence that drug-induced SLE, invariably accompanied by a positive ANA reaction with 90 percent having antihistone antibodies, may have a genetically determined basis. These symptoms of SLE, a relatively benign form of lupus, recede within days or weeks following the discontinuation of the responsible drug. Skin lesions occur in about 20 percent of cases. Drugs cause fewer than 8 percent of all cases of systemic LE.

The following drugs have been commonly associated with inducing, aggravating or unmasking SLE: beta-blockers, carbamazepine, chlorpromazine, estrogens, griseofulvin, hydralazine, isoniazid (INH), lithium, methyldopa, minoxidil, oral contraceptives, penicillamine, phenytoin (diphenylhydantoin), procainamide, propylthiouracil, quinidine, and testosterone.

Onycholysis

Onycholysis, the painless separation of the nail plate from the nail bed, is one of the most common nail disorders.

The unattached portion, which is white and opaque, usually begins at the free margin and proceeds proximally, causing part or most of the nail plate to become separated. The attached, healthy portion of the nail, by contrast, is pink and translucent.

Pemphigus vulgaris

Pemphigus vulgaris (PV) is a rare, serious, acute or chronic, blistering disease involving the skin and mucous membranes.

Characterized by thin-walled, easily-ruptured, flaccid bullae that are seen to arise on normal or erythematous skin and over mucous membranes, the lesions of PV appear initially in the mouth (in about 60 percent of the cases) and then spread, after weeks or months, to involve the axillae and groins, the scalp, face and neck. The lesions may become generalized.

Because of their fragile roofs, the bullae rupture leaving painful erosions and crusts may develop principally over the scalp.

Photosensitivity

A photosensitive reaction is a chemically induced change in the skin that makes an individual unusually sensitive to electromagnetic radiation (light). On absorbing light of a specific wavelength, an oral, injected or topical drug may be chemically altered to produce a reaction ranging from macules and papules, vesicles and bullae, edema, urticaria, or an acute eczematous reaction.

Any eruption that is prominent on the face, the dorsa of the hands, the "V" of the neck, and the presternal area should suggest an adverse reaction to light. The distribution is the key to the diagnosis.

Initially the eruption, which consists of erythema, edema, blisters, weeping and desquamation, involves the forehead, rims of the ears, the nose, the malar eminences and cheeks, the sides and back of the neck, the extensor surfaces of the forearms and the dorsa of the hands. These reactions commonly spare the shaded areas: those under the chin, under the nose, behind the ears and inside the fold of the upper eyelids. There is usually a sharp cut-off at the site of jewelry and at clothing margins. All light-exposed areas need not be affected equally.

There are two main types of photosensitive reactions: the phototoxic and the photoallergic reaction.

Phototoxic reactions, the most common type of drug-induced photosensitivity, resemble an exaggerated sunburn and occur within 5 to 20 hours after the skin has been exposed to a photosensitizing substance and light of the proper wavelength and intensity. It is not a form of allergy – prior sensitization is not required – and, theoretically, could occur in anyone given enough drug and light. Phototoxic reactions are dose-dependent both for drug and sunlight. Patients with phototoxicity reactions are commonly sensitive to ultraviolet A (UVA radiation), the so-called "tanning rays" at 320–400 nm. Phototoxic reactions may cause onycholysis, as the nailbed is particularly susceptible because of its lack of melanin protection.

Patients with a true photoallergy (the interaction of drug, light and the immune system), a less common form of drug-induced photosensitivity, are often sensitive to UVB radiation, the so-called "burning rays" at 290–320 nm. Photoallergic reactions, unlike phototoxic responses, represent an immunologic change and require a latent period of from 24 to 48 hours during which sensitization occurs. They are not dose-related.

If the photosensitizer acts internally, it is a photodrug reaction; if it acts externally, it is photocontact dermatitis.

Drugs that are likely to cause phototoxic reactions are: amiodarone, nalidixic acid, various NSAIDs, phenothiazines (especially chlorpromazine), and tetracyclines (particularly demeclocycline).

Photoallergic reactions may occur as a result of exposure to systemically-administered drugs such as griseofulvin, NSAIDs, phenothiazines, quinidine, sulfonamides, sulfonylureas, and thiazide diuretics as well as to external agents such as para-aminobenzoic acid (found in sunscreens), bithionol (used in soaps and cosmetics), paraphenylenediamine, and others.

Pigmentation

Drug-induced pigmentation on the skin, hair, nails, and mucous membranes is a result of either melanin synthesis, increased lipofuscin synthesis, or post-inflammatory pigmentation.

Color changes, which can be localized or widespread, can also be a result of a deposition of bile pigments (jaundice), exogenous metal compounds, and direct deposition of elements such as carotene or quinacrine.

Post-inflammatory pigmentation can follow a variety of drug-induced inflammatory cutaneous reactions; fixed eruptions are known to leave a residual pigmentation that can persist for months.

The following is a partial list of those drugs that can cause various pigmentary changes: anticonvulsants, antimalarials, cytostatics, hormones, metals, tetracyclines, phenothiazine tranquilizers, psoralens, amiodarone, etc.

Pityriasis rosea-like eruptions

Pityriasis rosea, commonly mistaken for ringworm, is a unique disorder that usually begins as a single, large, round or oval pinkish patch known as the "mother" or "herald" patch. The most common sites for this solitary lesion are the chest, the back, or the abdomen. This is followed in about 2 weeks by a blossoming of small, flat, round or oval, scaly patches of similar color, each with a central collarette scale, usually distributed in a Christmas tree pattern over the trunk and, to a lesser degree, the extremities. This eruption seldom itches and usually limits itself to areas from the neck to the knees.

While the etiology of idiopathic pityriasis rosea is unknown, we do know that various medications have been reported to give rise to this friendly disorder. These are: barbiturates, beta-blockers, bismuth, captopril, clonidine, gold, griseofulvin, isotretinoin, labetalol, meprobamate, metronidazole, penicillin, and tripelennamine.

In drug-induced pityriasis rosea, the "herald patch" is usually absent, and the eruption will often not follow the classic pattern.

Pruritus

Generalized itching, without any visible signs, is one of the least common adverse reactions to drugs. More frequently than not, drug-induced itching – moderate or severe – is fairly generalized.

For most drugs it is not known in what way they elicit pruritus; some drugs can cause itching directly or indirectly through cholestasis. Pruritus may develop by different pathogenetic mechanisms: allergic, pseudoallergic (histamine release), neurogenic, by vasodilatation, cholestatic effect, and others.

A partial list of those drugs that can cause pruritus are as follows: aspirin, NSAIDs, penicillins, sulfonamides, chloroquine, ACE-inhibitors, amiodarone, nicotinic acid derivatives, lithium, bleomycin, tamoxifen, interferons, gold, penicillamine, methoxsalen, isotretinoin, etc.

Psoriasis

Many drugs, as a result of their pharmacological action, have been implicated in the precipitation or exacerbation of psoriasis or psoriasiform eruptions.

Psoriasis is a common, chronic, papulosquamous disorder of unknown etiology with characteristic histopathological features and many biochemical, physiological, and immunological abnormalities.

Drugs that can precipitate psoriasis are, among others, beta-blockers and lithium. Drugs that are reported to aggravate psoriasis are antimalarials, beta-blockers, lithium, NSAIDs, quinidine, and photosensitizing drugs. The effect and extent of these drug-induced psoriatic eruptions are dose dependent.

Purpura

Purpura, a result of hemorrhage into the skin, can be divided into thrombocytopenic purpura and non-thrombocytopenic purpura (vascular purpura). Both thrombocytopenic and vascular purpura may be due to drugs, and most of the drugs producing purpura may do so by giving rise to vascular damage and thrombocytopenia. In both types of purpura, allergic or toxic (nonallergic) mechanisms may be involved.

Some drugs combine with platelets to form an antigen, stimulating formation of antibody to the platelet–drug combination. Thus the drug appears to act as a hapten; subsequent antigen–antibody reaction causes platelet destruction leading to thrombocytopenia.

The purpuric lesions are usually more marked over the lower portions of the body, notably the legs and dorsal aspects of the feet in ambulatory patients.

Other drug-induced cutaneous reactions – erythema multiforme, erythema nodosum, fixed eruption, necrotizing vasculitis, and others – can have a prominent purpuric component.

A whole host of drugs can give rise to purpura, the most common being: NSAIDs, thiazide diuretics, phenothiazines, cytostatics, gold, penicillamine, hydantoins, thiouracils, and sulfonamides.

Raynaud's phenomenon

Raynaud's phenomenon is the paroxysmal, cold-induced constriction of small arteries and arterioles of the fingers and, less often, the toes.

Occurring more frequently in women, Raynaud's phenomenon is characterized by blanching, pallor, and cyanosis. In severe cases, secondary changes may occur: thinning and ridging of the nails, telangiectases of the nail folds, and, in the later stages, sclerosis and atrophy of the digits.

Toxic epidermal necrolysis (TEN)

Also known as Lyell's syndrome and the scalded skin syndrome, toxic epidermal necrolysis is a rare, serious, acute exfoliative, bullous eruption of the skin and mucous membranes that usually develops as a reaction to diverse drugs. TEN can also be a result of a bacterial or viral infection and can develop after radiation therapy or vaccinations.

In the drug-induced form of TEN, a morbilliform eruption accompanied by large red, tender areas of the skin will develop shortly after the drug had been administered. This progresses rapidly to blistering, and a widespread exfoliation of the epidermis develops dramatically over a very short period accompanied by high fever. The hairy parts of the body are usually spared. The mucous membranes and eyes are often involved.

The clinical picture resembles an extensive second-degree burn; the patient is acutely ill. Fatigue, vomiting, diarrhea and angina are prodromal symptoms. In a few hours the condition becomes grave.

TEN is a medical emergency and unless the offending agent is discontinued immediately, the outcome may be fatal in the course of a few days.

Drugs that are the most common cause of TEN are: allopurinol, ampicillin, amoxicillin, carbamazepine, NSAIDs, phenobarbital, pentamidine, phenytoin (diphenylhydantoin), pyrazolons, and sulfonamides.

Urticaria

Urticaria induced by drugs is, after exanthems, the second most common type of drug reaction. Urticaria, or hives, is a vascular reaction of the skin characterized by pruritic, erythematous wheals. These welts – or wheals – caused by localized edema, can vary in size from one millimeter in diameter to large palm-sized swellings, favor the covered areas (trunk, buttocks, chest), and are, more often than not, generalized. Urticaria usually develops within 36 hours following the administration of the responsible drug. Individual lesions rarely persist for more than 24 hours.

Urticaria may be the only symptom of drug sensitivity, or it may be a concomitant or followed by the manifestations of serum sickness. Urticaria may be accompanied by angioedema of the lips or eyelids. It may, on rare occasions, progress to anaphylactoid reactions or to anaphylaxis.

The following are the most common causes of drug-induced urticaria: antibiotics, notably penicillin (more commonly following parenteral administration than by ingestion), barbiturates, captopril, levamisole, NSAIDs, quinine, rifampin, sulfonamides, thiopental, and vancomycin.

Vasculitis

Drug-induced cutaneous necrotizing vasculitis, a clinicopathologic process characterized by inflammation and necrosis of blood vessels, often presents with a variety of small, palpable purpuric lesions most frequently distributed over the lower extremities: urticaria-like lesions, small ulcerations, and occasional hemorrhagic vesicles and pustules. The basic process involves an immunologically mediated response to antigens that result in vessel-wall damage.

Beginning as small macules and papules, they ultimately eventuate into purpuric lesions and, in the more severe cases, into hemorrhagic blisters and frank ulcerations. A polymorphonuclear infiltrate and fibrinoid changes in the small dermal vessels characterize the vasculitic reaction.

Drugs that are commonly associated with vasculitis are: ACE-inhibitors, amiodarone, ampicillin, cimetidine, coumadin, furosemide, hydantoins, hydralazine, NSAIDs, pyrazolons, quinidine, sulfonamides, thiazides, and thiouracils.

Xerostomia

Xerostomia is a dryness of the oral cavity that makes speaking, chewing and swallowing difficult.

Resulting from a partial or complete absence of saliva production, xerostomia can be causedby a variety of medications.

DRUGS RESPONSIBLE FOR 80 REACTION PATTERNS

Acanthosis nigricans
- Azathioprine
- Corticosteroids
- Cortisone
- Diethylstilbestrol
- Gemfibrozil
- Heroin
- Lithium
- Mechlorethamine
- Methsuximide
- Methyltestosterone
- Niacin; niacinamide
- Oral contraceptives
- Thioridazine

Acne
- Acyclovir
- Alprazolam
- Amitriptyline
- Amoxapine
- Atorvastatin
- Azathioprine
- Betaxolol
- Bisoprolol
- Buspirone
- Cabergoline
- Carteolol
- Cefamandole
- Cefpodoxime
- Ceftazidime
- Cetirizine
- Chloral hydrate
- Ciprofloxacin
- Clofazimine
- Clomiphene
- Clomipramine
- Corticosteroids
- Cortisone
- Cyanocobalamin
- Cyclosporine
- Dactinomycin
- Danazol
- Dantrolene
- Deferoxamine
- Demeclocycline
- Desipramine
- Diazepam
- Diltiazem
- Disulfiram
- Erythromycin
- Estazolam
- Ethionamide
- Famotidine
- Felbamate
- Fenoprofen
- Fexofenadine
- Fluconazole
- Fluoxetine
- Fluoxymesterone
- Fluvoxamine
- Folic acid
- Foscarnet
- Gabapentin
- Ganciclovir
- Gold
- GCSF
- Grepafloxacin
- Haloperidol
- Halothane
- Heroin
- Interferons
- Isoniazid
- Isosorbide
- Isotretinoin
- Lamotrigine
- Lansoprazole
- Levothyroxine
- Lithium
- Maprotiline
- Medroxyprogesterone
- Mephenytoin
- Mesalamine
- Methotrexate
- Methoxsalen
- Methyltestosterone
- Minoxidil
- Nabumetone
- Nafarelin
- Naratriptan
- Nefazodone
- Nimodipine
- Nisoldipine
- Nizatidine
- Olsalazine
- Oral contraceptives
- Paramethadione
- Paroxetine
- Pentostatin
- Pergolide
- Phenobarbital
- Phenytoin
- Potassium iodide
- Primidone
- Propafenone
- Propranolol
- Psoralens
- Pyrazinamide
- Pyridoxine
- Quinidine
- Quinine
- Ramipril
- Riboflavin
- Rifampin
- Risperidone
- Ritonavir
- Saquinavir
- Sertraline
- Sibutramine
- Sparfloxacin
- Stanozolol
- Tacrine
- Testosterone
- Tetracycline
- Tiagabine
- Tizanidine
- Topiramate
- Trimethadione
- Trioxsalen
- Trovafloxacin
- Valproic acid
- Venlafaxine
- Verapamil
- Vinblastine
- Zalcitabine
- Zidovudine
- Zolpidem

Acral erythema
- Bleomycin
- Cyclophosphamide
- Cytarabine
- Didanosine
- Fluorouracil
- Hydroxyurea
- Idarubicin
- Lomustine
- Mercaptopurine

Acute febrile neutrophilic dermatosis
- Clofazimine
- Cotrimoxazole
- Cytarabine
- Furosemide
- Glucagon
- GCSF
- Hydralazine
- Minocycline
- Sulfamethoxazole

Verapamil

Acute generalized exanthematous pustulosis

Acetaminophen
Acetazolamide
Allopurinol
Amoxapine
Amoxicillin
Ampicillin
Aspirin
Carbamazepine
Cefaclor
Cefazolin
Cefuroxime
Cephalexin
Cephradine
Chloramphenicol
Chloroquine
Codeine
Cotrimoxazole
Diltiazem
Doxycycline
Erythromycin
Furosemide
Hydroxychloroquine
Imipenem/cilastatin
Isoniazid
Itraconazole
Metronidazole
Nifedipine
Nystatin
Penicillins
Phenytoin
Pyrimethamine
Quinidine
Ranitidine
Streptomycin
Sulfamethoxazole
Sulfasalazine
Terbinafine
Vancomycin

Ageusia

Acetazolamide
Amitriptyline
Atorvastatin
Azelastine
Betaxolol
Captopril
Cetirizine
Cisplatin
Clidinium
Clomipramine
Cocaine
Cyclobenzaprine
Diazoxide
Dicyclomine
Enalapril
Fluoxetine
Fluvoxamine
Fosinopril
Grepafloxacin
Indomethacin
Isotretinoin
Levodopa
Losartan
Methantheline
Methimazole
Nefazodone
Paroxetine
Penicillamine
Pentamidine
Propantheline
Propylthiouracil
Ramipril
Rifabutin
Rimantadine
Ritonavir
Spironolactone
Sulfadoxine
Sulindac
Terbinafine
Tiagabine
Topiramate
Venlafaxine
Zalcitabine

Anaphylactoid reaction

Acetaminophen
Acyclovir
Alteplase
Amiloride
Aminoglutethimide
Amitriptyline
Amoxicillin
Amphotericin B
Ampicillin
Asparaginase
Aspartame
Aspirin
Atenolol
Azathioprine
Azithromycin
Aztreonam
Bendroflumethiazide
Betaxolol
Bisoprolol
Bleomycin
Bromfenac
Bromocriptine
Butalbital
Calcitonin
Captopril
Carbenicillin
Carisoprodol
Carteolol
Cefaclor
Cefadroxil
Cefamandole
Cefazolin
Cefdinir
Cefixime
Cefotaxime
Cefoxitin
Cefpodoxime
Ceftazidime
Ceftriaxone
Cefuroxime
Cephalexin
Cephalothin
Cephradine
Cerivastatin
Cetirizine
Chloramphenicol
Chlorothiazide
Chlorpromazine
Chlorzoxazone
Cimetidine
Ciprofloxacin
Cisplatin
Clarithromycin
Clemastine
Clidinium
Clindamycin
Cloxacillin
Codeine
Colchicine
Corticosteroids
Cortisone
Cotrimoxazole
Cromolyn
Cyanocobalamin
Cyclobenzaprine
Cyclophosphamide
Cyclosporine
Cyproheptadine
Cytarabine
Dacarbazine
Dactinomycin
Dalteparin
Dantrolene
Daunorubicin
Deferoxamine
Demeclocycline
Diazepam
Diclofenac
Dicloxacillin
Dicyclomine
Didanosine
Diflunisal
Diphenhydramine
Diphenoxylate
Dipyridamole
Dirithromycin
Dolasetron
Doxorubicin
Doxycycline
Enalapril
Epoetin alfa
Erythromycin
Ethambutol
Ethanolamine
Etoposide
Felbamate
Fenoprofen

Fentanyl
Fluconazole
Flucytosine
Fluorouracil
Fluoxetine
Fluoxymesterone
Fluphenazine
Flurbiprofen
Fluvastatin
Fluvoxamine
Folic acid
Fosinopril
Furosemide
Ganciclovir
Gemcitabine
Gemfibrozil
Gentamicin
Granisetron
GCSF
Griseofulvin
Heparin
Ibuprofen
Ifosfamide
Indapamide
Indomethacin
Insulin
Ipodate
Ipratropium
Itraconazole
Ketoconazole
Ketoprofen
Ketorolac
Labetalol
Levamisole
Levofloxacin
Lidocaine
Lincomycin
Lisinopril
Loratadine
Marihuana
Mechlorethamine
Medroxyprogesterone
Mefenamic acid
Melphalan
Meprobamate
Mesoridazine
Metaxalone
Methantheline
Methicillin
Methocarbamol
Methohexital
Methotrexate
Methyclothiazide
Methyltestosterone
Metolazone
Mezlocillin
Midazolam
Minocycline
Misoprostol
Moexipril
Nabumetone
Nafcillin
Nalidixic acid
Naproxen
Neomycin
Niacin; niacinamide
Nitrofurantoin
Norfloxacin
Octreotide
Ofloxacin
Ondansetron
Orphenadrine
Oxacillin
Oxaprozin
Oxytetracycline
Penicillins
Pentostatin
Perphenazine
Phenazopyridine
Phytonadione
Piperacillin
Piroxicam
Pravastatin
Prazosin
Probenecid
Prochlorperazine
Progestins
Promethazine
Propantheline
Propofol
Propranolol
Protamine
Pyrilamine
Ramipril
Ranitidine
Repaglinide
Rifampin
Risperidone
Ritonavir
Ritordine
Salsalate
Scopolamine
Simvastatin
Sparfloxacin
Spectinomycin
Spironolactone
Streptokinase
Streptomycin
Succinylcholine
Sulfadoxine
Sulfamethoxazole
Sulfasalazine
Sulfisoxazole
Sulindac
Sumatriptan
Temazepam
Terazosin
Terbinafine
Terfenadine
Testosterone
Tetracycline
Thiabendazole
Thiamine
Thiopental
Thioridazine
Thiotepa
Thiothixene
Ticarcillin
Timolol
Tolmetin
Triamterene
Trichlormethiazide
Trifluoperazine
Trimeprazine
Tripelennamine
Troleandomycin
Trovafloxacin
Urokinase
Vancomycin
Vasopressin
Vincristine
Vitamin A
Zalcitabine
Zolpidem

Angioedema

Acetaminophen
Aldesleukin
Allopurinol
Alteplase
Aminoglutethimide
Aminosalicylate sodium
Amitriptyline
Amobarbital
Amoxicillin
Ampicillin
Aprobarbital
Ascorbic acid
Asparaginase
Aspartame
Aspirin
Astemizole
Azatadine
Azathioprine
Azithromycin
Aztreonam
Benactyzine
Benazepril
Betaxolol
Bisoprolol
Bleomycin
Brompheniramine
Butabarbital
Captopril
Carbamazepine
Carbenicillin
Carisoprodol
Carteolol
Carvedilol
Cefaclor
Cefadroxil
Cefoxitin
Ceftazidime
Ceftriaxone

Risperidone
Ritonavir
Salmeterol
Salsalate
Secobarbital
Sertraline
Simvastatin
Sparfloxacin
Streptokinase
Streptomycin
Sucralfate
Sulfamethoxazole
Sulfasalazine
Sulfisoxazole
Sulindac
Sumatriptan
Terbinafine
Terfenadine
Tetracycline
Thiabendazole
Thiamine
Thiopental
Thioridazine
Thiotepa
Ticarcillin
Ticlopidine
Timolol
Tiopronin
Tolmetin
Torsemide
Tramadol
Trandolapril
Trifluoperazine
Trimeprazine
Trimetrexate
Tripelennamine
Triprolidine
Troleandomycin
Trovafloxacin
Urokinase
Valsartan
Vancomycin
Vasopressin
Verapamil
Vincristine
Warfarin
Zalcitabine

Anosmia

Acetazolamide
Ciprofloxacin
Cocaine
Cromolyn
Doxycycline
Enalapril
Ganciclovir
Interferons
Minoxidil
Paroxetine
Pentamidine
Sparfloxacin
Terbinafine

Aphthous stomatitis

Aldesleukin
Asparaginase
Aspirin
Azathioprine
Azelastine
Captopril
Cotrimoxazole
Cyclosporine
Delavirdine
Diclofenac
Diflunisal
Doxepin
Fenoprofen
Fluoxetine
Flurbiprofen
Gold
Ibuprofen
Indinavir
Indomethacin
Ketoprofen
Ketorolac
Meclofenamate
Naproxen
Olanzapine
Paroxetine
Penicillamine
Piroxicam
Sertraline
Sulfamethoxazole
Sulfasalazine
Sulfisoxazole
Sulindac
Terbinafine
Tolmetin
Trientine
Zalcitabine

Black hairy tongue

Amoxicillin
Ampicillin
Chloramphenicol
Corticosteroids
Cortisone
Cotrimoxazole
Isocarboxazid
Minocycline
Nortriptyline
Oxytetracycline
Penicillins
Protriptyline
Streptomycin
Sulfamethoxazole
Tetracycline

Black tongue

Amitriptyline
Amoxapine
Carbenicillin
Clarithromycin
Clomipramine
Cloxacillin
Desipramine
Dicloxacillin
Griseofulvin
Imipramine
Lansoprazole
Maprotiline
Methicillin
Methyldopa
Mezlocillin
Minocycline
Nafcillin
Oxacillin
Phenelzine
Ticarcillin
Tranylcypromine

Bullous eruption

Acetazolamide
Acitretin
Aldesleukin
Aminocaproic acid
Aminosalicylate sodium
Amitriptyline
Ampicillin
Aspirin
Atropine sulfate
Benactyzine
Bleomycin
Bumetanide
Buspirone
Busulfan
Butabarbital
Butalbital
Captopril
Carbamazepine
Cetirizine
Chloral hydrate
Chloramphenicol
Chlorothiazide
Chlorpromazine
Chlorpropamide
Ciprofloxacin
Clopidogrel
Cocaine
Codeine
Colchicine
Cotrimoxazole
Cyanocobalamin
Cyclamate
Cyclosporine
Cytarabine
Dalteparin
Dapsone
Demeclocycline
Dexfenfluramine
Dextromethorphan
Diazepam
Diclofenac
Dicumarol
Diethylstilbestrol
Diflunisal
Digoxin
Dirithromycin

Disulfiram
Ephedrine
Ethambutol
Ethchlorvynol
Ethotoin
Felbamate
Fluconazole
Fluorouracil
Fluoxetine
Flutamide
Fluvoxamine
Furosemide
Ganciclovir
Glyburide
Gold
Griseofulvin
Hydralazine
Hydrochlorothiazide
Hydroxychloroquine
Ibuprofen
Idarubicin
Imipramine
Indapamide
Indomethacin
Insulin
Interferons
Isoniazid
Ketoprofen
Lidocaine
Lisinopril
Lithium
Mechlorethamine
Mephenytoin
Meprobamate
Methicillin
Methotrexate
Methoxsalen
Miconazole
Minoxidil
Mitomycin
Nabumetone
Nalidixic acid
Naproxen
Neomycin
Nifedipine
Nitrofurantoin
Norfloxacin
Ofloxacin
Omeprazole
Oral contraceptives
Oxacillin
Penicillamine
Pentamidine
Pentobarbital
Pentostatin
Phenobarbital
Phenolphthalein
Phenytoin
Promethazine
Propranolol
Pyridoxine
Pyrimethamine
Quinapril
Quinethazone
Quinidine
Quinine
Reserpine
Rifampin
Risperidone
Ritonavir
Sertraline
Sparfloxacin
Streptomycin
Sulfadoxine
Sulfamethoxazole
Sulfasalazine
Sulfisoxazole
Tacrine
Tetracycline
Thalidomide
Thiopental
Tolbutamide
Trimethadione
Trioxsalen
Urokinase
Vancomycin
Vasopressin
Vinblastine
Warfarin
Zalcitabine
Zidovudine
Zolpidem

Bullous pemphigoid

Aldesleukin
Amoxicillin
Ampicillin
Bumetanide
Captopril
Dactinomycin
Enalapril
Fosinopril
Furosemide
Gold
Ibuprofen
Mefenamic acid
Methoxsalen
Nadolol
Omeprazole
Penicillamine
Penicillins
Potassium iodide
Psoralens
Risperidone
Sulfasalazine
Tiopronin
Tolbutamide

Cheilitis

Acitretin
Atorvastatin
Busulfan
Clofazimine
Clomipramine
Cyanocobalamin
Dactinomycin
Gold
Grepafloxacin
Indinavir
Isotretinoin
Methoxsalen
Methyldopa
Psoralens
Ritonavir
Saquinavir
Streptomycin
Sulfasalazine
Tetracycline
Trovafloxacin
Vitamin A

Contact dermatitis

Acetaminophen
Acyclovir
Albendazole
Albuterol
Amantadine
Aminocaproic acid
Aminophylline
Amoxicillin
Ampicillin
Apraclonidine
Atorvastatin
Atropine sulfate
Azathioprine
Azelastine
Bendroflumethiazide
Betaxolol
Biperiden
Bumetanide
Captopril
Carbamazepine
Carmustine
Cephalexin
Chloramphenicol
Chloroquine
Chlorpromazine
Chlorpropamide
Cisplatin
Clindamycin
Clomipramine
Clonidine
Cloxacillin
Codeine
Corticosteroids
Cromolyn
Cyanocobalamin
Cyclophosphamide
Cyproheptadine
Daunorubicin
Diazepam
Diclofenac
Diphenhydramine
Disulfiram
Doxepin
Doxorubicin

Ephedrine
Epinephrine
Epoetin alfa
Erythromycin
Ethambutol
Ethanolamine
Famotidine
Fluorouracil
Fluoxetine
Fluoxymesterone
Furazolidone
Gentamicin
Gold
Haloperidol
Heparin
Heroin
Ibuprofen
Indinavir
Indomethacin
Insulin
Interferons
Ipratropium
Isoniazid
Isosorbide
Ketoconazole
Ketoprofen
Labetalol
Levobunolol
Lidocaine
Lincomycin
Mechlorethamine
Mesoridazine
Methoxsalen
Methyltestosterone
Metronidazole
Mezlocillin
Miconazole
Minoxidil
Mitomycin
Neomycin
Niacin; niacinamide
Nitrofurantoin
Nitroglycerin
Nizatidine
Nystatin
Olanzapine
Oxytetracycline
Paroxetine
Penicillamine
Penicillins
Pentostatin
Perphenazine
Phytonadione
Piroxicam
Promethazine
Propantheline
Propranolol
Psoralens
Pyridoxine
Quinidine
Quinine
Ranitidine
Rifampin
Ritonavir
Scopolamine
Sildenafil
Sparfloxacin
Spectinomycin
Spironolactone
Streptomycin
Succinylcholine
Terbutaline
Testosterone
Thiabendazole
Thiamine
Tiagabine
Timolol
Tiopronin
Tobramycin
Tolazoline
Tolbutamide
Valproic acid
Venlafaxine
Vitamin A
Vitamin E

Dermatitis herpetiformis

Amitriptyline
Aspirin
Cyclophosphamide
Diclofenac
Doxorubicin
Flurbiprofen
Ibuprofen
Indomethacin
Interferons
Levothyroxine
Lithium
Oral contraceptives
Potassium iodide
Vincristine

Dysgeusia

Acetaminophen
Acetazolamide
Acyclovir
Albuterol
Aldesleukin
Alendronate
Alprazolam
Amiloride
Amiodarone
Amitriptyline
Amlodipine
Amoxapine
Amoxicillin
Apraclonidine
Aspirin
Astemizole
Atorvastatin
Atovaquone
Azelastine
Aztreonam
Benazepril
Benzthiazide
Betaxolol
Bisoprolol
Bromfenac
Buspirone
Busulfan
Butorphanol
Calcitonin
Captopril
Carbamazepine
Carbenicillin
Carbidopa
Carteolol
Cefaclor
Cefamandole
Cefpodoxime
Ceftazidime
Ceftibuten
Ceftriaxone
Cerivastatin
Cetirizine
Chloral hydrate
Chlormezanone
Chlorothiazide
Cholestyramine
Ciprofloxacin
Clarithromycin
Clidinium
Clindamycin
Clofazimine
Clofibrate
Clomipramine
Clonidine
Clozapine
Codeine
Cotrimoxazole
Cromolyn
Cyclobenzaprine
Cyproheptadine
Dacarbazine
Dantrolene
Delavirdine
Desipramine
Dexfenfluramine
Dextroamphetamine
Diazoxide
Diclofenac
Dicloxacillin
Diethylpropion
Diltiazem
Dipyridamole
Dirithromycin
Disulfiram
Divalproex
Docusate
Dolasetron
Donepezil
Doxazosin
Doxepin
Doxycycline
Enalapril

Ergocalciferol
Esmolol
Estazolam
Ethchlorvynol
Ethionamide
Etidronate
Etoposide
Famotidine
Felbamate
Fenfluramine
Fenoprofen
Fentanyl
Flecainide
Fluconazole
Fluorouracil
Fluoxetine
Flurazepam
Flurbiprofen
Fluvastatin
Fluvoxamine
Foscarnet
Fosinopril
Ganciclovir
Gemfibrozil
Gold
Granisetron
Grepafloxacin
Griseofulvin
Guanabenz
Guanfacine
Hydroflumethiazide
Hydromorphone
Hydroxychloroquine
Imipenem/cilastatin
Imipramine
Indinavir
Interferons
Ipratropium
Isotretinoin
Ketoprofen
Ketorolac
Labetalol
Lamotrigine
Lansoprazole
Leuprolide
Levamisole
Levodopa
Levofloxacin
Lisinopril
Lithium
Lomefloxacin
Loratadine
Losartan
Lovastatin
Maprotiline
Mazindol
Mechlorethamine
Meclofenamate
Mesalamine
Mesna
Metformin
Methamphetamine
Methantheline
Methazolamide
Methicillin
Methimazole
Methocarbamol
Methotrexate
Methyclothiazide
Metolazone
Metoprolol
Metronidazole
Mexiletine
Mezlocillin
Midazolam
Minoxidil
Moexipril
Moricizine
Nadolol
Nafcillin
Naratriptan
Nefazodone
Nifedipine
Nisoldipine
Norfloxacin
Nortriptyline
Ofloxacin
Olanzapine
Omeprazole
Oxacillin
Oxaprozin
Pamidronate
Paroxetine
Penbutolol
Penicillamine
Pentamidine
Pentazocine
Pentostatin
Pentoxifylline
Pergolide
Phendimetrazine
Phentermine
Phytonadione
Pimozide
Pindolol
Potassium iodide
Pramipexole
Pravastatin
Procainamide
Propafenone
Propantheline
Propofol
Propranolol
Propylthiouracil
Protriptyline
Pyrimethamine
Quazepam
Quinapril
Quinidine
Ramipril
Ranitidine
Rifabutin
Rimantadine
Risperidone
Ritonavir
Saccharin
Saquinavir
Selegiline
Sertraline
Sibutramine
Simvastatin
Sparfloxacin
Sulfamethoxazole
Sulfasalazine
Sulfisoxazole
Sulindac
Sumatriptan
Tacrine
Tamoxifen
Temazepam
Terbinafine
Terbutaline
Tiagabine
Ticarcillin
Tolazamide
Tolbutamide
Tolmetin
Topiramate
Tramadol
Trazodone
Triamterene
Triazolam
Trimipramine
Trovafloxacin
Ursodiol
Vancomycin
Venlafaxine
Vinblastine
Vincristine
Vinorelbine
Zalcitabine
Zidovudine
Zolpidem

Ecchymoses

Allopurinol
Alprostadil
Alteplase
Amiodarone
Amoxicillin
Atorvastatin
Benactyzine
Beta-carotene
Bromfenac
Buspirone
Carbenicillin
Chlorzoxazone
Cholestyramine
Cloxacillin
Corticosteroids
Cortisone
Delavirdine
Desipramine
Dexfenfluramine

Dicloxacillin
Dicumarol
Diethylpropion
Divalproex
Donepezil
Enoxaparin
Etodolac
Etoposide
Fluvoxamine
Heparin
Indomethacin
Interferons
Irbesartan
Lamotrigine
Latanoprost
Leuprolide
Losartan
Meprobamate
Mesalamine
Methicillin
Methotrexate
Mezlocillin
Nafcillin
Naproxen
Nefazodone
Nisoldipine
Ofloxacin
Olanzapine
Oxacillin
Oxaprozin
Paroxetine
Pentostatin
Piroxicam
Plicamycin
Ritonavir
Sibutramine
Sparfloxacin
Sulindac
Tacrolimus
Thiotepa
Tiagabine
Ticarcillin
Ticlopidine
Tiopronin
Tizanidine
Vasopressin
Venlafaxine
Verapamil
Warfarin
Zidovudine
Zolmitriptan

Erythema annulare centrifugum

Ampicillin
Chloroquine
Cimetidine
Gold
Hydrochlorothiazide
Hydroxychloroquine
Penicillins
Piroxicam
Spironolactone

Erythema multiforme

Acebutolol
Acetaminophen
Acetazolamide
Allopurinol
Aminosalicylate sodium
Amlodipine
Amoxapine
Amoxicillin
Ampicillin
Aspirin
Atenolol
Atropine sulfate
Azathioprine
Aztreonam
Benactyzine
Bumetanide
Busulfan
Butabarbital
Butalbital
Captopril
Carbamazepine
Carbenicillin
Carisoprodol
Cefaclor
Cefadroxil
Cefamandole
Cefazolin
Cefdinir
Cefepime
Cefixime
Cefotaxime
Cefpodoxime
Ceftazidime
Ceftriaxone
Cefuroxime
Cephalexin
Cephalothin
Cephradine
Cerivastatin
Chloral hydrate
Chlorambucil
Chloramphenicol
Chlordiazepoxide
Chloroquine
Chlorothiazide
Chlorotrianisene
Chlorpromazine
Chlorpropamide
Chlorzoxazone
Cimetidine
Ciprofloxacin
Clindamycin
Clofibrate
Clomiphene
Cloxacillin
Clozapine
Codeine
Cotrimoxazole
Cyclophosphamide
Dactinomycin
Danazol
Dapsone
Deferoxamine
Delavirdine
Dexfenfluramine
Diclofenac
Dicloxacillin
Didanosine
Diethylpropion
Diethylstilbestrol
Diflunisal
Diltiazem
Dipyridamole
Divalproex
Doxycycline
Enalapril
Enoxacin
Erythromycin
Ethambutol
Ethosuximide
Etodolac
Etoposide
Fenoprofen
Fluconazole
Fluorouracil
Fluoxetine
Flurbiprofen
Fluvastatin
Furazolidone
Furosemide
Gemfibrozil
Glucagon
Gold
Griseofulvin
Hydrochlorothiazide
Hydroxychloroquine
Hydroxyurea
Hydroxyzine
Ibuprofen
Imipenem/cilastatin
Indapamide
Indomethacin
Isoniazid
Isotretinoin
Itraconazole
Ketoprofen
Lamotrigine
Levamisole
Levofloxacin
Lidocaine
Lincomycin
Lithium
Loracarbef
Loratadine
Lorazepam
Lovastatin
Maprotiline
Mechlorethamine
Meclofenamate
Mefenamic acid

Mefloquine
Mephenytoin
Meprobamate
Methenamine
Methicillin
Methotrexate
Methsuximide
Methyclothiazide
Methyldopa
Methylphenidate
Metoprolol
Mezlocillin
Minocycline
Minoxidil
Mitomycin
Mitotane
Nabumetone
Nadolol
Nafcillin
Nalidixic acid
Naproxen
Neomycin
Nifedipine
Nitrofurantoin
Norfloxacin
Nystatin
Ofloxacin
Omeprazole
Oral contraceptives
Oxacillin
Oxaprozin
Oxazepam
Paramethadione
Penicillamine
Penicillins
Pentobarbital
Phenobarbital
Phenolphthalein
Phensuximide
Phenytoin
Pindolol
Piroxicam
Pravastatin
Primidone
Probenecid
Progestins
Promethazine
Propranolol
Pyrazinamide
Pyrimethamine
Quinidine
Quinine
Ramipril
Ranitidine
Ribavirin
Rifampin
Ritordine
Scopolamine
Sertraline
Simvastatin
Spironolactone
Streptomycin
Sulfadoxine
Sulfamethoxazole
Sulfasalazine
Sulfisoxazole
Sulindac
Terbinafine
Tetracycline
Thiabendazole
Thiopental
Thioridazine
Ticarcillin
Ticlopidine
Timolol
Tiopronin
Tobramycin
Tolbutamide
Tolcapone
Tolmetin
Trazodone
Trimethadione
Troleandomycin
Valproic acid
Vancomycin
Verapamil
Vinblastine
Vitamin A
Vitamin E
Zalcitabine
Zidovudine

Erythema nodosum

Acetaminophen
Acyclovir
Aldesleukin
Amiodarone
Aspirin
Azathioprine
Busulfan
Carbamazepine
Cefdinir
Chlordiazepoxide
Chlorotrianisene
Chlorpropamide
Ciprofloxacin
Clomiphene
Codeine
Cotrimoxazole
Dapsone
Diclofenac
Diethylstilbestrol
Disopyramide
Enoxacin
Fluoxetine
Furosemide
Glucagon
Gold
GCSF
Hydralazine
Ibuprofen
Indomethacin
Isotretinoin
Levofloxacin
Meclofenamate
Medroxyprogesterone
Meprobamate
Mesalamine
Methyldopa
Minocycline
Naproxen
Nifedipine
Nitrofurantoin
Ofloxacin
Omeprazole
Oral contraceptives
Paroxetine
Penicillamine
Penicillins
Progestins
Propylthiouracil
Sparfloxacin
Streptomycin
Sulfamethoxazole
Sulfasalazine
Sulfisoxazole
Thalidomide
Verapamil

Erythroderma

Aldesleukin
Aspirin
Captopril
Carbamazepine
Chloroquine
Ciprofloxacin
Clofazimine
Colchicine
Cotrimoxazole
Cytarabine
Dapsone
Dicloxacillin
Diflunisal
Hydroxychloroquine
Meclofenamate
Methotrexate
Minoxidil
Nitroglycerin
Nystatin
Phenobarbital
Phenytoin
Piroxicam
Sulfamethoxazole
Sulfasalazine
Terbinafine
Thalidomide
Timolol
Vincristine
Zalcitabine (ddC)
Zidovudine

Exanthems

Acebutolol
Acetaminophen
Acetazolamide
Acetohexamide

Acitretin
Acyclovir
Aldesleukin
Allopurinol
Alprazolam
Altretamine
Amantadine
Amikacin
Amiloride
Aminocaproic acid
Aminoglutethimide
Aminophylline
Aminosalicylate sodium
Amiodarone
Amitriptyline
Amlodipine
Amobarbital
Amoxapine
Amoxicillin
Amphotericin B
Ampicillin
Aprobarbital
Asparaginase
Aspartame
Aspirin
Astemizole
Atenolol
Atorvastatin
Atovaquone
Atropine sulfate
Azatadine
Azathioprine
Azelastine
Azithromycin
Aztreonam
Benactyzine
Benazepril
Bendroflumethiazide
Benztropine
Betaxolol
Bicalutamide
Biperiden
Bisacodyl
Bisoprolol
Bleomycin
Bromfenac
Bromocriptine
Brompheniramine
Bumetanide
Buspirone
Busulfan
Butabarbital
Butalbital
Butorphanol
Calcitonin
Captopril
Carbamazepine
Carbenicillin
Carbidopa
Carboplatin
Carisoprodol
Carmustine
Carteolol
Carvedilol
Cefaclor
Cefadroxil
Cefamandole
Cefazolin
Cefdinir
Cefepime
Cefoxitin
Ceftazidime
Ceftriaxone
Cefuroxime
Cephalexin
Cephalothin
Cephradine
Cetirizine
Chloral hydrate
Chlorambucil
Chloramphenicol
Chlordiazepoxide
Chlormezanone
Chloroquine
Chlorothiazide
Chlorpromazine
Chlorpropamide
Chlorthalidone
Chlorzoxazone
Cholestyramine
Cimetidine
Ciprofloxacin
Cisapride
Cisplatin
Cladribine
Clarithromycin
Clemastine
Clindamycin
Clofazimine
Clofibrate
Clomiphene
Clomipramine
Clonazepam
Clonidine
Clopidogrel
Clorazepate
Cloxacillin
Clozapine
Codeine
Colchicine
Colestipol
Corticosteroids
Cortisone
Cotrimoxazole
Cromolyn
Cyanocobalamin
Cyclamate
Cyclophosphamide
Cycloserine
Cyclosporine
Cyclothiazide
Cyproheptadine
Cytarabine
Dacarbazine
Dactinomycin
Dalteparin
Danazol
Dantrolene
Dapsone
Daunorubicin
Deferoxamine
Delavirdine
Demeclocycline
Desipramine
Dexfenfluramine
Diazepam
Diazoxide
Diclofenac
Dicloxacillin
Dicumarol
Dicyclomine
Didanosine
Diethylpropion
Diethylstilbestrol
Diflunisal
Digoxin
Diltiazem
Dimenhydrinate
Diphenhydramine
Dipyridamole
Disopyramide
Disulfiram
Divalproex
Docetaxel
Docusate
Dopamine
Doxazosin
Doxepin
Doxorubicin
Doxycycline
Enalapril
Enoxacin
Ephedrine
Epinephrine
Epoetin alfa
Erythromycin
Estramustine
Ethacrynic acid
Ethambutol
Ethionamide
Ethosuximide
Etodolac
Etoposide
Famotidine
Felodipine
Fenfluramine
Fenofibrate
Fenoprofen
Fentanyl
Finasteride
Flavoxate
Flecainide
Fluconazole

Flucytosine
Fluorouracil
Fluoxetine
Fluoxymesterone
Fluphenazine
Flurazepam
Flurbiprofen
Flutamide
Fluvoxamine
Folic acid
Foscarnet
Fosfomycin
Furazolidone
Furosemide
Gabapentin
Ganciclovir
Gemcitabine
Gemfibrozil
Gentamicin
Glimepiride
Glipizide
Glucagon
Glyburide
Gold
Granisetron
GCSF
Grepafloxacin
Griseofulvin
Guanethidine
Guanfacine
Haloperidol
Halothane
Heparin
Heroin
Hydralazine
Hydrochlorothiazide
Hydromorphone
Hydroxychloroquine
Hydroxyurea
Hydroxyzine
Ibuprofen
Idarubicin
Imipenem/cilastatin
Imipramine
Indapamide
Indomethacin
Insulin
Interferons
Ipodate
Ipratropium
Isocarboxazid
Isoniazid
Isosorbide
Isotretinoin
Isradipine
Itraconazole
Ivermectin
Kanamycin
Ketoconazole
Ketoprofen
Ketorolac
Labetalol
Lamivudine
Lamotrigine
Lansoprazole
Letrozole
Leuprolide
Levamisole
Levodopa
Lidocaine
Lincomycin
Lisinopril
Lithium
Lomefloxacin
Loratadine
Lorazepam
Lovastatin
Loxapine
Maprotiline
Marihuana
Mazindol
Mebendazole
Mechlorethamine
Meclizine
Meclofenamate
Medroxyprogesterone
Mefenamic acid
Mefloquine
Melphalan
Mephenytoin
Mephobarbital
Meprobamate
Mercaptopurine
Mesalamine
Mesna
Metformin
Methadone
Methantheline
Methazolamide
Methenamine
Methicillin
Methimazole
Methocarbamol
Methohexital
Methotrexate
Methoxsalen
Methsuximide
Methyclothiazide
Methyldopa
Methylphenidate
Methyltestosterone
Methysergide
Metoclopramide
Metolazone
Metoprolol
Metronidazole
Mexiletine
Mezlocillin
Miconazole
Midazolam
Minocycline
Minoxidil
Misoprostol
Mitomycin
Mitotane
Moexipril
Moricizine
Nabumetone
Nadolol
Nafarelin
Nafcillin
Nalidixic acid
Naloxone
Naproxen
Naratriptan
Nefazodone
Neomycin
Nevirapine
Niacin; niacinamide
Nicardipine
Nifedipine
Nimodipine
Nisoldipine
Nitrofurantoin
Nitroglycerin
Nizatidine
Norfloxacin
Nortriptyline
Nystatin
Octreotide
Ofloxacin
Olanzapine
Olsalazine
Omeprazole
Ondansetron
Oral contraceptives
Orphenadrine
Oxacillin
Oxaprozin
Oxazepam
Oxytetracycline
Pamidronate
Paramethadione
Paroxetine
Pemoline
Penbutolol
Penicillamine
Penicillins
Pentagastrin
Pentamidine
Pentazocine
Pentobarbital
Pentostatin
Pentoxifylline
Pergolide
Perphenazine
Phenazopyridine
Phenelzine
Phenobarbital
Phenolphthalein
Phenytoin
Phytonadione
Pimozide

Pindolol
Piperacillin
Piroxicam
Plicamycin
Polythiazide
Potassium iodide
Pravastatin
Prazepam
Prazosin
Primaquine
Primidone
Procainamide
Procarbazine
Prochlorperazine
Progestins
Promazine
Promethazine
Propafenone
Propantheline
Propofol
Propoxyphene
Propranolol
Protamine
Protriptyline
Pseudoephedrine
Pyrazinamide
Pyrimethamine
Quinacrine
Quinapril
Quinethazone
Quinidine
Quinine
Ramipril
Ranitidine
Reserpine
Ribavirin
Rifampin
Ritonavir
Ritordine
Ropinirole
Saccharin
Salmeterol
Salsalate
Saquinavir
Scopolamine
Secobarbital
Sertraline
Simvastatin
Sotalol
Sparfloxacin
Spectinomycin
Spironolactone
Stanozolol
Streptokinase
Streptomycin
Streptozocin
Succinylcholine
Sucralfate
Sulfadoxine
Sulfamethoxazole
Sulfasalazine
Sulfinpyrazone
Sulfisoxazole
Sulindac
Sumatriptan
Tacrine
Tamoxifen
Temazepam
Terazosin
Terbinafine
Terbutaline
Terfenadine
Testosterone
Tetracycline
Thalidomide
Thiabendazole
Thiamine
Thioguanine
Thiopental
Thioridazine
Thiothixene
Tiagabine
Ticarcillin
Ticlopidine
Timolol
Tiopronin
Tizanidine
Tobramycin
Tolazamide
Tolazoline
Tolbutamide
Tolmetin
Topiramate
Torsemide
Tramadol
Tranylcypromine
Trazodone
Triamterene
Triazolam
Trichlormethiazide
Trifluoperazine
Trimeprazine
Trimethadione
Trimetrexate
Trimipramine
Triprolidine
Troleandomycin
Urokinase
Valproic acid
Vancomycin
Vasopressin
Venlafaxine
Verapamil
Vinblastine
Vincristine
Vitamin A
Vitamin E
Warfarin
Zalcitabine
Zidovudine

Exfoliative dermatitis

Acetaminophen
Aldesleukin
Allopurinol
Aminoglutethimide
Aminophylline
Aminosalicylate sodium
Amiodarone
Amitriptyline
Amobarbital
Amoxicillin
Amphotericin B
Ampicillin
Aprobarbital
Aspirin
Atropine sulfate
Aztreonam
Benactyzine
Bendroflumethiazide
Betaxolol
Bisoprolol
Bumetanide
Butabarbital
Butalbital
Captopril
Carbamazepine
Carbenicillin
Carbidopa
Carteolol
Cefdinir
Cefoxitin
Chlorambucil
Chloroquine
Chlorothiazide
Chlorpromazine
Chlorpropamide
Cimetidine
Ciprofloxacin
Cisplatin
Clofazimine
Clofibrate
Cloxacillin
Codeine
Cotrimoxazole
Cromolyn
Cytarabine
Dapsone
Demeclocycline
Desipramine
Diazepam
Diclofenac
Dicloxacillin
Diethylstilbestrol
Diflunisal
Diltiazem
Doxorubicin
Doxycycline
Enalapril
Ephedrine
Ethambutol
Ethosuximide
Etodolac
Fenoprofen

Fentanyl
Flecainide
Fluconazole
Fluoxetine
Fluphenazine
Flurbiprofen
Fluvoxamine
Fosinopril
Furosemide
Ganciclovir
Gemfibrozil
Gentamicin
Gold
GCSF
Grepafloxacin
Griseofulvin
Guanfacine
Haloperidol
Hydroxychloroquine
Imipramine
Indomethacin
Isoniazid
Isosorbide
Ketoconazole
Ketoprofen
Ketorolac
Levamisole
Lidocaine
Lincomycin
Lithium
Meclofenamate
Mefenamic acid
Mefloquine
Mephenytoin
Mephobarbital
Meprobamate
Mesoridazine
Methantheline
Methicillin
Methsuximide
Methylphenidate
Mexiletine
Mezlocillin
Mibefradil
Minocycline
Mitomycin
Nafcillin
Nalidixic acid
Naproxen
Nifedipine
Nisoldipine
Nitrofurantoin
Nitroglycerin
Nizatidine
Norfloxacin
Ofloxacin
Omeprazole
Oxacillin
Oxaprozin
Oxytetracycline
Paramethadione
Penicillamine
Penicillins
Pentobarbital
Pentostatin
Perphenazine
Phenobarbital
Phenolphthalein
Phenytoin
Piroxicam
Primidone
Procarbazine
Prochlorperazine
Propranolol
Propylthiouracil
Pseudoephedrine
Pyrimethamine
Quinacrine
Quinapril
Quinidine
Quinine
Rifampin
Risperidone
Secobarbital
Sildenafil
Sparfloxacin
Streptomycin
Sulfadoxine
Sulfamethoxazole
Sulfasalazine
Sulfisoxazole
Sulindac
Tetracycline
Thalidomide
Tiagabine
Ticarcillin
Ticlopidine
Timolol
Tizanidine
Tobramycin
Trazodone
Trifluoperazine
Trimethadione
Vancomycin
Venlafaxine
Verapamil
Vitamin A
Warfarin
Yohimbine
Zalcitabine

Fixed eruption

Acetaminophen
Acyclovir
Alendronate
Allopurinol
Aminosalicylate sodium
Amitriptyline
Amoxicillin
Amphotericin B
Ampicillin
Aspirin
Atropine sulfate
Azathioprine
Benactyzine
Bisacodyl
Butabarbital
Butalbital
Cabergoline
Carbamazepine
Carisoprodol
Cefazolin
Cephalexin
Chloral hydrate
Chloramphenicol
Chlordiazepoxide
Chlormezanone
Chloroquine
Chlorothiazide
Chlorpromazine
Chlorpropamide
Cimetidine
Ciprofloxacin
Clarithromycin
Codeine
Colchicine
Cortisone
Cotrimoxazole
Dacarbazine
Dapsone
Demeclocycline
Dextromethorphan
Diazepam
Diflunisal
Dimenhydrinate
Diphenhydramine
Disulfiram
Doxycycline
Ephedrine
Epinephrine
Erythromycin
Ethchlorvynol
Ethotoin
Etodolac
Fluconazole
Flurbiprofen
Foscarnet
Ganciclovir
Gold
Griseofulvin
Guanethidine
Heparin
Heroin
Hydralazine
Hydrochlorothiazide
Hydroxychloroquine
Hydroxyurea
Hydroxyzine
Ibuprofen
Imipramine
Indomethacin
Isotretinoin
Itraconazole
Ketoconazole

Levamisole
Lidocaine
Lorazepam
Meclofenamate
Mefenamic acid
Meprobamate
Mesna
Methenamine
Methimazole
Methyldopa
Methylphenidate
Metronidazole
Minocycline
Naproxen
Neomycin
Niacin; niacinamide
Nifedipine
Nitrofurantoin
Norfloxacin
Nystatin
Ofloxacin
Ondansetron
Oral contraceptives
Oxazepam
Oxytetracycline
Penicillins
Pentobarbital
Phenobarbital
Phenolphthalein
Phenytoin
Piroxicam
Procarbazine
Prochlorperazine
Promethazine
Propofol
Pyrazinamide
Pyridoxine
Pyrimethamine
Quinacrine
Quinidine
Quinine
Ranitidine
Ribavirin
Rifampin
Saccharin
Scopolamine
Sertraline
Sildenafil
Streptomycin
Sulfamethoxazole
Sulfasalazine
Sulfisoxazole
Sulindac
Temazepam
Terbinafine
Terfenadine
Tetracycline
Thiabendazole
Thiopental
Tolbutamide
Trifluoperazine
Trimethadione
Trimetrexate
Tripelennamine
Triprolidine
Valproic acid

Galactorrhea

Alprazolam
Amitriptyline
Amoxapine
Buspirone
Chlordiazepoxide
Chlorpromazine
Cimetidine
Clomipramine
Cyclobenzaprine
Desipramine
Divalproex
Doxepin
Fluphenazine
Haloperidol
Imipramine
Isotretinoin
Loxapine
Maprotiline
Medroxyprogesterone
Mesoridazine
Methyldopa
Metoclopramide
Minocycline
Molindone
Nitrofurantoin
Nortriptyline
Octreotide
Oral contraceptives
Paroxetine
Perphenazine
Pimozide
Prochlorperazine
Progestins
Promazine
Protriptyline
Risperidone
Sertraline
Tamoxifen
Terfenadine
Thalidomide
Thioridazine
Trazodone
Trifluoperazine
Trimipramine
Valproic acid
Verapamil

Gingival hyperplasia

Amlodipine
Cotrimoxazole
Cyclosporine
Diltiazem
Erythromycin
Ethosuximide
Ethotoin
Felodipine
Ketoconazole
Lamotrigine
Lithium
Mephenytoin
Methsuximide
Nifedipine
Nisoldipine
Oral contraceptives
Phensuximide
Phenytoin
Primidone
Sertraline
Tiagabine
Topiramate
Valproic acid
Verapamil

Gynecomastia

Alprazolam
Amiloride
Amitriptyline
Amlodipine
Amoxapine
Atorvastatin
Bendroflumethiazide
Bicalutamide
Busulfan
Captopril
Cerivastatin
Chlordiazepoxide
Chlorotrianisene
Chlorpromazine
Cimetidine
Ciprofloxacin
Clofibrate
Clomiphene
Clomipramine
Clonidine
Cyclobenzaprine
Cyclosporine
Delavirdine
Desipramine
Dexfenfluramine
Diazepam
Diethylpropion
Diethylstilbestrol
Digoxin
Diltiazem
Disopyramide
Divalproex
Doxepin
Enalapril
Estazolam
Estramustine
Ethionamide
Etodolac
Famotidine
Finasteride
Fluoxetine
Fluoxymesterone
Fluphenazine
Flutamide

Fluvastatin
Foscarnet
Griseofulvin
Guanabenz
Haloperidol
Ibuprofen
Imipramine
Indinavir
Indomethacin
Isotretinoin
Itraconazole
Ketoconazole
Ketoprofen
Lansoprazole
Latanoprost
Leuprolide
Loratadine
Lovastatin
Loxapine
Maprotiline
Medroxyprogesterone
Meprobamate
Mesoridazine
Methotrexate
Methyldopa
Methyltestosterone
Metoclopramide
Metronidazole
Minocycline
Misoprostol
Molindone
Nafarelin
Nefazodone
Nifedipine
Nizatidine
Nortriptyline
Octreotide
Omeprazole
Penicillamine
Pentostatin
Perphenazine
Phenytoin
Pimozide
Pravastatin
Procarbazine
Prochlorperazine
Progestins
Promazine
Protriptyline
Pyrilamine
Quinestrol
Ranitidine
Reserpine
Risperidone
Ropinirole
Sertraline
Sildenafil
Simvastatin
Spironolactone
Stanozolol
Sulindac
Terfenadine
Testosterone
Thioridazine
Thiothixene
Tiagabine
Tolmetin
Topiramate
Trazodone
Triamterene
Trifluoperazine
Trimeprazine
Trimipramine
Valproic acid
Venlafaxine
Verapamil
Vitamin E

Hair – alopecia

Acebutolol
Acetaminophen
Acetohexamide
Acitretin
Acyclovir
Albendazole
Aldesleukin
Allopurinol
Altretamine
Amantadine
Amiloride
Aminophylline
Aminosalicylate sodium
Amiodarone
Amitriptyline
Amlodipine
Amoxapine
Asparaginase
Aspirin
Astemizole
Atenolol
Atorvastatin
Azathioprine
Bendroflumethiazide
Betaxolol
Bicalutamide
Bisoprolol
Bleomycin
Bromfenac
Bromocriptine
Buspirone
Busulfan
Captopril
Carbamazepine
Carbidopa
Carboplatin
Carmustine
Carteolol
Carvedilol
Cerivastatin
Cetirizine
Chlorambucil
Chloramphenicol
Chlordiazepoxide
Chloroquine
Chlorothiazide
Chlorotrianisene
Chlorpropamide
Cimetidine
Cisplatin
Clofibrate
Clomiphene
Clomipramine
Clonazepam
Clonidine
Colchicine
Cyclobenzaprine
Cyclophosphamide
Cyclosporine
Cytarabine
Dacarbazine
Dactinomycin
Danazol
Daunorubicin
Delavirdine
Desipramine
Dexfenfluramine
Diazoxide
Diclofenac
Dicumarol
Didanosine
Diethylpropion
Diethylstilbestrol
Diflunisal
Diltiazem
Disopyramide
Divalproex
Docetaxel
Donepezil
Dopamine
Doxazosin
Doxepin
Doxorubicin
Enalapril
Epinephrine
Estramustine
Ethambutol
Ethionamide
Ethosuximide
Etidronate
Etodolac
Etoposide
Famotidine
Felbamate
Fenfluramine
Fenofibrate
Fenoprofen
Flecainide
Fluconazole
Fluorouracil
Fluoxetine
Fluoxymesterone
Flurbiprofen
Fluvastatin
Fluvoxamine

Foscarnet
Gabapentin
Ganciclovir
Gemcitabine
Gemfibrozil
Gentamicin
Gold
Granisetron
GCSF
Grepafloxacin
Guanethidine
Guanfacine
Haloperidol
Halothane
Heparin
Hydromorphone
Hydroxychloroquine
Hydroxyurea
Ibuprofen
Idarubicin
Ifosfamide
Imipramine
Indinavir
Indomethacin
Interferons
Ipratropium
Isoniazid
Isotretinoin
Itraconazole
Ketoconazole
Ketoprofen
Labetalol
Lamivudine
Lamotrigine
Lansoprazole
Letrozole
Leuprolide
Levamisole
Levobunolol
Levodopa
Levothyroxine
Liothyronine
Lisinopril
Lithium
Lomustine
Loratadine
Lorazepam
Losartan
Lovastatin
Loxapine
Maprotiline
Mebendazole
Mechlorethamine
Meclofenamate
Medroxyprogesterone
Mefloquine
Melphalan
Mephenytoin
Mercaptopurine
Mesalamine
Mesoridazine
Methimazole
Methotrexate
Methsuximide
Methyldopa
Methylphenidate
Methyltestosterone
Methysergide
Metoprolol
Mexiletine
Minoxidil
Misoprostol
Mitomycin
Mitotane
Moexipril
Nabumetone
Nadolol
Nalidixic acid
Naproxen
Naratriptan
Nefazodone
Neomycin
Nifedipine
Nimodipine
Nisoldipine
Nitrofurantoin
Nortriptyline
Octreotide
Olanzapine
Omeprazole
Ondansetron
Oral contraceptives
Oxaprozin
Paramethadione
Paroxetine
Penbutolol
Penicillamine
Penicillins
Pentostatin
Pergolide
Phensuximide
Phentermine
Phenytoin
Pindolol
Piroxicam
Pravastatin
Prazepam
Prazosin
Probenecid
Procarbazine
Progestins
Propafenone
Propranolol
Propylthiouracil
Protriptyline
Pyrimethamine
Quazepam
Quinacrine
Quinidine
Ramipril
Ranitidine
Risperidone
Selegiline
Sertraline
Simvastatin
Sotalol
Sparfloxacin
Spironolactone
Stanozolol
Sulfasalazine
Sulfisoxazole
Sulindac
Tacrine
Tacrolimus
Tamoxifen
Terfenadine
Testosterone
Thalidomide
Thioguanine
Thioridazine
Thiotepa
Thiothixene
Timolol
Tiopronin
Tizanidine
Tolcapone
Topiramate
Topotecan
Trazodone
Triazolam
Trimethadione
Trimipramine
Ursodiol
Valproic acid
Vasopressin
Venlafaxine
Verapamil
Vinblastine
Vincristine
Vinorelbine
Vitamin A
Warfarin
Zalcitabine
Zidovudine

Hair – alopecia areata

Clomipramine
Cyclosporine
Fluvoxamine
Haloperidol
Imipramine
Lithium
Oral contraceptives
Terbinafine

Hair – hirsutism

Acetazolamide
Aminoglutethimide
Chlorotrianisene
Clonazepam
Corticosteroids
Danazol
Dexfenfluramine
Diethylstilbestrol
Diltiazem

Donepezil
Ethosuximide
Fluoxetine
Fluoxymesterone
Gemfibrozil
Isotretinoin
Lamotrigine
Lorazepam
Medroxyprogesterone
Methsuximide
Methyltestosterone
Minoxidil
Nafarelin
Olanzapine
Oral contraceptives
Penicillamine
Pergolide
Phensuximide
Phenytoin
Prazepam
Progestins
Quazepam
Sertraline
Spironolactone
Stanozolol
Tamoxifen
Testosterone
Triazolam
Venlafaxine

Hair – hypertrichosis

Amantadine
Amiodarone
Betaxolol
Cetirizine
Clomiphene
Clomipramine
Corticosteroids
Cortisone
Cyclosporine
Diazoxide
Epoetin alfa
Interferons
Latanoprost
Methoxsalen
Minoxidil
Phenytoin
Psoralens
Risperidone
Selegiline
Streptomycin
Tamoxifen
Thioridazine
Tiopronin
Trioxsalen
Verapamil
Zidovudine

Herpes simplex

Azathioprine
Azelastine
Butabarbital
Butalbital
Chlorambucil
Clonidine
Corticosteroids
Cyclosporine
Fluoxetine
Flurbiprofen
Foscarnet
Grepafloxacin
Indinavir
Interferons
Methotrexate
Methoxsalen
Nisoldipine
Pentobarbital
Pentostatin
Phenobarbital
Psoralens
Ribavirin
Ropinirole
Saquinavir
Sibutramine
Sildenafil
Sparfloxacin
Tacrine
Tiagabine
Tizanidine
Tolcapone
Trioxsalen
Venlafaxine
Zolpidem

Herpes zoster

Acyclovir
Azathioprine
Chlorambucil
Corticosteroids
Cyclosporine
Cytarabine
Enalapril
Fluoxetine
Flurbiprofen
Gold
Griseofulvin
Indinavir
Isoniazid
Mechlorethamine
Methoxsalen
Nisoldipine
Pentostatin
Procarbazine
Psoralens
Ropinirole
Saquinavir
Tacrine
Tiagabine
Tizanidine
Tolcapone
Trioxsalen
Venlafaxine
Zolpidem

Hyperhidrosis

Acebutolol
Acetaminophen
Acitretin
Acyclovir
Albuterol
Allopurinol
Alprazolam
Amiloride
Aminophylline
Amiodarone
Amitriptyline
Amlodipine
Amoxapine
Aspirin
Atenolol
Atorvastatin
Atovaquone
Azatadine
Aztreonam
Benazepril
Bendroflumethiazide
Betaxolol
Bethanechol
Bicalutamide
Bisoprolol
Bromfenac
Bumetanide
Buspirone
Butorphanol
Carbidopa
Carisoprodol
Carteolol
Carvedilol
Cefamandole
Cefpodoxime
Ceftazidime
Ceftriaxone
Cetirizine
Chlordiazepoxide
Ciprofloxacin
Cisplatin
Clemastine
Clofibrate
Clomiphene
Clomipramine
Clonazepam
Clonidine
Clorazepate
Clozapine
Codeine
Cortisone
Cyclobenzaprine
Cyclophosphamide
Cyproheptadine
Danazol
Dantrolene
Desipramine
Desmopressin
Dexfenfluramine
Dextroamphetamine
Diazepam
Diazoxide

Diclofenac
Diethylpropion
Diflunisal
Diltiazem
Dimenhydrinate
Diphenhydramine
Diphenoxylate
Dirithromycin
Dolasetron
Doxapram
Doxazosin
Doxepin
Dronabinol
Edrophonium
Enalapril
Enoxacin
Ephedrine
Epinephrine
Estazolam
Ethambutol
Ethchlorvynol
Etodolac
Felodipine
Fenfluramine
Fenoprofen
Fentanyl
Flecainide
Flumazenil
Fluoxetine
Fluphenazine
Flurazepam
Flurbiprofen
Flutamide
Fluvoxamine
Foscarnet
Fosinopril
Gemcitabine
Grepafloxacin
Guanabenz
Guanfacine
Haloperidol
Hydrochlorothiazide
Hydroxyzine
Ibuprofen
Imipenem/cilastatin
Imipramine
Indapamide
Indinavir
Indomethacin
Insulin
Interferons
Isocarboxazid
Isoproterenol
Isosorbide
Isotretinoin
Isradipine
Ketoprofen
Ketorolac
Labetalol
Lamotrigine
Letrozole
Levodopa
Levofloxacin
Levothyroxine
Liothyronine
Lomefloxacin
Loratadine
Lorazepam
Losartan
Loxapine
Maprotiline
Mazindol
Medroxyprogesterone
Mefenamic acid
Mesalamine
Mesoridazine
Methadone
Methamphetamine
Methylphenidate
Metoprolol
Mexiletine
Mibefradil
Misoprostol
Moexipril
Moricizine
Nabumetone
Nadolol
Naloxone
Naproxen
Naratriptan
Nifedipine
Nimodipine
Nisoldipine
Nitroglycerin
Nizatidine
Norfloxacin
Nortriptyline
Octreotide
Ofloxacin
Olanzapine
Omeprazole
Oxaprozin
Oxazepam
Paroxetine
Penbutolol
Penicillins
Pentagastrin
Pentazocine
Pentostatin
Pentoxifylline
Pergolide
Phendimetrazine
Phenelzine
Phenindamine
Phentermine
Phytonadione
Pimozide
Pindolol
Piroxicam
Potassium iodide
Pramipexole
Prazepam
Prazosin
Procarbazine
Progestins
Promethazine
Propantheline
Propoxyphene
Propranolol
Protriptyline
Pseudoephedrine
Pyrilamine
Quazepam
Quinapril
Quinine
Raloxifene
Ramipril
Rifampin
Risperidone
Ritonavir
Ritordine
Ropinirole
Saquinavir
Selegiline
Sertraline
Sibutramine
Sildenafil
Simvastatin
Sotalol
Sparfloxacin
Streptokinase
Sulfasalazine
Sulindac
Sumatriptan
Tacrine
Tacrolimus
Tamoxifen
Temazepam
Terazosin
Terbutaline
Terfenadine
Tetracycline
Thalidomide
Thiamine
Thiothixene
Tiagabine
Ticlopidine
Timolol
Tizanidine
Tolazamide
Tolcapone
Topiramate
Toremifene
Tramadol
Tranylcypromine
Trazodone
Triamterene
Triazolam
Trimeprazine
Trimipramine
Tripelennamine
Triprolidine
Trovafloxacin

Urokinase
Ursodiol
Vasopressin
Venlafaxine
Verapamil
Yohimbine
Zalcitabine
Zidovudine
Zolmitriptan
Zolpidem

Hyperpigmentation

Ciprofloxacin
Clonidine
Corticosteroids
Cortisone
Cyclosporine
Doxorubicin
Enoxacin
Etodolac
Isotretinoin
Mechlorethamine
Niacin; niacinamide
Pentazocine
Pimozide
Quinine
Stanozolol
Thiotepa
Vinblastine

Hypersensitivity

Acetaminophen
Alendronate
Allopurinol
Aminophylline
Amoxicillin
Ampicillin
Asparaginase
Azathioprine
Bleomycin
Carbamazepine
Carboplatin
Cefaclor
Cefuroxime
Cerivastatin
Chlorambucil
Chloramphenicol
Cimetidine
Ciprofloxacin
Clarithromycin
Cortisone
Cotrimoxazole
Cromolyn
Cyanocobalamin
Cyclophosphamide
Cytarabine
Dacarbazine
Dapsone
Diazoxide
Dicumarol
Didanosine
Diflunisal
Diltiazem
Docetaxel
Edrophonium
Enoxacin
Enoxaparin
Epoetin alfa
Erythromycin
Ethambutol
Etidronate
Etoposide
Flavoxate
Fluconazole
Fluoxetine
Fluoxymesterone
Flurbiprofen
Glyburide
Gold
Granisetron
Heparin
Heroin
Hydroxyzine
Ibuprofen
Imipenem/cilastatin
Indomethacin
Insulin
Isoniazid
Ketoconazole
Ketorolac
Lamotrigine
Levobunolol
Lidocaine
Lomefloxacin
Mechlorethamine
Meclofenamate
Melphalan
Mesalamine
Methyldopa
Methylphenidate
Methyltestosterone
Metronidazole
Mezlocillin
Minocycline
Nafarelin
Nafcillin
Nitrofurantoin
Nystatin
Ondansetron
Orphenadrine
Oxytetracycline
Pamidronate
Penicillamine
Penicillins
Pentagastrin
Phenobarbital
Phenytoin
Phytonadione
Piperacillin
Probenecid
Procarbazine
Promethazine
Protamine
Pyridoxine
Pyrimethamine
Quinethazone
Quinine
Ramipril
Ranitidine
Salmeterol
Sparfloxacin
Spectinomycin
Succinylcholine
Sulfadoxine
Sulfamethoxazole
Sulfasalazine
Sulindac
Terbinafine
Testosterone
Tetracycline
Thiabendazole
Ticarcillin
Tobramycin
Tolbutamide
Trimetrexate
Valproic acid
Vancomycin
Vitamin A
Warfarin

Jarisch-Herxheimer reaction

Amoxicillin
Carbenicillin
Ceftriaxone
Cefuroxime
Cloxacillin
Dicloxacillin
Griseofulvin
Ketoconazole
Methicillin
Mezlocillin
Nafcillin
Oxacillin
Penicillins
Pentamidine
Piperacillin
Thiabendazole
Ticarcillin

Kaposi's sarcoma

Aldesleukin
Aminocaproic acid
Azathioprine
Busulfan
Captopril
Chlorambucil
Corticosteroids
Cortisone
Cyclosporine
Heroin
Interferons

Lichen planus

Allopurinol
Captopril
Doxazosin
Felbamate
Gemfibrozil

Gold
Hydroxyurea
Imipramine
Indomethacin
Interferons
Labetalol
Levobunolol
Lithium
Mesalamine
Methyldopa
Naproxen
Omeprazole
Penicillamine
Phenytoin
Prazosin
Procainamide
Psoralens
Quinidine
Quinine
Simvastatin
Spironolactone
Sulfasalazine
Sulindac
Ursodiol

Lichenoid eruption

Acebutolol
Acetohexamide
Acyclovir
Aminosalicylate sodium
Aspirin
Atenolol
Azathioprine
Captopril
Carbamazepine
Chloral hydrate
Chloroquine
Chlorothiazide
Chlorpromazine
Chlorpropamide
Colchicine
Cotrimoxazole
Cycloserine
Cyclosporine
Cyproheptadine
Dapsone
Demeclocycline
Diazoxide
Diflunisal
Diltiazem
Enalapril
Epoetin alfa
Ethambutol
Fluoxetine
Fluoxymesterone
Furosemide
Glipizide
Gold
Griseofulvin
Hydrochlorothiazide
Hydroxychloroquine
Hydroxyurea
Isoniazid
Labetalol
Levamisole
Lisinopril
Mercaptopurine
Metformin
Methamphetamine
Methyldopa
Methyltestosterone
Metoprolol
Minocycline
Nadolol
Naproxen
Nifedipine
Oral contraceptives
Penicillamine
Phenytoin
Pindolol
Piroxicam
Pravastatin
Prazosin
Propranolol
Propylthiouracil
Pyrimethamine
Quinacrine
Quinidine
Quinine
Ranitidine
Risperidone
Simvastatin
Sotalol
Sparfloxacin
Spironolactone
Streptomycin
Sulfamethoxazole
Temazepam
Terazosin
Testosterone
Tetracycline
Timolol
Tiopronin
Tolazamide
Tolbutamide
Torsemide
Tripelennamine
Triprolidine
Venlafaxine
Verapamil

Linear IgA bullous dermatosis

Aldesleukin
Amiodarone
Ampicillin
Captopril
Cefamandole
Diclofenac
Glyburide
Interferons
Lithium
Penicillins
Phenytoin
Piroxicam
Rifampin
Sulfisoxazole
Vancomycin

Livedo reticularis

Amantadine
Bromocriptine
Dihydrotachysterol
Diphenhydramine
Felbamate
Heparin
Ibuprofen
Quinidine
Warfarin

Lupus erythematosus

Acebutolol
Acetazolamide
Albuterol
Allopurinol
Aminoglutethimide
Aminosalicylate sodium
Amiodarone
Amitriptyline
Atenolol
Betaxolol
Bisoprolol
Butabarbital
Butalbital
Captopril
Carbamazepine
Carteolol
Cerivastatin
Chlorambucil
Chlordiazepoxide
Chlorothiazide
Chlorpromazine
Chlorpropamide
Chlorthalidone
Cimetidine
Clofibrate
Clonidine
Clozapine
Corticosteroids
Cortisone
Cotrimoxazole
Cyclosporine
Cyproheptadine
Danazol
Dapsone
Demeclocycline
Diclofenac
Diethylstilbestrol
Diltiazem
Disopyramide
Divalproex
Doxazosin
Doxycycline
Enalapril
Ethambutol
Ethionamide
Ethosuximide
Ethotoin

Felbamate
Fluoxetine
Fluoxymesterone
Fluphenazine
Flutamide
Fluvastatin
Furosemide
Gemfibrozil
Gold
Griseofulvin
Guanethidine
Hydralazine
Hydrochlorothiazide
Hydroxyurea
Ibuprofen
Imipramine
Interferons
Isoniazid
Labetalol
Lamotrigine
Leuprolide
Levodopa
Lidocaine
Lithium
Lovastatin
Meclofenamate
Mephenytoin
Meprobamate
Mercaptopurine
Mesalamine
Mesoridazine
Methimazole
Methoxsalen
Methsuximide
Methyldopa
Methyltestosterone
Methysergide
Metoprolol
Minocycline
Minoxidil
Nadolol
Nalidixic acid
Naproxen
Nifedipine
Nitrofurantoin
Olsalazine
Omeprazole
Oral contraceptives
Oxytetracycline
Paramethadione
Penicillamine
Penicillins
Pentobarbital
Perphenazine
Phenelzine
Phenindamine
Phenobarbital
Phenolphthalein
Phensuximide
Phenytoin
Pindolol
Piroxicam
Potassium iodide
Pravastatin
Prazosin
Primidone
Procainamide
Prochlorperazine
Promethazine
Propafenone
Propranolol
Propylthiouracil
Psoralens
Pyrilamine
Quinidine
Quinine
Reserpine
Rifabutin
Simvastatin
Spironolactone
Streptomycin
Sulfadoxine
Sulfamethoxazole
Sulfasalazine
Sulfisoxazole
Terfenadine
Testosterone
Tetracycline
Thioridazine
Ticlopidine
Timolol
Tiopronin
Tolazamide
Triamterene
Trichlormethiazide
Trientine
Trifluoperazine
Trimeprazine
Trimethadione
Trioxsalen
Tripelennamine
Valproic acid
Vancomycin
Vitamin E
Yohimbine

Melanoma

Carbidopa
Clomiphene
Cyclosporine
Diazepam
Gemfibrozil
Interferons
Levodopa
Methotrexate
Oral contraceptives
Paroxetine
Psoralens
Tacrine
Trioxsalen

Nails – onycholysis

Acebutolol
Allopurinol
Atenolol
Bleomycin
Captopril
Clofazimine
Cloxacillin
Demeclocycline
Diflunisal
Docetaxel
Doxorubicin
Doxycycline
Etoposide
Fluorouracil
Gold
Hydroxyurea
Ibuprofen
Indomethacin
Isoniazid
Isotretinoin
Ketoprofen
Methotrexate
Metoprolol
Minocycline
Nadolol
Nitrofurantoin
Oral contraceptives
Pindolol
Piroxicam
Propranolol
Tetracycline
Timolol

Nails – pigmentation

Betaxolol
Bleomycin
Busulfan
Chloroquine
Chlorpromazine
Cyclophosphamide
Dacarbazine
Daunorubicin
Demeclocycline
Docetaxel
Doxorubicin
Fluorouracil
Flurbiprofen
Gold
Hydroxychloroquine
Hydroxyurea
Ketoconazole
Methotrexate
Methoxsalen
Minocycline
Oxytetracycline
Phenytoin
Psoralens
Quinacrine
Timolol
Trioxsalen
Zidovudine

Paresthesias

Acetazolamide
Acitretin

Acyclovir
Allopurinol
Alprazolam
Amikacin
Amiloride
Amiodarone
Amitriptyline
Amlodipine
Amoxapine
Amphotericin B
Apraclonidine
Astemizole
Atorvastatin
Azatadine
Aztreonam
Benactyzine
Benazepril
Bendroflumethiazide
Benzthiazide
Benztropine
Betaxolol
Bicalutamide
Biperiden
Bisoprolol
Bromfenac
Bromocriptine
Brompheniramine
Buspirone
Butorphanol
Cabergoline
Calcitonin
Captopril
Carisoprodol
Carteolol
Carvedilol
Cefaclor
Cefamandole
Cefpodoxime
Ceftazidime
Ceftibuten
Cerivastatin
Cetirizine
Chloramphenicol
Chlordiazepoxide
Chlorothiazide
Chlorthalidone
Cholestyramine
Ciprofloxacin
Clemastine
Clomipramine
Clonazepam
Clopidogrel
Clorazepate
Codeine
Cromolyn
Cyclamate
Cyclobenzaprine
Cycloserine
Cyclosporine
Cyclothiazide
Cyproheptadine

Dacarbazine
Danazol
Delavirdine
Demeclocycline
Desipramine
Dexfenfluramine
Diazepam
Diazoxide
Diclofenac
Didanosine
Diflunisal
Diltiazem
Dimenhydrinate
Diphenhydramine
Dipyridamole
Dirithromycin
Disopyramide
Disulfiram
Divalproex
Docetaxel
Dolasetron
Donepezil
Doxapram
Doxazosin
Doxepin
Doxycycline
Enalapril
Enoxacin
Epoetin alfa
Esmolol
Estazolam
Ethambutol
Ethchlorvynol
Etidronate
Etodolac
Etoposide
Famciclovir
Famotidine
Felbamate
Felodipine
Fentanyl
Flecainide
Fluconazole
Flucytosine
Flumazenil
Fluorouracil
Fluoxetine
Fluoxymesterone
Flurazepam
Flurbiprofen
Flutamide
Fluvastatin
Fluvoxamine
Foscarnet
Fosfomycin
Fosinopril
Furosemide
Gabapentin
Ganciclovir
Gemcitabine
Gemfibrozil

Gentamicin
Glipizide
Glyburide
Grepafloxacin
Griseofulvin
Guanadrel
Guanethidine
Guanfacine
Hydralazine
Hydrochlorothiazide
Hydroflumethiazide
Hydromorphone
Ibuprofen
Imipenem/cilastatin
Imipramine
Indapamide
Indinavir
Indomethacin
Interferons
Ipratropium
Irbesartan
Isoniazid
Isradipine
Kanamycin
Ketoconazole
Ketoprofen
Ketorolac
Labetalol
Lamivudine
Lamotrigine
Lansoprazole
Leuprolide
Levamisole
Levofloxacin
Lidocaine
Lisinopril
Lomefloxacin
Loratadine
Lorazepam
Losartan
Lovastatin
Loxapine
Mazindol
Meclofenamate
Medroxyprogesterone
Meprobamate
Mesalamine
Mesoridazine
Methazolamide
Methimazole
Methyclothiazide
Methyldopa
Methyltestosterone
Methysergide
Metoclopramide
Metolazone
Metoprolol
Metronidazole
Mexiletine
Mibefradil
Midazolam

Minocycline
Minoxidil
Mitomycin
Moricizine
Nabumetone
Nadolol
Nafarelin
Nalidixic acid
Naratriptan
Nefazodone
Nelfinavir
Nevirapine
Niacin; niacinamide
Nicardipine
Nifedipine
Nisoldipine
Nitrofurantoin
Nizatidine
Norfloxacin
Nortriptyline
Ofloxacin
Omeprazole
Ondansetron
Orphenadrine
Oxazepam
Oxytetracycline
Paramethadione
Paroxetine
Pentagastrin
Pentazocine
Pentostatin
Pentoxifylline
Pergolide
Phenytoin
Pindolol
Piroxicam
Polythiazide
Potassium iodide
Pramipexole
Pravastatin
Prazepam
Prazosin
Procarbazine
Promethazine
Propafenone
Propranolol
Propylthiouracil
Protriptyline
Pyridoxine
Pyrilamine
Quazepam
Quetiapine
Quinapril
Quinethazone
Ramipril
Repaglinide
Rifabutin
Risperidone
Ritonavir
Ropinirole
Salmeterol
Saquinavir
Selegiline
Sertraline
Sibutramine
Sildenafil
Simvastatin
Sotalol
Sparfloxacin
Spironolactone
Streptomycin
Sulindac
Sumatriptan
Tacrine
Tacrolimus
Temazepam
Terazosin
Terfenadine
Testosterone
Tetracycline
Thiabendazole
Thiamine
Thioridazine
Thiothixene
Tiagabine
Timolol
Tizanidine
Tobramycin
Tolazamide
Tolbutamide
Tolcapone
Tolterodine
Topiramate
Topotecan
Tramadol
Trandolapril
Tranylcypromine
Trazodone
Triamterene
Triazolam
Trichlormethiazide
Trihexyphenidyl
Trimeprazine
Trimethadione
Trimipramine
Tripelennamine
Triprolidine
Trovafloxacin
Valproic acid
Valsartan
Vancomycin
Venlafaxine
Verapamil
Vinblastine
Vincristine
Vinorelbine
Zalcitabine
Zidovudine
Zolmitriptan
Zolpidem

Pemphigus

Acetaminophen
Aldesleukin
Amoxicillin
Ampicillin
Aspirin
Captopril
Cefadroxil
Cefazolin
Ceftriaxone
Cefuroxime
Cephalexin
Enalapril
Glyburide
Gold
Heroin
Indomethacin
Interferons
Isotretinoin
Levamisole
Levodopa
Meprobamate
Moexipril
Penicillamine
Penicillins
Phenobarbital
Phenytoin
Piroxicam
Propranolol
Ramipril
Rifampin
Tiopronin

Periorbital edema

Aspirin
Cabergoline
Chlorambucil
Clozapine
Diltiazem
Donepezil
Ethosuximide
Famotidine
Foscarnet
Furosemide
Ibuprofen
Indomethacin
Levamisole
Methsuximide
Moricizine
Nifedipine
Phensuximide
Pimozide
Sertraline
Streptokinase
Sulfadoxine
Trovafloxacin
Urokinase
Zolpidem

Peripheral edema

Abciximab
Acyclovir
Aldesleukin
Amantadine
Amlodipine

Benazepril
Bicalutamide
Cabergoline
Carteolol
Carvedilol
Cerivastatin
Chlorpromazine
Cyproheptadine
Delavirdine
Diethylstilbestrol
Diltiazem
Dirithromycin
Divalproex
Dolasetron
Enoxaparin
Etodolac
Felodipine
Fenoprofen
Fluoxetine
Fluphenazine
Foscarnet
Gabapentin
Gemcitabine
GCSF
Grepafloxacin
Guanadrel
Guanfacine
Heparin
Indapamide
Isocarboxazid
Leuprolide
Lisinopril
Loratadine
Meprobamate
Mesalamine
Methyldopa
Methysergide
Metoprolol
Midazolam
Moexipril
Nefazodone
Nicardipine
Nifedipine
Nimodipine
Nisoldipine
Olanzapine
Paroxetine
Pentostatin
Pergolide
Perphenazine
Phenelzine
Pramipexole
Prochlorperazine
Quinapril
Quinestrol
Raloxifene
Reserpine
Ritonavir
Ropinirole
Selegiline
Sertraline
Sibutramine
Sildenafil
Sparfloxacin
Tacrine
Tacrolimus
Tamoxifen
Terazosin
Terbinafine
Thiothixene
Tiagabine
Trifluoperazine
Trimeprazine
Tripelennamine
Troglitazone
Trovafloxacin
Verapamil

Petechiae

Abciximab
Alendronate
Allopurinol
Amitriptyline
Amlodipine
Amoxapine
Amoxicillin
Aspirin
Atorvastatin
Aztreonam
Benactyzine
Carbamazepine
Chlorzoxazone
Cladribine
Clozapine
Danazol
Delavirdine
Desipramine
Diltiazem
Divalproex
Fluconazole
Fluoxetine
Gemcitabine
Gemfibrozil
Griseofulvin
Heparin
Imipramine
Indomethacin
Lamotrigine
Maprotiline
Melphalan
Meprobamate
Mercaptopurine
Methyldopa
Nisoldipine
Nortriptyline
Octreotide
Ofloxacin
Pentostatin
Piroxicam
Plicamycin
Procarbazine
Protriptyline
Simvastatin
Sparfloxacin
Tacrine
Thioguanine
Tiagabine
Ticlopidine
Tizanidine
Trimethadione
Trimipramine
Valproic acid

Peyronie's disease

Acebutolol
Atenolol
Betaxolol
Bisoprolol
Carteolol
Labetalol
Methotrexate
Metoprolol
Nadolol
Penbutolol
Phenytoin
Pindolol
Propranolol
Ropinirole
Timolol

Photoallergic reaction

Chlorothiazide
Enoxacin
Fenofibrate
Hydrochlorothiazide
Ibuprofen
Imipramine
Indomethacin
Itraconazole
Methoxsalen
Nalidixic acid
Pentobarbital
Phenobarbital
Piroxicam
Promazine
Promethazine
Psoralens
Quinethazone
Quinidine
Quinine
Sulfisoxazole
Thioridazine
Tolbutamide
Trioxsalen

Photosensitivity

Acetazolamide
Acetohexamide
Aldesleukin
Allopurinol
Alprazolam
Amantadine
Amiloride
Aminosalicylate sodium
Amiodarone
Amitriptyline
Amoxapine

Astemizole
Atenolol
Atorvastatin
Azatadine
Azathioprine
Azithromycin
Benazepril
Bendroflumethiazide
Benzthiazide
Betaxolol
Bisoprolol
Brompheniramine
Bumetanide
Butabarbital
Butalbital
Captopril
Carbamazepine
Carisoprodol
Carteolol
Cefazolin
Ceftazidime
Cerivastatin
Cetirizine
Chlorambucil
Chlordiazepoxide
Chloroquine
Chlorothiazide
Chlorpromazine
Chlorpropamide
Chlorthalidone
Ciprofloxacin
Clemastine
Clofazimine
Clofibrate
Clomipramine
Clorazepate
Clozapine
Cotrimoxazole
Cromolyn
Cyclamate
Cyclobenzaprine
Cyclothiazide
Cyproheptadine
Dacarbazine
Danazol
Dapsone
Demeclocycline
Desipramine
Diazoxide
Diclofenac
Diflunisal
Diltiazem
Dimenhydrinate
Diphenhydramine
Disopyramide
Divalproex
Docetaxel
Doxepin
Doxycycline
Enalapril
Enoxacin
Epoetin alfa
Estazolam
Ethacrynic acid
Ethambutol
Ethionamide
Etodolac
Felbamate
Fenofibrate
Flucytosine
Fluorouracil
Fluphenazine
Flurbiprofen
Flutamide
Fluvastatin
Fluvoxamine
Fosinopril
Furazolidone
Furosemide
Ganciclovir
Gentamicin
Glimepiride
Glipizide
Glyburide
Gold
Grepafloxacin
Griseofulvin
Haloperidol
Heroin
Hydralazine
Hydrochlorothiazide
Hydroflumethiazide
Hydroxychloroquine
Hydroxyurea
Hydroxyzine
Ibuprofen
Imipramine
Indapamide
Interferons
Isocarboxazid
Isoniazid
Isotretinoin
Kanamycin
Ketoconazole
Ketoprofen
Levofloxacin
Lincomycin
Lisinopril
Lomefloxacin
Loratadine
Losartan
Loxapine
Maprotiline
Meclizine
Meclofenamate
Mefenamic acid
Meprobamate
Mercaptopurine
Mesalamine
Mesoridazine
Metformin
Methazolamide
Methenamine
Methotrexate
Methoxsalen
Methyclothiazide
Methyldopa
Methylphenidate
Metolazone
Minocycline
Mitomycin
Moexipril
Molindone
Nabumetone
Nalidixic acid
Naproxen
Naratriptan
Nefazodone
Nifedipine
Nisoldipine
Nitrofurantoin
Norfloxacin
Nortriptyline
Ofloxacin
Olanzapine
Oral contraceptives
Oxytetracycline
Paroxetine
Pentostatin
Perphenazine
Phenelzine
Phenindamine
Pimozide
Piroxicam
Polythiazide
Pravastatin
Procarbazine
Prochlorperazine
Promazine
Promethazine
Propranolol
Protriptyline
Psoralens
Pyrazinamide
Pyridoxine
Pyrilamine
Pyrimethamine
Quetiapine
Quinacrine
Quinapril
Quinethazone
Quinidine
Quinine
Ramipril
Ranitidine
Risperidone
Ritonavir
Ropinirole
Saccharin
Saquinavir
Selegiline
Sertraline
Sildenafil

Simvastatin
Sotalol
Sparfloxacin
Spironolactone
Streptomycin
Sulfadoxine
Sulfamethoxazole
Sulfasalazine
Sulfisoxazole
Sulindac
Sumatriptan
Tacrolimus
Terbinafine
Terfenadine
Tetracycline
Thioguanine
Thiothixene
Tiagabine
Timolol
Tiopronin
Tolazamide
Tolbutamide
Topiramate
Torsemide
Tranylcypromine
Trazodone
Triamterene
Triazolam
Trichlormethiazide
Trifluoperazine
Trimeprazine
Trimethadione
Trimetrexate
Trimipramine
Trioxsalen
Tripelennamine
Triprolidine
Trovafloxacin
Valproic acid
Venlafaxine
Verapamil
Vinblastine
Vitamin A
Zalcitabine
Zolmitriptan
Zolpidem

Phototoxic reaction

Alprazolam
Captopril
Cetirizine
Chlorpromazine
Ciprofloxacin
Demeclocycline
Doxycycline
Enoxacin
Fenofibrate
Fluorouracil
Fluoxetine
Furosemide
Grepafloxacin
Hydrochlorothiazide
Itraconazole
Lomefloxacin
Methoxsalen
Nabumetone
Naproxen
Norfloxacin
Nortriptyline
Ofloxacin
Oxaprozin
Prochlorperazine
Promazine
Propranolol
Protriptyline
Psoralens
Sparfloxacin
Sulfisoxazole
Sulindac
Terazosin
Tetracycline
Thioridazine
Trioxsalen
Vinblastine

Pigmentation

Amiodarone
Amitriptyline
Azathioprine
Betaxolol
Bisoprolol
Bleomycin
Busulfan
Captopril
Carbidopa
Carboplatin
Carmustine
Carteolol
Cerivastatin
Chloroquine
Chlorpromazine
Cisplatin
Clofazimine
Clomipramine
Corticosteroids
Cyclophosphamide
Dactinomycin
Dapsone
Daunorubicin
Deferoxamine
Demeclocycline
Desipramine
Diazepam
Dicumarol
Donepezil
Doxorubicin
Doxycycline
Esmolol
Etoposide
Fluorouracil
Fluoxetine
Fluphenazine
Fluvoxamine
Foscarnet
Ganciclovir
Gold
Griseofulvin
Haloperidol
Heroin
Hydroxychloroquine
Hydroxyurea
Ifosfamide
Imipramine
Insulin
Ketoconazole
Ketoprofen
Labetalol
Leuprolide
Lidocaine
Loxapine
Mephenytoin
Mercaptopurine
Mesoridazine
Methamphetamine
Methimazole
Methotrexate
Methoxsalen
Methyldopa
Minocycline
Mitomycin
Molindone
Nisoldipine
Ofloxacin
Olanzapine
Oral contraceptives
Oxytetracycline
Paroxetine
Pentostatin
Perphenazine
Phenazopyridine
Phenolphthalein
Phenytoin
Procarbazine
Prochlorperazine
Promazine
Propylthiouracil
Psoralens
Pyrimethamine
Quinacrine
Quinidine
Quinine
Rifabutin
Risperidone
Ropinirole
Sparfloxacin
Spironolactone
Sulfasalazine
Tetracycline
Thioridazine
Thiothixene
Tiagabine
Timolol
Tolcapone
Topiramate
Toremifene

Trifluoperazine
Trioxsalen
Vinorelbine
Vitamin A
Zidovudine

Pityriasis rosea

Acetaminophen
Ampicillin
Aspirin
Captopril
Clonidine
Codeine
Corticosteroids
Cortisone
Dexfenfluramine
Gold
Griseofulvin
Isotretinoin
Meprobamate
Metronidazole
Mitomycin
Naproxen
Omeprazole
Penicillins
Terbinafine
Tiopronin
Tripelennamine

Pruritus

Abciximab
Acebutolol
Acetaminophen
Acetazolamide
Acetohexamide
Acitretin
Acyclovir
Albendazole
Albuterol
Aldesleukin
Alendronate
Allopurinol
Alprazolam
Altretamine
Amantadine
Amikacin
Amiloride
Aminocaproic acid
Aminoglutethimide
Aminophylline
Aminosalicylate sodium
Amiodarone
Amitriptyline
Amlodipine
Amoxapine
Amoxicillin
Amphotericin B
Ampicillin
Apraclonidine
Asparaginase
Aspartame
Aspirin
Astemizole
Atenolol
Atorvastatin
Atovaquone
Atropine sulfate
Aztreonam
Benactyzine
Benazepril
Bendroflumethiazide
Benztropine
Betaxolol
Bisoprolol
Bleomycin
Bromfenac
Bumetanide
Buspirone
Butabarbital
Butalbital
Butorphanol
Cabergoline
Calcitonin
Captopril
Carbamazepine
Carbenicillin
Carbidopa
Carboplatin
Carisoprodol
Carteolol
Carvedilol
Cefaclor
Cefadroxil
Cefamandole
Cefazolin
Cefdinir
Cefepime
Cefixime
Cefotaxime
Cefoxitin
Cefpodoxime
Ceftazidime
Ceftibuten
Ceftriaxone
Cefuroxime
Cephalexin
Cephalothin
Cephradine
Cerivastatin
Cetirizine
Chloral hydrate
Chlorambucil
Chloramphenicol
Chlordiazepoxide
Chlormezanone
Chloroquine
Chlorothiazide
Chlorpromazine
Chlorpropamide
Chlorzoxazone
Cimetidine
Ciprofloxacin
Cisapride
Cisplatin
Cladribine
Clarithromycin
Clindamycin
Clofazimine
Clofibrate
Clomiphene
Clomipramine
Clonazepam
Clonidine
Clopidogrel
Clorazepate
Cloxacillin
Clozapine
Codeine
Colchicine
Corticosteroids
Cotrimoxazole
Cromolyn
Cyanocobalamin
Cyclamate
Cyclobenzaprine
Cyclophosphamide
Cycloserine
Cyclosporine
Cytarabine
Dactinomycin
Dalteparin
Danazol
Dantrolene
Dapsone
Deferoxamine
Delavirdine
Demeclocycline
Desipramine
Dexfenfluramine
Diazepam
Diazoxide
Diclofenac
Dicloxacillin
Dicumarol
Dicyclomine
Didanosine
Diethylpropion
Diethylstilbestrol
Diflunisal
Digoxin
Diltiazem
Diphenhydramine
Diphenoxylate
Dipyridamole
Dirithromycin
Disopyramide
Divalproex
Docetaxel
Donepezil
Dopamine
Doxapram
Doxazosin
Doxepin
Doxorubicin
Enalapril

Epoetin alfa
Ergocalciferol
Erythromycin
Estazolam
Estramustine
Ethambutol
Ethchlorvynol
Ethosuximide
Etidronate
Etodolac
Etoposide
Famciclovir
Famotidine
Felbamate
Felodipine
Fenfluramine
Fenofibrate
Fenoprofen
Fentanyl
Flecainide
Fluconazole
Flucytosine
Fluorouracil
Fluoxetine
Fluoxymesterone
Fluphenazine
Flurazepam
Flurbiprofen
Fluvastatin
Fluvoxamine
Folic acid
Foscarnet
Fosfomycin
Fosinopril
Furazolidone
Furosemide
Gabapentin
Ganciclovir
Gemcitabine
Gemfibrozil
Gentamicin
Glimepiride
Glipizide
Glyburide
Gold
GCSF
Grepafloxacin
Griseofulvin
Guanabenz
Guanfacine
Haloperidol
Heparin
Heroin
Hydralazine
Hydrochlorothiazide
Hydromorphone
Hydroxychloroquine
Hydroxyurea
Ibuprofen
Imipenem/cilastatin
Imipramine
Indapamide
Indinavir
Indomethacin
Insulin
Interferons
Ipodate
Ipratropium
Irbesartan
Isocarboxazid
Isoniazid
Isoproterenol
Isosorbide
Isotretinoin
Isradipine
Itraconazole
Ivermectin
Kanamycin
Ketoconazole
Ketoprofen
Ketorolac
Labetalol
Lamotrigine
Lansoprazole
Latanoprost
Letrozole
Leuprolide
Levamisole
Levobunolol
Levofloxacin
Levothyroxine
Lidocaine
Lincomycin
Lisinopril
Lithium
Lomefloxacin
Loracarbef
Loratadine
Lorazepam
Losartan
Lovastatin
Loxapine
Maprotiline
Marihuana
Mechlorethamine
Meclofenamate
Medroxyprogesterone
Mefenamic acid
Mefloquine
Melphalan
Meperidine
Mephenytoin
Meprobamate
Mercaptopurine
Mesalamine
Mesna
Mesoridazine
Metaxalone
Metformin
Methadone
Methenamine
Methicillin
Methimazole
Methocarbamol
Methotrexate
Methoxsalen
Methsuximide
Methyldopa
Methyltestosterone
Methysergide
Metolazone
Metoprolol
Metronidazole
Mexiletine
Mezlocillin
Miconazole
Midazolam
Minocycline
Minoxidil
Mitomycin
Mitotane
Moexipril
Molindone
Moricizine
Nabumetone
Nadolol
Nafarelin
Nafcillin
Nalidixic acid
Naloxone
Naproxen
Nefazodone
Nelfinavir
Neomycin
Niacin; niacinamide
Nifedipine
Nimodipine
Nisoldipine
Nitrofurantoin
Nizatidine
Norfloxacin
Nortriptyline
Nystatin
Octreotide
Ofloxacin
Olanzapine
Olsalazine
Omeprazole
Ondansetron
Oral contraceptives
Orphenadrine
Oxacillin
Oxaprozin
Oxazepam
Oxytetracycline
Paramethadione
Paroxetine
Penbutolol
Penicillamine
Penicillins
Pentagastrin
Pentamidine
Pentazocine

Pentobarbital
Pentostatin
Pentoxifylline
Pergolide
Perphenazine
Phenazopyridine
Phenelzine
Phenobarbital
Phenolphthalein
Phensuximide
Phenytoin
Pimozide
Pindolol
Piperacillin
Piroxicam
Pramipexole
Pravastatin
Prazepam
Prazosin
Primaquine
Probenecid
Procainamide
Procarbazine
Prochlorperazine
Progestins
Propafenone
Propofol
Propoxyphene
Propranolol
Propylthiouracil
Protriptyline
Psoralens
Pyrazinamide
Pyrimethamine
Quazepam
Quinacrine
Quinapril
Quinethazone
Quinidine
Quinine
Ramipril
Ranitidine
Reserpine
Rifampin
Risperidone
Ritonavir
Ropinirole
Saccharin
Salmeterol
Salsalate
Sertraline
Sibutramine
Sildenafil
Simvastatin
Sotalol
Sparfloxacin
Spectinomycin
Spironolactone
Streptokinase
Streptomycin
Streptozocin
Succinylcholine
Sucralfate
Sulfadoxine
Sulfamethoxazole
Sulfasalazine
Sulfisoxazole
Sulindac
Sumatriptan
Tacrine
Tacrolimus
Tamoxifen
Temazepam
Terazosin
Terbinafine
Terbutaline
Terfenadine
Testosterone
Tetracycline
Thalidomide
Thiabendazole
Thiamine
Thioguanine
Thiopental
Thiotepa
Thiothixene
Tiagabine
Ticarcillin
Ticlopidine
Timolol
Tiopronin
Tizanidine
Tobramycin
Tolazamide
Tolbutamide
Tolcapone
Tolmetin
Tolterodine
Topiramate
Toremifene
Tramadol
Trandolapril
Tranylcypromine
Trazodone
Triamterene
Triazolam
Trifluoperazine
Trimeprazine
Trimethadione
Trimetrexate
Trimipramine
Trioxsalen
Troleandomycin
Trovafloxacin
Urokinase
Ursodiol
Valproic acid
Valsartan
Vancomycin
Venlafaxine
Verapamil
Vincristine
Vitamin A
Warfarin
Zalcitabine
Zidovudine
Zileuton
Zolmitriptan
Zolpidem

Pruritus ani

Aspartame
Cefazolin
Clindamycin
Demeclocycline
Doxycycline
Foscarnet
Lincomycin
Tetracycline
Trovafloxacin

Pseudolymphoma

Alprazolam
Amitriptyline
Atenolol
Carbamazepine
Cefixime
Chlorpromazine
Cimetidine
Clarithromycin
Clonazepam
Cotrimoxazole
Cyclosporine
Desipramine
Diltiazem
Doxepin
Fluoxetine
Furosemide
Gemfibrozil
Gold
Lamotrigine
Lithium
Lorazepam
Methotrexate
Nizatidine
Perphenazine
Phenytoin
Ranitidine
Sulfamethoxazole
Sulfasalazine
Terfenadine
Thioridazine

Psoriasis

Acebutolol
Acitretin
Aldesleukin
Amiodarone
Amoxicillin
Ampicillin
Aspirin
Atenolol
Betaxolol
Bisoprolol
Captopril
Carbamazepine

Carteolol
Carvedilol
Chlorambucil
Chloroquine
Chlorthalidone
Cimetidine
Clarithromycin
Clomipramine
Clonidine
Cotrimoxazole
Cyclosporine
Dexfenfluramine
Diclofenac
Digoxin
Diltiazem
Dipyridamole
Doxycycline
Enalapril
Flecainide
Fluoxetine
Fluoxymesterone
Foscarnet
Ganciclovir
Gemfibrozil
Glimepiride
Glipizide
Glyburide
Gold
GCSF
Hydroxychloroquine
Ibuprofen
Indomethacin
Interferons
Ketoprofen
Labetalol
Letrozole
Levamisole
Lithium
Meclofenamate
Mesalamine
Methyltestosterone
Metoprolol
Nadolol
Omeprazole
Oral contraceptives
Penbutolol
Penicillamine
Pentostatin
Pindolol
Primaquine
Propranolol
Psoralens
Quinidine
Quinine
Ranitidine
Risperidone
Ritonavir
Ropinirole
Sotalol
Sulfamethoxazole
Sulfasalazine
Tacrine
Terbinafine
Terfenadine
Testosterone
Tetracycline
Thiabendazole
Tiagabine
Timolol
Trazodone
Valproic acid
Venlafaxine

Purpura

Acetaminophen
Acetazolamide
Acitretin
Aldesleukin
Allopurinol
Alprazolam
Alteplase
Amiloride
Aminocaproic acid
Aminoglutethimide
Aminosalicylate sodium
Amiodarone
Amitriptyline
Amlodipine
Amobarbital
Amoxapine
Amphotericin B
Ampicillin
Aprobarbital
Aspartame
Aspirin
Atenolol
Azatadine
Azathioprine
Aztreonam
Bendroflumethiazide
Benzthiazide
Betaxolol
Bisoprolol
Bromocriptine
Bumetanide
Buspirone
Busulfan
Butabarbital
Butalbital
Captopril
Carbamazepine
Carbenicillin
Carbidopa
Carteolol
Cefaclor
Cefamandole
Cefdinir
Cefoxitin
Ceftriaxone
Cefuroxime
Cephalexin
Cephalothin
Cephradine
Cerivastatin
Cetirizine
Chloral hydrate
Chlorambucil
Chloramphenicol
Chlordiazepoxide
Chlorothiazide
Chlorpromazine
Chlorpropamide
Chlorthalidone
Cimetidine
Ciprofloxacin
Cladribine
Clemastine
Clindamycin
Clofibrate
Clomiphene
Clomipramine
Clonazepam
Clopidogrel
Clorazepate
Clozapine
Colchicine
Corticosteroids
Cortisone
Cotrimoxazole
Cyclobenzaprine
Cyclophosphamide
Cyclosporine
Cyclothiazide
Cyproheptadine
Danazol
Dapsone
Deferoxamine
Delavirdine
Demeclocycline
Desipramine
Dexfenfluramine
Diazepam
Diazoxide
Diclofenac
Dicumarol
Didanosine
Diethylpropion
Diethylstilbestrol
Diflunisal
Digoxin
Diltiazem
Diphenhydramine
Dipyridamole
Disopyramide
Disulfiram
Dolasetron
Doxazosin
Doxepin
Doxorubicin
Doxycycline
Enalapril
Enoxacin
Ephedrine
Estazolam

Estramustine
Ethacrynic acid
Ethambutol
Ethchlorvynol
Ethionamide
Ethosuximide
Ethotoin
Etodolac
Etoposide
Famotidine
Felbamate
Felodipine
Fenoprofen
Fluconazole
Flucytosine
Fluoxetine
Fluoxymesterone
Fluphenazine
Flurazepam
Flurbiprofen
Fluvastatin
Fluvoxamine
Furosemide
Gabapentin
Ganciclovir
Gentamicin
Glipizide
Glyburide
Gold
Griseofulvin
Guanethidine
Guanfacine
Haloperidol
Heparin
Heroin
Hydralazine
Hydrochlorothiazide
Hydroflumethiazide
Hydroxychloroquine
Hydroxyurea
Hydroxyzine
Ibuprofen
Imipramine
Indapamide
Indomethacin
Insulin
Interferons
Ipodate
Isoniazid
Itraconazole
Ketoconazole
Ketoprofen
Ketorolac
Labetalol
Leuprolide
Levamisole
Levodopa
Levofloxacin
Lidocaine
Lincomycin
Lisinopril
Lithium
Lomefloxacin
Loratadine
Lorazepam
Losartan
Loxapine
Maprotiline
Mechlorethamine
Meclofenamate
Mefenamic acid
Melphalan
Mephenytoin
Mephobarbital
Meprobamate
Mercaptopurine
Metformin
Methadone
Methazolamide
Methimazole
Methotrexate
Methoxsalen
Methsuximide
Methyclothiazide
Methyldopa
Methylphenidate
Methyltestosterone
Metolazone
Metoprolol
Mexiletine
Miconazole
Minocycline
Mitomycin
Nalidixic acid
Naproxen
Naratriptan
Nifedipine
Nimodipine
Nitrofurantoin
Nitroglycerin
Nortriptyline
Octreotide
Ofloxacin
Omeprazole
Oral contraceptives
Oxaprozin
Oxazepam
Oxytetracycline
Paroxetine
Penbutolol
Penicillamine
Penicillins
Pentagastrin
Pentamidine
Pentobarbital
Pentostatin
Pentoxifylline
Perphenazine
Phenindamine
Phenobarbital
Phensuximide
Phentermine
Phenytoin
Pindolol
Piroxicam
Plicamycin
Polythiazide
Pravastatin
Prazepam
Procainamide
Procarbazine
Prochlorperazine
Promazine
Promethazine
Propafenone
Propranolol
Propylthiouracil
Protriptyline
Pyrazinamide
Pyridoxine
Pyrilamine
Pyrimethamine
Quazepam
Quinethazone
Quinidine
Quinine
Ramipril
Ranitidine
Reserpine
Rifampin
Risperidone
Ropinirole
Salsalate
Secobarbital
Sertraline
Simvastatin
Sparfloxacin
Spironolactone
Streptokinase
Streptomycin
Streptozocin
Sulfadoxine
Sulfamethoxazole
Sulfasalazine
Sulfinpyrazone
Sulfisoxazole
Sulindac
Tacrine
Tacrolimus
Tamoxifen
Temazepam
Terfenadine
Tetracycline
Thalidomide
Thiamine
Thioguanine
Thiopental
Thioridazine
Ticlopidine
Timolol
Tizanidine
Tobramycin
Tolazamide

Tolbutamide
Tolmetin
Topiramate
Topotecan
Torsemide
Trazodone
Triamterene
Triazolam
Trichlormethiazide
Trifluoperazine
Trimeprazine
Trimethadione
Trimipramine
Tripelennamine
Triprolidine
Urokinase
Valproic acid
Vancomycin
Vasopressin
Verapamil
Vinblastine
Warfarin
Zidovudine
Zolpidem

Pustular psoriasis
Acetazolamide
Aminoglutethimide
Amiodarone
Amoxicillin
Ampicillin
Aspirin
Atenolol
Chloroquine
Cimetidine
Corticosteroids
Cyclosporine
Diclofenac
Diltiazem
Hydroxychloroquine
Indomethacin
Lithium
Methicillin
Penicillins
Potassium iodide
Propranolol
Terbinafine

Radiation recall
Bleomycin
Buspirone
Codeine
Cotrimoxazole
Dactinomycin
Doxorubicin
Etoposide
Fluorouracil
Hydroxyurea
Idarubicin
Mercaptopurine
Methotrexate
Simvastatin
Sulfamethoxazole
Tamoxifen
Vinblastine

Raynaud's phenomenon
Acebutolol
Amphotericin B
Atenolol
Azathioprine
Betaxolol
Bisoprolol
Bleomycin
Bromocriptine
Carteolol
Cisplatin
Clonidine
Cyclosporine
Dopamine
Doxorubicin
Ethosuximide
Gemfibrozil
Interferons
Labetalol
Methysergide
Metoprolol
Minocycline
Nadolol
Octreotide
Phentermine
Pindolol
Propranolol
Sotalol
Spironolactone
Sulfasalazine
Sulindac
Thiothixene
Timolol
Vinblastine
Vincristine

Scleroderma
Aldesleukin
Azathioprine
Bleomycin
Bromocriptine
Carbidopa
Cocaine
Dapsone
Diethylpropion
Docetaxel
Heparin
Medroxyprogesterone
Mephenytoin
Methoxsalen
Methysergide
Metoprolol
Penicillamine
Pentazocine
Phenytoin
Phytonadione
Psoralens
Sotalol
Trioxsalen
Valproic acid

Seborrhea
Acitretin
Atorvastatin
Bromfenac
Cetirizine
Clomipramine
Danazol
Delavirdine
Divalproex
Doxycycline
Fluoxetine
Fluoxymesterone
Fluphenazine
Flurbiprofen
Fluvoxamine
Foscarnet
Gemfibrozil
Indinavir
Loxapine
Mesoridazine
Methyltestosterone
Nafarelin
Olanzapine
Oral contraceptives
Pentostatin
Pergolide
Risperidone
Ritonavir
Tacrine
Testosterone
Tolcapone
Topiramate
Trovafloxacin

Seborrheic dermatitis
Buspirone
Chlorpromazine
Cimetidine
Ethionamide
Fluorouracil
Fluoxymesterone
Gold
Griseofulvin
Haloperidol
Interferons
Lithium
Methoxsalen
Methyldopa
Methyltestosterone
Psoralens
Saquinavir
Stanozolol
Testosterone
Thiothixene
Trioxsalen

Serum sickness
Amobarbital
Amoxicillin
Ampicillin
Aprobarbital
Asparaginase
Carbenicillin

Cefaclor
Cefadroxil
Cefamandole
Cefazolin
Cefixime
Cefoxitin
Cefpodoxime
Ceftazidime
Ceftriaxone
Cefuroxime
Cephalexin
Cephalothin
Cephradine
Ciprofloxacin
Cloxacillin
Cotrimoxazole
Cromolyn
Diclofenac
Dicloxacillin
Fluoxetine
Furazolidone
Griseofulvin
Heroin
Ibuprofen
Indomethacin
Isoniazid
Lincomycin
Meclofenamate
Mephobarbital
Methicillin
Methimazole
Metronidazole
Mezlocillin
Minocycline
Nafcillin
Nizatidine
Ofloxacin
Oxacillin
Penicillamine
Penicillins
Pentoxifylline
Phenytoin
Piperacillin
Piroxicam
Propranolol
Rifampin
Secobarbital
Sparfloxacin
Streptokinase
Sulfamethoxazole
Sulfasalazine
Sulfisoxazole
Sulindac
Terbinafine
Tetracycline
Ticarcillin
Ticlopidine
Tolmetin
Verapamil

Sialorrhea

Acitretin
Alprazolam
Amiodarone
Amitriptyline
Amoxapine
Betaxolol
Bethanechol
Buspirone
Cetirizine
Chlordiazepoxide
Clomipramine
Clonazepam
Clorazepate
Clozapine
Delavirdine
Diazepam
Diazoxide
Edrophonium
Estazolam
Ethionamide
Etodolac
Fluoxetine
Fluphenazine
Flurazepam
Fluvoxamine
Gabapentin
Gentamicin
Guanabenz
Guanethidine
Guanfacine
Haloperidol
Ifosfamide
Imipenem/cilastatin
Kanamycin
Ketamine
Ketoprofen
Lamotrigine
Levodopa
Lithium
Loratadine
Lorazepam
Maprotiline
Mesoridazine
Methohexital
Midazolam
Molindone
Nefazodone
Olanzapine
Oxazepam
Paroxetine
Pentoxifylline
Perphenazine
Pimozide
Potassium iodide
Pramipexole
Prazepam
Propofol
Quazepam
Quetiapine
Ramipril
Risperidone
Ropinirole
Sertraline
Succinylcholine
Tacrine
Temazepam
Thiothixene
Tiagabine
Tobramycin
Tolcapone
Trazodone
Triazolam
Trovafloxacin
Valproic acid
Venlafaxine

Stevens-Johnson syndrome

Acetaminophen
Acetazolamide
Acyclovir
Albendazole
Allopurinol
Aminophylline
Amiodarone
Amobarbital
Amoxicillin
Ampicillin
Aprobarbital
Aspirin
Astemizole
Atropine sulfate
Bleomycin
Butabarbital
Butalbital
Captopril
Carbamazepine
Carbenicillin
Carvedilol
Cefaclor
Cefadroxil
Cefamandole
Cefazolin
Cefdinir
Cefepime
Cefixime
Cefpodoxime
Ceftazidime
Ceftriaxone
Cefuroxime
Cephalexin
Cephradine
Cerivastatin
Chlorambucil
Chloramphenicol
Chlormezanone
Chloroquine
Chlorothiazide
Chlorpropamide
Cimetidine
Ciprofloxacin
Cisplatin
Clarithromycin
Clindamycin
Clofibrate

Cloxacillin
Clozapine
Cotrimoxazole
Cyclophosphamide
Cycloserine
Danazol
Dapsone
Delavirdine
Dexfenfluramine
Diclofenac
Dicloxacillin
Didanosine
Diflunisal
Diltiazem
Dipyridamole
Divalproex
Doxycycline
Enalapril
Enoxacin
Erythromycin
Ethambutol
Ethosuximide
Etidronate
Etodolac
Etoposide
Felbamate
Fenoprofen
Fluconazole
Fluoxetine
Flurbiprofen
Fluvastatin
Fluvoxamine
Furosemide
Ganciclovir
Griseofulvin
Ibuprofen
Indapamide
Indomethacin
Isoniazid
Itraconazole
Ketoprofen
Ketorolac
Lamotrigine
Levofloxacin
Lidocaine
Lincomycin
Lomefloxacin
Lorazepam
Lovastatin
Maprotiline
Mechlorethamine
Meclofenamate
Mefenamic acid
Mefloquine
Mephenytoin
Mephobarbital
Meprobamate
Methazolamide
Methicillin
Methotrexate
Methsuximide
Methyclothiazide
Methyldopa
Mexiletine
Mezlocillin
Minocycline
Minoxidil
Nabumetone
Nafcillin
Naproxen
Nevirapine
Nifedipine
Nitrofurantoin
Norfloxacin
Nystatin
Ofloxacin
Omeprazole
Oral contraceptives
Oxacillin
Oxaprozin
Penicillamine
Penicillins
Pentamidine
Pentobarbital
Phenobarbital
Phenolphthalein
Phensuximide
Phenytoin
Piperacillin
Piroxicam
Pravastatin
Promethazine
Propranolol
Pyrimethamine
Quinine
Rifampin
Ritonavir
Secobarbital
Simvastatin
Sparfloxacin
Streptomycin
Sulfadoxine
Sulfamethoxazole
Sulfasalazine
Sulfisoxazole
Sulindac
Terbinafine
Tetracycline
Thiabendazole
Thiopental
Ticarcillin
Ticlopidine
Tolmetin
Torsemide
Trimethadione
Valproic acid
Vancomycin
Verapamil
Vitamin A
Zidovudine

Stomatitis

Acitretin
Aldesleukin
Allopurinol
Amitriptyline
Amoxapine
Amoxicillin
Ampicillin
Atorvastatin
Azathioprine
Azelastine
Benactyzine
Bleomycin
Bromfenac
Busulfan
Carbamazepine
Carbenicillin
Carboplatin
Carmustine
Cefdinir
Cetirizine
Chloral hydrate
Chlorambucil
Chloramphenicol
Chloroquine
Ciprofloxacin
Clarithromycin
Clofibrate
Clomipramine
Cloxacillin
Cotrimoxazole
Cyclobenzaprine
Cyclophosphamide
Cyclosporine
Cytarabine
Dacarbazine
Dactinomycin
Daunorubicin
Delavirdine
Desipramine
Diclofenac
Dicloxacillin
Diflunisal
Divalproex
Docetaxel
Doxepin
Doxorubicin
Enalapril
Enoxacin
Ethionamide
Etodolac
Etoposide
Fenoprofen
Fluorouracil
Fluoxetine
Fluoxymesterone
Fluvoxamine
Foscarnet
Gabapentin
Gemcitabine
Gentamicin
Gold
GCSF

Grepafloxacin
Hydroxyurea
Ibuprofen
Idarubicin
Ifosfamide
Imipramine
Interferons
Ipratropium
Ketoprofen
Ketorolac
Lamotrigine
Lansoprazole
Levamisole
Lidocaine
Lincomycin
Lithium
Lomustine
Loratadine
Lovastatin
Maprotiline
Meclofenamate
Melphalan
Mephenytoin
Meprobamate
Mercaptopurine
Methenamine
Methicillin
Methotrexate
Methyltestosterone
Metronidazole
Mezlocillin
Mitomycin
Nabumetone
Nafcillin
Naproxen
Nefazodone
Norfloxacin
Nortriptyline
Olanzapine
Olsalazine
Oxacillin
Oxaprozin
Pamidronate
Paroxetine
Penicillamine
Pentostatin
Piroxicam
Plicamycin
Pravastatin
Procarbazine
Protriptyline
Pyrilamine
Quetiapine
Rifampin
Rimantadine
Risperidone
Ropinirole
Saquinavir
Sertraline
Sildenafil
Sparfloxacin
Streptokinase
Streptomycin
Sulfadoxine
Sulfamethoxazole
Sulfasalazine
Sulfisoxazole
Sulindac
Tacrine
Terbinafine
Terfenadine
Testosterone
Thioguanine
Thiotepa
Tiagabine
Ticarcillin
Tiopronin
Tolmetin
Topiramate
Topotecan
Tramadol
Triazolam
Trimeprazine
Trimetrexate
Trimipramine
Tripelennamine
Trovafloxacin
Ursodiol
Valproic acid
Venlafaxine
Vinblastine
Vinorelbine
Zalcitabine

Telangiectases

Amlodipine
Carmustine
Corticosteroids
Felodipine
Hydroxyurea
Interferons
Isocarboxazid
Isotretinoin
Lithium
Methotrexate
Methysergide
Nifedipine
Oral contraceptives
Phenelzine
Progestins
Thiothixene

Toxic epidermal necrolysis

Acebutolol
Acetaminophen
Acetazolamide
Aldesleukin
Allopurinol
Alprostadil
Aminosalicylate sodium
Amiodarone
Amobarbital
Amoxapine
Amoxicillin
Ampicillin
Asparaginase
Aspirin
Atenolol
Atorvastatin
Azathioprine
Aztreonam
Betaxolol
Butabarbital
Butalbital
Captopril
Carbamazepine
Carbenicillin
Cefaclor
Cefadroxil
Cefamandole
Cefazolin
Cefdinir
Cefepime
Cefoxitin
Cefpodoxime
Ceftazidime
Ceftibuten
Cefuroxime
Cephalexin
Cephalothin
Cephradine
Cerivastatin
Chlorambucil
Chloramphenicol
Chlormezanone
Chloroquine
Chlorothiazide
Chlorpromazine
Chlorpropamide
Chlorthalidone
Cimetidine
Ciprofloxacin
Cladribine
Clindamycin
Clofibrate
Codeine
Colchicine
Cotrimoxazole
Cyclophosphamide
Cyclosporine
Cytarabine
Dactinomycin
Dapsone
Deferoxamine
Demeclocycline
Dextroamphetamine
Diclofenac
Diflunisal
Diltiazem
Diphenhydramine
Dipyridamole
Disulfiram
Divalproex
Doxycycline
Enalapril

Enoxacin
Erythromycin
Ethambutol
Etidronate
Etodolac
Famotidine
Felbamate
Fenoprofen
Fluconazole
Fluoxetine
Fluphenazine
Flurbiprofen
Flutamide
Fluvastatin
Fluvoxamine
Foscarnet
Gentamicin
Gold
Grepafloxacin
Griseofulvin
Heparin
Heroin
Hydrochlorothiazide
Hydroxychloroquine
Ibuprofen
Imipenem/cilastatin
Indapamide
Indomethacin
Isoniazid
Isotretinoin
Ketoprofen
Ketorolac
Lamotrigine
Lovastatin
Meclofenamate
Mefenamic acid
Mefloquine
Meperidine
Mephenytoin
Meprobamate
Mercaptopurine
Methazolamide
Methotrexate
Methyldopa
Metolazone
Metoprolol
Metronidazole
Nabumetone
Nadolol
Nalidixic acid
Naproxen
Neomycin
Nifedipine
Nitrofurantoin
Norfloxacin
Ofloxacin
Omeprazole
Paroxetine
Penicillamine
Penicillins
Pentamidine
Pentazocine
Pentobarbital
Phenobarbital
Phenolphthalein
Phenytoin
Pindolol
Piroxicam
Plicamycin
Pravastatin
Primidone
Procarbazine
Prochlorperazine
Promethazine
Propranolol
Pyridoxine
Pyrimethamine
Quinidine
Quinine
Ranitidine
Reserpine
Rifampin
Simvastatin
Sparfloxacin
Streptomycin
Streptozocin
Sulfadoxine
Sulfamethoxazole
Sulfasalazine
Sulfisoxazole
Sulindac
Terbinafine
Tetracycline
Thiabendazole
Thiopental
Thioridazine
Timolol
Tiopronin
Tolbutamide
Tolmetin
Valproic acid
Vancomycin
Vinorelbine
Zidovudine

Urticaria

Acebutolol
Acetaminophen
Acetazolamide
Acetohexamide
Acitretin
Acyclovir
Albendazole
Albuterol
Aldesleukin
Allopurinol
Alprazolam
Alteplase
Amantadine
Amikacin
Amiloride
Aminocaproic acid
Aminoglutethimide
Aminophylline
Aminosalicylate sodium
Amiodarone
Amitriptyline
Amlodipine
Amobarbital
Amoxapine
Amoxicillin
Amphotericin B
Ampicillin
Aprobarbital
Asparaginase
Aspartame
Aspirin
Astemizole
Atenolol
Atorvastatin
Atropine sulfate
Azatadine
Azathioprine
Azithromycin
Aztreonam
Benactyzine
Benazepril
Bendroflumethiazide
Benzthiazide
Benztropine
Betaxolol
Biperiden
Bisacodyl
Bisoprolol
Bleomycin
Bromfenac
Bromocriptine
Bumetanide
Buspirone
Busulfan
Butabarbital
Butalbital
Butorphanol
Calcitonin
Captopril
Carbamazepine
Carbenicillin
Carbidopa
Carboplatin
Carisoprodol
Cefaclor
Cefadroxil
Cefamandole
Cefazolin
Cefepime
Cefixime
Cefotaxime
Cefoxitin
Ceftazidime
Ceftibuten
Ceftriaxone
Cefuroxime
Cephalexin
Cephalothin

Cephradine
Cerivastatin
Cetirizine
Chloral hydrate
Chlorambucil
Chloramphenicol
Chlordiazepoxide
Chlormezanone
Chloroquine
Chlorothiazide
Chlorotrianisene
Chlorpromazine
Chlorpropamide
Chlorthalidone
Chlorzoxazone
Cholestyramine
Cimetidine
Ciprofloxacin
Cisapride
Cisplatin
Clarithromycin
Clemastine
Clidinium
Clindamycin
Clofazimine
Clofibrate
Clomiphene
Clomipramine
Clonazepam
Clonidine
Clopidogrel
Clorazepate
Cloxacillin
Clozapine
Codeine
Colchicine
Colestipol
Corticosteroids
Cortisone
Cotrimoxazole
Cromolyn
Cyanocobalamin
Cyclamate
Cyclobenzaprine
Cyclophosphamide
Cycloserine
Cyclosporine
Cyclothiazide
Cyproheptadine
Cytarabine
Dacarbazine
Dactinomycin
Danazol
Dantrolene
Dapsone
Daunorubicin
Deferoxamine
Delavirdine
Demeclocycline
Desipramine
Dexfenfluramine
Dextroamphetamine
Diazepam
Diazoxide
Diclofenac
Dicloxacillin
Dicumarol
Dicyclomine
Didanosine
Diethylpropion
Diethylstilbestrol
Diflunisal
Digoxin
Diltiazem
Dimenhydrinate
Diphenhydramine
Diphenoxylate
Dipyridamole
Dirithromycin
Disopyramide
Disulfiram
Docetaxel
Dolasetron
Donepezil
Dopamine
Doxazosin
Doxepin
Doxorubicin
Doxycycline
Enalapril
Enoxacin
Enoxaparin
Ephedrine
Epinephrine
Epoetin alfa
Erythromycin
Estazolam
Estramustine
Ethacrynic acid
Ethambutol
Ethchlorvynol
Ethionamide
Ethosuximide
Etidronate
Etodolac
Etoposide
Famotidine
Felbamate
Felodipine
Fenfluramine
Fenofibrate
Fenoprofen
Fentanyl
Finasteride
Flavoxate
Flecainide
Fluconazole
Flucytosine
Fluorouracil
Fluoxetine
Fluoxymesterone
Fluphenazine
Flurazepam
Flurbiprofen
Flutamide
Fluvastatin
Fluvoxamine
Folic acid
Foscarnet
Fosinopril
Furazolidone
Furosemide
Gabapentin
Ganciclovir
Gemfibrozil
Gentamicin
Glimepiride
Glipizide
Glucagon
Glyburide
Gold
Granisetron
GCSF
Grepafloxacin
Griseofulvin
Guanethidine
Guanfacine
Haloperidol
Halothane
Heparin
Heroin
Hydralazine
Hydrochlorothiazide
Hydroflumethiazide
Hydromorphone
Hydroxychloroquine
Hydroxyurea
Hydroxyzine
Ibuprofen
Idarubicin
Imipenem/cilastatin
Imipramine
Indapamide
Indinavir
Indomethacin
Insulin
Interferons
Ipodate
Ipratropium
Isoniazid
Isoproterenol
Isosorbide
Isotretinoin
Isradipine
Itraconazole
Ivermectin
Kanamycin
Ketoconazole
Ketoprofen
Ketorolac
Labetalol
Lamivudine
Lamotrigine

Lansoprazole
Leuprolide
Levamisole
Levobunolol
Levodopa
Levofloxacin
Levothyroxine
Lidocaine
Lincomycin
Liothyronine
Lisinopril
Lithium
Lomefloxacin
Loracarbef
Loratadine
Lorazepam
Losartan
Lovastatin
Loxapine
Maprotiline
Marihuana
Mazindol
Mebendazole
Mechlorethamine
Meclizine
Meclofenamate
Medroxyprogesterone
Mefenamic acid
Mefloquine
Melphalan
Meperidine
Mephenytoin
Mephobarbital
Meprobamate
Mercaptopurine
Mesalamine
Mesna
Mesoridazine
Metaxalone
Metformin
Methadone
Methamphetamine
Methantheline
Methazolamide
Methenamine
Methicillin
Methimazole
Methocarbamol
Methohexital
Methotrexate
Methoxsalen
Methsuximide
Methyclothiazide
Methyldopa
Methylphenidate
Methyltestosterone
Methysergide
Metoclopramide
Metolazone
Metoprolol
Metronidazole
Mexiletine
Mezlocillin
Miconazole
Midazolam
Minocycline
Minoxidil
Mitomycin
Mitotane
Moexipril
Moricizine
Nabumetone
Nadolol
Nafarelin
Nafcillin
Nalidixic acid
Naloxone
Naproxen
Naratriptan
Nefazodone
Nelfinavir
Neomycin
Niacin; niacinamide
Nicardipine
Nifedipine
Nisoldipine
Nitrofurantoin
Nitroglycerin
Nizatidine
Norfloxacin
Nortriptyline
Nystatin
Octreotide
Ofloxacin
Olanzapine
Olsalazine
Omeprazole
Ondansetron
Oral contraceptives
Orphenadrine
Oxacillin
Oxaprozin
Oxazepam
Oxytetracycline
Paroxetine
Penicillamine
Penicillins
Pentagastrin
Pentamidine
Pentazocine
Pentobarbital
Pentostatin
Pentoxifylline
Pergolide
Perphenazine
Phendimetrazine
Phenelzine
Phenindamine
Phenobarbital
Phenolphthalein
Phentermine
Phenytoin
Phytonadione
Pimozide
Pindolol
Piperacillin
Piroxicam
Polythiazide
Potassium iodide
Pravastatin
Prazepam
Praziquantel
Prazosin
Primaquine
Primidone
Probenecid
Procainamide
Procarbazine
Prochlorperazine
Progestins
Promazine
Promethazine
Propafenone
Propantheline
Propofol
Propoxyphene
Propranolol
Propylthiouracil
Protamine
Protriptyline
Pseudoephedrine
Psoralens
Pyrazinamide
Pyrilamine
Pyrimethamine
Quazepam
Quinacrine
Quinapril
Quinestrol
Quinethazone
Quinidine
Quinine
Ramipril
Ranitidine
Reserpine
Riboflavin
Rifampin
Risperidone
Ritonavir
Ritordine
Ropinirole
Saccharin
Salmeterol
Salsalate
Saquinavir
Secobarbital
Secretin
Sertraline
Sildenafil
Simvastatin
Sotalol
Sparfloxacin
Spectinomycin

Spironolactone
Stanozolol
Streptokinase
Streptomycin
Succinylcholine
Sucralfate
Sulfadoxine
Sulfamethoxazole
Sulfasalazine
Sulfisoxazole
Sulindac
Sumatriptan
Tacrine
Tamoxifen
Temazepam
Terbinafine
Terbutaline
Terfenadine
Testosterone
Tetracycline
Thalidomide
Thiabendazole
Thiamine
Thiopental
Thioridazine
Thiotepa
Thiothixene
Tiagabine
Ticarcillin
Ticlopidine
Timolol
Tiopronin
Tizanidine
Tobramycin
Tolazamide
Tolazoline
Tolbutamide
Tolcapone
Tolmetin
Topiramate
Torsemide
Tramadol
Tranylcypromine
Trazodone
Triamterene
Triazolam
Trichlormethiazide
Trifluoperazine
Trihexyphenidyl
Trimeprazine
Trimethadione
Trimipramine
Tripelennamine
Triprolidine
Troleandomycin
Trovafloxacin
Urokinase
Ursodiol
Valproic acid
Vancomycin
Vasopressin
Venlafaxine
Verapamil
Vinblastine
Vincristine
Vitamin E
Warfarin
Zalcitabine
Zidovudine
Zolmitriptan
Zolpidem

Vasculitis

Acebutolol
Acetaminophen
Acyclovir
Allopurinol
Amiloride
Aminosalicylate sodium
Amiodarone
Amitriptyline
Amlodipine
Amoxapine
Ampicillin
Aspirin
Atenolol
Azathioprine
Bendroflumethiazide
Benzthiazide
Bromocriptine
Bumetanide
Busulfan
Butabarbital
Butalbital
Captopril
Carbamazepine
Cefdinir
Cerivastatin
Chloramphenicol
Chlordiazepoxide
Chloroquine
Chlorothiazide
Chlorpromazine
Chlorpropamide
Chlorthalidone
Cimetidine
Ciprofloxacin
Clarithromycin
Clindamycin
Clomipramine
Clorazepate
Clozapine
Colchicine
Corticosteroids
Cortisone
Cotrimoxazole
Cromolyn
Cyclophosphamide
Cyclosporine
Cyclothiazide
Cyproheptadine
Cytarabine
Delavirdine
Diclofenac
Didanosine
Diflunisal
Digoxin
Diltiazem
Diphenhydramine
Disulfiram
Divalproex
Doxycycline
Enalapril
Ephedrine
Erythromycin
Ethacrynic acid
Etodolac
Famotidine
Fluoxetine
Flurbiprofen
Fluvastatin
Fosinopril
Furosemide
Gemfibrozil
Gentamicin
Glucagon
Glyburide
Gold
GCSF
Griseofulvin
Guanethidine
Heparin
Heroin
Hydralazine
Hydrochlorothiazide
Hydroflumethiazide
Hydroxychloroquine
Hydroxyurea
Ibuprofen
Imipenem/cilastatin
Imipramine
Indapamide
Indomethacin
Insulin
Interferons
Isoniazid
Isotretinoin
Itraconazole
Ketoconazole
Levamisole
Lisinopril
Lithium
Lomefloxacin
Lovastatin
Maprotiline
Meclofenamate
Mefenamic acid
Mefloquine
Melphalan
Meprobamate
Mesalamine
Metformin
Methazolamide
Methimazole

Methotrexate
Methoxsalen
Methyldopa
Methylphenidate
Metolazone
Minocycline
Mitotane
Nabumetone
Naproxen
Nifedipine
Nizatidine
Norfloxacin
Ofloxacin
Oxytetracycline
Penicillamine
Penicillins
Pentamidine
Pentobarbital
Pergolide
Phenobarbital
Phenytoin
Phytonadione
Piroxicam
Polythiazide
Potassium iodide
Pravastatin
Procainamide
Propylthiouracil
Psoralens
Pyridoxine
Quinapril
Quinethazone
Quinidine
Quinine
Ramipril
Ranitidine
Rifampin
Ritordine
Simvastatin
Sparfloxacin
Spironolactone
Streptokinase
Streptomycin
Sulfamethoxazole
Sulfasalazine
Sulfisoxazole
Sulindac
Tamoxifen
Terbutaline
Tetracycline
Thalidomide
Thiamine
Ticlopidine
Torsemide
Trazodone
Triamterene
Trichlormethiazide
Trimethadione
Trioxsalen
Valproic acid
Vancomycin
Verapamil
Warfarin
Zidovudine

Xerosis

Acebutolol
Acitretin
Aldesleukin
Alprazolam
Amlodipine
Amoxapine
Atenolol
Atorvastatin
Benztropine
Betaxolol
Bisoprolol
Bleomycin
Buspirone
Busulfan
Captopril
Carteolol
Cerivastatin
Cetirizine
Cimetidine
Clofazimine
Clofibrate
Clomipramine
Delavirdine
Diazoxide
Dicyclomine
Doxazosin
Estazolam
Estramustine
Famotidine
Fluorouracil
Fluoxetine
Flurbiprofen
Fluvastatin
Fluvoxamine
Foscarnet
Gemfibrozil
Gold
Grepafloxacin
Hydroxyurea
Indinavir
Interferons
Isotretinoin
Ketoconazole
Lamotrigine
Leuprolide
Levamisole
Lithium
Loratadine
Losartan
Mechlorethamine
Medroxyprogesterone
Mesalamine
Mesoridazine
Methantheline
Metolazone
Metoprolol
Mexiletine
Moricizine
Nabumetone
Nadolol
Naratriptan
Nefazodone
Niacin; niacinamide
Nisoldipine
Nizatidine
Olanzapine
Omeprazole
Paroxetine
Penicillamine
Pentamidine
Pentostatin
Pergolide
Pindolol
Promazine
Propantheline
Quetiapine
Ranitidine
Risperidone
Ritonavir
Saquinavir
Scopolamine
Sertraline
Sparfloxacin
Spironolactone
Sulfasalazine
Tacrine
Tamoxifen
Thalidomide
Tiagabine
Timolol
Tizanidine
Tolterodine
Topiramate
Trihexyphenidyl
Ursodiol
Venlafaxine
Vitamin A
Zalcitabine

Xerostomia

Acebutolol
Acetazolamide
Acitretin
Albendazole
Albuterol
Alprazolam
Alprostadil
Amantadine
Amiloride
Amitriptyline
Amlodipine
Amoxapine
Amoxicillin
Apraclonidine
Astemizole
Atropine sulfate
Azatadine
Azathioprine
Azelastine

Benactyzine
Bendroflumethiazide
Benztropine
Betaxolol
Bicalutamide
Biperiden
Bisoprolol
Bromfenac
Bromocriptine
Brompheniramine
Buclizine
Bumetanide
Buspirone
Butorphanol
Cabergoline
Captopril
Carbamazepine
Carbenicillin
Carbidopa
Carisoprodol
Carteolol
Carvedilol
Cefixime
Ceftibuten
Cerivastatin
Cetirizine
Chloramphenicol
Chlordiazepoxide
Chlormezanone
Chlorpromazine
Cimetidine
Ciprofloxacin
Cisapride
Clemastine
Clidinium
Clomipramine
Clonazepam
Clonidine
Clorazepate
Clozapine
Codeine
Cromolyn
Cyclobenzaprine
Cyproheptadine
Delavirdine
Desipramine
Dexfenfluramine
Dextroamphetamine
Diazepam
Diazoxide
Diclofenac
Dicloxacillin
Dicyclomine
Didanosine
Diethylpropion
Diflunisal
Diltiazem
Dimenhydrinate
Diphenhydramine
Diphenoxylate
Dirithromycin
Disopyramide
Divalproex
Donepezil
Doxazosin
Doxepin
Dronabinol
Enalapril
Ephedrine
Epinephrine
Ergocalciferol
Esmolol
Estazolam
Ethionamide
Etodolac
Famotidine
Felbamate
Felodipine
Fenfluramine
Fenoprofen
Fentanyl
Flavoxate
Flecainide
Fluconazole
Flucytosine
Flumazenil
Fluoxetine
Fluphenazine
Flurazepam
Flurbiprofen
Fluvoxamine
Fosfomycin
Fosinopril
Furosemide
Gabapentin
Ganciclovir
Grepafloxacin
Griseofulvin
Guanabenz
Guanadrel
Guanethidine
Guanfacine
Haloperidol
Hydrochlorothiazide
Hydromorphone
Hydroxyzine
Ibuprofen
Imipramine
Indapamide
Indinavir
Indomethacin
Interferons
Ipratropium
Isocarboxazid
Isoproterenol
Isosorbide
Isotretinoin
Isradipine
Itraconazole
Ketoprofen
Ketorolac
Labetalol
Lamotrigine
Lansoprazole
Levodopa
Levofloxacin
Lisinopril
Lithium
Lomefloxacin
Loratadine
Lorazepam
Lovastatin
Loxapine
Maprotiline
Mazindol
Mebendazole
Meclizine
Meclofenamate
Meperidine
Meprobamate
Mesoridazine
Methadone
Methamphetamine
Methantheline
Methicillin
Methyldopa
Methylphenidate
Metoclopramide
Metolazone
Metronidazole
Mexiletine
Mezlocillin
Moexipril
Molindone
Moricizine
Nabumetone
Nadolol
Nafcillin
Naproxen
Nefazodone
Nicardipine
Nifedipine
Nisoldipine
Nitrofurantoin
Nitroglycerin
Nizatidine
Norfloxacin
Nortriptyline
Octreotide
Ofloxacin
Olanzapine
Omeprazole
Ondansetron
Orphenadrine
Oxacillin
Oxazepam
Paroxetine
Pentamidine
Pentazocine
Pentoxifylline
Pergolide
Perphenazine
Phendimetrazine

Phenelzine
Phenindamine
Phenobarbital
Phentermine
Pimozide
Piroxicam
Pramipexole
Prazepam
Prazosin
Procarbazine
Prochlorperazine
Procyclidine
Promazine
Promethazine
Propafenone
Propantheline
Propofol
Propoxyphene
Propranolol
Protriptyline
Pyrilamine
Pyrimethamine
Quazepam
Quetiapine
Quinapril
Quinethazone
Ramipril
Reserpine
Rimantadine
Risperidone
Ritonavir
Ropinirole
Saquinavir
Scopolamine
Selegiline
Sertraline
Sibutramine
Sildenafil
Sparfloxacin
Spironolactone
Sulfasalazine
Sulindac
Sumatriptan
Tacrine
Tamoxifen
Temazepam
Terazosin
Terbutaline
Terfenadine
Thalidomide
Thiabendazole
Thioridazine
Thiothixene
Tiagabine
Ticarcillin
Tiopronin
Tizanidine
Tolcapone
Tolmetin
Tolterodine
Topiramate
Tramadol
Trandolapril
Tranylcypromine
Trazodone
Triamterene
Triazolam
Trichlormethiazide
Trifluoperazine
Trihexyphenidyl
Trimeprazine
Trimipramine
Tripelennamine
Triprolidine
Trovafloxacin
Valsartan
Venlafaxine
Verapamil
Vitamin A
Zalcitabine
Zolmitriptan
Zolpidem